Gastrointestinal Nursing

The human body is made up of trillions of cells, each of which requires access to nutrients to survive. These include carbohydrates, proteins, fats, vitamins and minerals. These nutrients provide energy for metabolic processes and the building blocks for cell growth and repair, and they exist within the food we eat.

This essential guide to the gastrointestinal system will enable nurses and allied health professionals to apply principles of anatomy and physiology to clinical practice. Taking a practical and evidence-based approach, each chapter explores associated anatomy, function, abnormalities and diseases.

The accessible writing style and full colour illustrations make this an ideal introduction for students and professionals new to gastrointestinal care.

Paul Ong is a senior lecturer on the adult nursing undergraduate programme at Oxford Brookes University. He has earned a BA (Hons) in health and community studies from Chester College and completed his Registered General Nurse training at Charing Cross Hospital, London. Paul started his nursing career in neurosurgery at the Radcliffe Infirmary. He then spent six years in gastrointestinal surgery at the John Radcliffe Hospital.

Rachel Skittrall is a principal lecturer and programme lead for the undergraduate nursing programme at Oxford Brookes University. She earned a degree in podiatric medicine at the University of Westminster and MSc in applied microbiology from Birkbeck College, University of London. Since practicing as a podiatrist and lecturer at the London Foot Hospital, Rachel has been teaching anatomy and physiology to pre-registration nursing students at Oxford Brookes University.

Gastrointestinal Nursing

Paul Ong and Rachel Skittrall

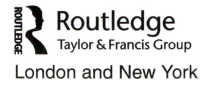

Routledge
Taylor & Francis Group

London and New York

First published 2018
by Routledge
2 Park Square, Milton Park, Abingdon, Oxon OX14 4RN

and by Routledge
711 Third Avenue, New York, NY 10017

Routledge is an imprint of the Taylor & Francis Group, an informa business

© 2018 by Taylor & Francis Group

British Library Cataloguing-in-Publication Data
A catalogue record for this book is available from the British Library

Library of Congress Cataloguing-in-Publication Data
A catalogue record for this book is available from the Library of
Congress

ISBN: 978-1-138-62717-8 (hbk)
ISBN: 978-1-4987-6956-3 (pbk)
ISBN: 978-1-4987-6957-0 (ebk)

Typeset in Bembo
by Nova Techset Private Limited, Bengaluru & Chennai, India

Printed in Canada

Contents

Chapter 1

INTRODUCTION

Specific learning outcomes
- Describe the embryonic development and gross anatomy of the gastrointestinal tract and accessory organs.
- Describe the general histology and physiological functions of the gastrointestinal tract and accessory organs.
- Identify and describe the neuroendocrine systems involved in the control and regulation of mechanical and chemical digestion.
- Discuss the neuroendocrine interface and its role in control and regulation of digestion.

OVERVIEW OF THE DIGESTIVE SYSTEM

The human body is made up of trillions of cells, each of which requires access to nutrients to survive. These include carbohydrates, proteins, fats, vitamins and minerals. These nutrients provide energy for metabolic processes and are the building blocks for cell growth and repair, existing within the food we eat (*macromolecules*). For the cells to be able to gain access to these nutrients, the food material must be broken down into much smaller *micromolecules* (amino acids, fatty acids, glucose) that are absorbed via the small intestine and transported via the circulatory system to the cells. Conversion of large molecules to small molecules is achieved through the action of two interrelated processes: *mechanical* digestion and *chemical* digestion. This is carried out by the gastrointestinal tract, which can be defined as a hollow tube running from the mouth to the anus.

- *Mechanical digestion* is the use of muscles to mix and break up food to increase the surface area for the action of enzymes. Mechanical digestion starts with chewing where the teeth and the tongue break up the food material. This is assisted by saliva that helps dissolve the nutrients within the food. Mechanical digestion continues in the stomach where a churning action, generated by smooth muscle contractions, pushes the gastric contents in different directions. Mechanical digestion is also assisted by the process of *segmentation,* which consists of localised rhythmic constrictions of the intestines which helps mix the food material with enzymes.

- *Chemical digestion* is provided by the action of *enzymes* that break the chemical bonds from complex food materials, helping to produce the small micromolecules ready for absorption. Chemical digestion begins in the mouth with the action of the enzymes *amylase* and *lipase*, continues in the stomach with the action of *pepsin* and is then completed in the small intestine with the assistance of enzymes from the pancreas.

The digestive system is divided into two parts: the *gastrointestinal tract* and the *accessory organs*. The gastrointestinal (GI) tract is made up of a number of organs that are directly involved in the process of digestion: mouth, *pharynx, oesophagus, stomach, small intestine, large intestine* and *rectum* (Figure 1.1). The accessory organs are a group of organs that assist in the process of digestion, and they include the teeth, tongue and *gallbladder,* which facilitate digestion. There are also a number of digestive glands such as the *salivary glands*, *liver* and *pancreas* that produce secretions that assist in the process of digestion but are not considered part of the gastrointestinal tract. This is why they are termed *accessory organs* (Figure 1.2). These organs are constructed of specialised cells that perform different complex functions. How the cells are specialised is dependent upon the function they perform.

There are a number of complex processes that take place within the gastrointestinal tract and associated accessory organs; however, most of the sections of the gastrointestinal tract will share three fundamental processes: *secretion, absorption* and *motility*. The

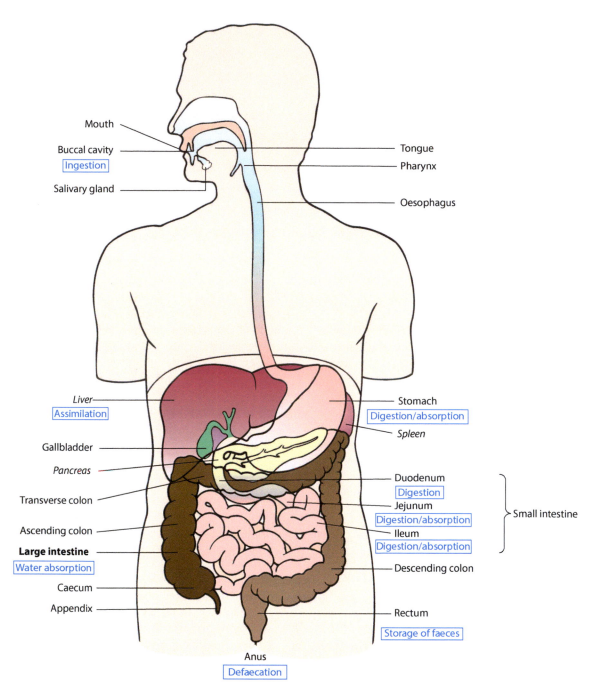

Figure 1.1 General picture of GI tract.

level of specialism in each of these three areas will be dependent upon the function to be carried out:

- *Secretion – mucous from goblet cells* to aid protection and lubrication; enzymes from the glandular cells of the salivary glands and pancreas as well as the *epithelial* cells of the stomach and small intestine; *hormones* from the *enteroendocrine* cells which line the stomach and duodenum; bile from the gallbladder to aid in the digestion of fats.

Main organs	Accessory organs
Mouth	Lips, teeth, tongue, salivary glands, palate
Pharynx	
Oesophagus	
Stomach	
Small intestine	Pancreas, gallbladder, liver
Large intestine	

Figure 1.2 Main organs and accessory organs.

- *Absorption* – water, *electrolytes*, *monosaccharides* (e.g. glucose), *amino acids* and *fats* from the lumen of the small intestine cross the *plasma membrane* into *enterocytes* via the processes of *diffusion*, *co-transport* and *osmosis* and then move into the blood circulation by diffusion.
- *Motility* – the movement of *smooth muscle* contractions during peristalsis and segmentation in the wall of the gastrointestinal tract mix and propel food material.

INTRODUCTION TO THE DIGESTIVE SYSTEM

Disorders of the *gastrointestinal tract* make up some of the most common illnesses experienced across the *lifespan* affecting individuals in infancy, childhood and adulthood. *Ingestion*, transportation, *digestion* and *absorption* can be affected by a number of disorders that relate to factors such as structural changes, inflammatory disorders, *malabsorption* and motility disorders. Any changes to the structure and function of the specialised areas of the gastrointestinal tract can also have an impact on the accessory organs that assist digestion. This book will explore normal anatomy and physiology and look at the changes associated with each stage of the lifespan from the developing embryo to old age. These developmental elements will be considered at the point where the general anatomy, physiology and function are explored for each section of the gastrointestinal tract and related accessory organs. An understanding of anatomy and physiology through the lifespan is essential to the understanding of disorders associated with the digestive system.

Practitioners need an understanding of normal anatomy and function so that they are equipped to understand the impact of dysfunction and disease within the body. Selected *pathology* and associated *pathophysiology*, from across the lifespan, will be used to support understanding of how disorders can disrupt the development and function of the gastrointestinal tract.

Overview of prenatal development of the digestive system

Very early on in embryonic development the embryo consists of three germ layers: endoderm, mesoderm and ectoderm (Figure 1.3a). This is called the *embryonic disc*. The majority of the digestive system develops from the endoderm layer during embryonic development (*embryogenesis*). These endodermal cells *differentiate* to form the many different types of epithelial and glandular cells that make up the organs of the gastrointestinal tract. These include the oesophagus, stomach, and small and large intestine.

During the third week of embryonic development the embryo starts to fold. As the folding progresses it eventually causes a section of the yolk sac to become separated. This separated section becomes the primitive gut (Figure 1.3b).

The primitive gut can be described as a hollow tube made up of *endodermal cells*. This digestive tube extends from the *oropharyngeal (buccopharyngeal) membrane* to the *cloacal membrane*. Breakdown of these membranes form the precursors of the mouth (stomadeum) and anus (proctadeum), respectively. Towards the end of the third week the digestive tube starts to elongate and can be divided into three sections – *foregut*, *midgut* and *hindgut* (Figure 1.3b,c) – from which the specialised structures of the tract and accessory organs emerge (see Chapters 5 and 7 for more details about the embryonic development of the small and large intestine).

The foregut stretches from the mouth to the duodenum at the entrance of the *bile duct*. It is from the foregut that the accessory organs, the liver, biliary system (gallbladder and ducts) and the pancreas, will develop. The foregut develops rapidly, dilating and rotating to form the primitive stomach. As the stomach grows it

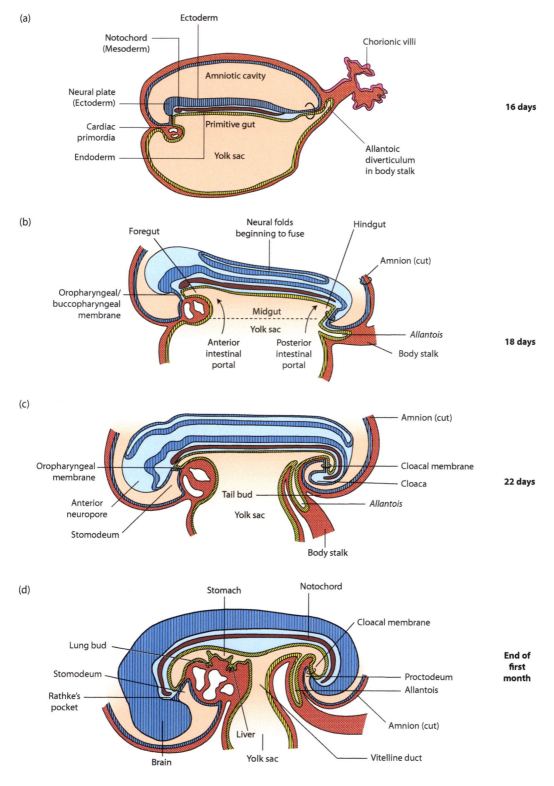

Figure 1.3 Embryonic development.

generates curvatures, peritoneal sacs and an omentum (Figure 1.3d). (See Chapter 4 for more details about the embryonic development of the stomach.)

The midgut stretches from the liver to about two thirds along what will become the transverse colon (*posterior intestinal portal*). During embryonic development the majority of the midgut develops outside the abdomen. This allows for rotation of the midgut, which must occur so that the gastrointestinal tract is in the correct position in relation to the mesentry. The hindgut stretches from what will become the final third of the transverse colon to the rectum and cloaca.

The *mesoderm* layer divides into the *somatic* and *splanchnic* layers which eventually leads to the primitive gut being completely surrounded. The muscles, vascular system and fibrous elements that make up the gastrointestinal tract are derived from the somatic mesoderm. The splanchnic mesoderm gives rise to the *visceral peritoneum*. The development of the mesoderm gives rise to *coelom* which will eventually become the ventral body cavity (abdominal cavity).

Foetal swallowing of *amniotic fluid* is a vital part of the normal development of the gut. Swallowed amniotic fluid provides the growing foetus with *protein* requirements and also contributes to the normal growth and development of the liver, pancreas and *gastric mucosa*.

Peristalsis can be observed from 14 weeks but it is not until 34 weeks that coordination of gut motility is evident. This includes sucking, swallowing and peristalsis. Gut activity leads to the accumulation of *meconium*.

During the development of the digestive system a number of abnormalities can occur and examples of these will be introduced as each element of the digestive system is introduced and explored.

Although the gastrointestinal tract is active before birth, the *foetus* relies upon the *placenta* to provide nutrients and remove waste products. At birth the *neonate* has to adapt from *passive* provision of nutrition to a more active system that involves ingestion, digestion and absorption via the gastrointestinal tract.

Functional histology of the gastrointestinal tract

The gastrointestinal tract is made up of a hollow tube that travels through the body from the mouth to the anus. The tube is open to the exterior at both ends, and although it passes through body cavities, it is separate to the internal body environment. The wall of the tube is made up of four main layers: the *mucosa, submucosa, muscularis externa* and *serosa* (Figure 1.4). Each of these components is adapted throughout the length of the gastrointestinal tract according to its function to provide

- Physical and mechanical protection
- Movement
- Secretion
- Absorption

Mucosa

The mucosa is the innermost layer of the gastrointestinal tract wall, being exposed to the lumen and contents of the tract. The mucosa is further subdivided into three layers – the *mucosal epithelium, lamina propria* and *muscularis mucosae* (Figure 1.4):

- The *mucosal epithelium* varies according to the specific function of a segment of the tract. *Stratified squamous epithelium* forms the mucosal epithelial lining in areas such as the oral cavity, pharynx, oesophagus and anus where the epithelium is subject to increased trauma and abrasion from food or wastes that are passed through the lumen. *Simple columnar epithelium* forms the rest of the digestive tract in structures such as the stomach and small and large intestines. This provides a thin layer through which nutrients can be absorbed and secretions released.
- The *lamina propria* is formed of a layer of loose connective tissue inside which capillaries and lymphatic vessels supply and drain nutrients and wastes. Nerve fibres within the mucosa provide sensory information regarding the gastrointestinal tract contents which are relayed to nerve plexuses within the gastrointestinal tract wall and to the central nervous system.
- As the name suggests the *muscularis mucosae* is a thin layer of smooth muscle tissue which can contract to form convolutions of the mucosal layer. These provide increases in surface area in parts of the tract, such as the small intestine, to facilitate the absorption of nutrients.

Submucosa

The submucosa consists of a thick connective tissue layer. This holds the main blood and lymphatic vessels which communicate with those of the underlying mucosa. The submucosa also contains the

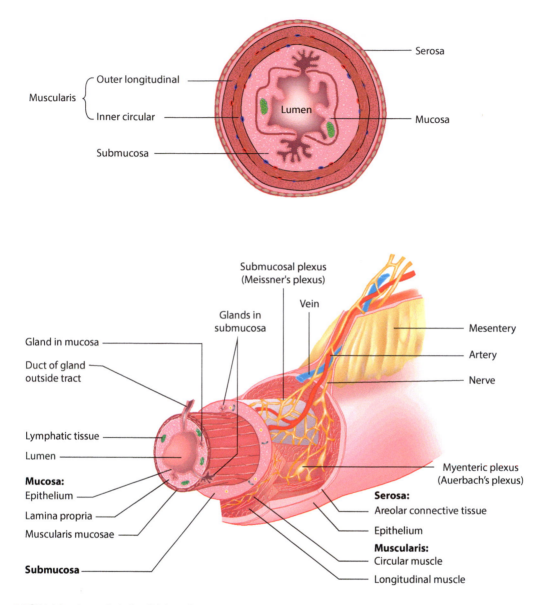

Figure 1.4 GI histology layers, including divisions of mucosa.

submucosal or Meissner nerve plexus that forms part of the enteric nervous system (Figure 1.4).

Muscularis externa

The muscularis externa consists of a thick layer of smooth muscle tissue covering the circumference of the tube. It lies external to the mucosa and submucosa and is generally arranged in two layers: circular positioned fibres internally and longitudinal fibres externally (Figure 1.4). Thickening of the circular fibres forms *sphincters* at points throughout the gastrointestinal tract where control of movement of tract contents is required. The sphincters divide the gastrointestinal tract into segments, maintaining a higher resting tone than the segments it separates. For example the pyloric sphincter contracts and relaxes to allow the controlled passage of chyme between the stomach and the duodenum.

Adaptions to the muscularis externa occur along the gastrointestinal tract. In the stomach there is an additional oblique smooth muscle layer. This allows the production of forceful contractions that are required to mix ingested food with stomach digestive secretions. In the large intestine or colon, the longitudinal fibres form 'ribbons' of muscle tissue called '*taenia coli*'. These lie longitudinally in three bands rather than around the whole circumference of the gastrointestinal tract. When contracted they form pouches or *haustra* along the length of the colon.

The muscularis externa is supplied by the myenteric or Auerbach's nerve plexus. This is responsible for controlling movements such as peristalsis and segmentation within the tract. This ensures that the contents are constantly mixed and moved along the tract in order that digestion, absorption and elimination occur in a timely fashion.

Serosa

The *serosa* is the outermost layer of the gastrointestinal tract (Figure 1.4). It consists of a thin layer of *mesothelium* supported by a thin layer of connective tissue. The serosa refers to a layer of peritoneum that covers the digestive organs inside the abdominopelvic cavity.

- The *peritoneum* is divided into the
  - *Parietal layer* which lines the abdominopelvic cavity walls.
  - *Visceral layer* which covers the surface of the organs within the peritoneal cavity. It is equivalent to the serosa.

  The two layers are continuous with one another. Between the two layers is the peritoneal cavity, separated by a film of peritoneal fluid. This lubricates the layers, prevents friction and allows movement between gastrointestinal tract organs. Organs within the peritoneal cavity that are completely surrounded by peritoneum are called *intraperitoneal*. Those organs where only part of the surface is covered in peritoneum are classed as *retroperitoneal*. This includes the ascending and descending colon, parts of the duodenum and pancreas.

- *Mesenteries* – In some areas there is a double layer of peritoneum. This is called a mesentery. Mesenteries are used as a pathway for blood vessels, nerves and lymph vessels to travel to and from an organ within the peritoneal cavity. Mesenteries are often associated with large amounts of adipose tissue. Mesenteries attach to the anterior and posterior abdominal walls securing digestive organs in place.

Overview of control and regulation of the digestive system

In order for digestion and absorption to take place the transit of nutrients through the gastrointestinal tract must be coordinated. This is achieved by a combination of neural, hormonal and local mechanisms. These controls respond to sensory stimuli via the central nervous system and to the environment within the lumen of the gastrointestinal tract. Normal functioning of the gastrointestinal tract is dependent on communication between the central nervous system (CNS), the autonomic nervous system (ANS), the enteric nervous system (ENS) and neurohormonal responses.

Neural regulation

Neural regulation of the gastrointestinal tract occurs as a result of both intrinsic and extrinsic neural control. Intrinsic or independent control is via internal enteric nerve plexuses within the smooth muscle wall, while extrinsic control is via the central nervous system, which exerts its effects of regulation, adjustment and control. The ability of different structures within the gastrointestinal tract to function independently varies. The stomach and oesophagus require more external CNS input, whereas the intestines can function more independently.

The *central nervous system* (CNS) provides overall control of digestive tract activity and can influence homeostatic control through cognitive and behavioural factors. The CNS can also provide influence from emotional responses in the control of the digestive system via the limbic system of the brain. The sight or smell of food stimulates long reflexes from the central nervous system via the hypothalamus and medulla to the gastrointestinal tract to increase gastric and intestinal tone, motility or secretions. Sensory receptors in the wall of the gastrointestinal tract can also stimulate long reflexes in the opposing direction towards the CNS, which integrate with the autonomic nervous system to effect changes in secretion and motility within the gastrointestinal tract.

- The *autonomic nervous system* (ANS) is divided into two parts: parasympathetic nervous system (PNS) innervation has a stimulatory response, increasing motility and secretions and relaxing sphincters. This is mediated through the vagus nerve (cranial nerve X). Sympathetic nervous system (SNS) innervation has an inhibitory effect decreasing blood flow to the digestive tract, decreasing secretions and motility and contracting sphincters. Efferent motor nerves of the sympathetic and parasympathetic pathways of the ANS synapse with the ENS plexuses.
- The intrinsic control of the gastrointestinal tract is via the *enteric nervous system* (ENS). The ENS

consists of two defined nerve plexuses within the walls of the digestive tract; the myenteric (or Auerbach's) plexus and the submucosal (Meissner's) plexus (Figure 1.4). The two plexuses are interconnected and can communicate with the CNS via long reflexes or provide short local reflex responses within the gastrointestinal tract wall.

The enteric nervous system is also able to function independently of the ANS and CNS and is often called the gut 'mini brain'. The ENS does this through *short reflexes* that are programmed with specific responses to stimuli from sensory receptors in the mucosal wall of the tract (Figure 1.5).

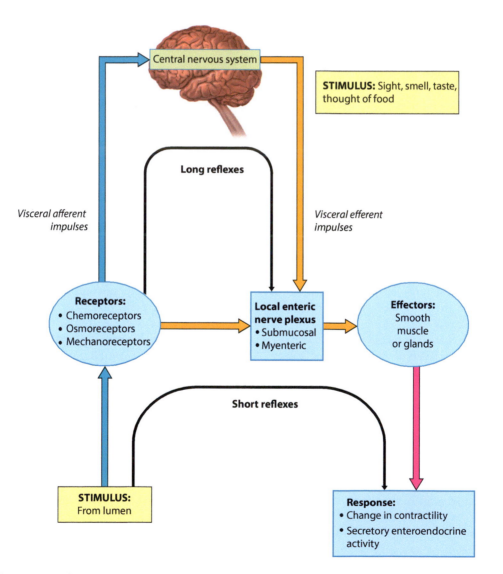

Figure 1.5 Neural control of GI tract.

The sensory stimuli can be mechanical via mechanoreceptors that respond to distension as nutrients enter parts of the tract, or caused by the movement of contents as they brush the mucosal surface. Chemical or *chemoreceptors* are stimulated as a result of nutrient concentrations, *pH* and *osmolarity* of luminal contents. There are also *nociceptors* able to stimulate pain and *thermoreceptors* that supply the brain with temperature regulatory information. The sensory information from these receptors is converted into action potentials that are transmitted via *afferent nerve fibres* or neurons to synapse with *interneurons*. The interneurons process the information and organise a response through motor or efferent neurons to endocrine cells, blood vessels, muscle tissue and epithelial transport mechanisms.

Hormonal regulation

Gastrointestinal tract motility and secretion are also controlled by hormonal mechanisms. The digestive tract wall contains hormone-secreting cells called *entero-endocrine (enterochromaffin) cells*. These are dispersed among the mucosal cells of the gastrointestinal tract and can be stimulated by luminal content and physical variables similar to those described above. In response to this, hormones are released into the circulation surrounding the gastrointestinal tract. The hormones stimulate secretory cells in the mucosal lining of the tract to secrete digestive acids and enzymes. Hormone secretions can also be stimulated directly via the ENS and ANS reflexes. (Table 1.1 shows the main hormones acting on the gastrointestinal tract.)

The interaction between the nervous and endocrine systems in the regulation of gastrointestinal activity can be seen during the cephalic, gastric and intestinal phases of gastric secretion (Figure 1.6).

Cephalic phase ('getting ready for food') – The CNS receives sensory information from the olfactory nerve (smell), the gustatory nerve (taste) and the optic nerve (sight). Interpretation of this information by the CNS, and the anticipation of food, leads to nerve impulses being sent from the CNS to the gastrointestinal tract in preparation for the imminent arrival of food. This is mediated via the vagus nerve of the PNS to the submucosal plexuses innervating secretory cells within the stomach.

Gastric phase ('arrival of food') – When food arrives in the stomach distension of the stomach wall,

a change in pH and specific food content stimulates mechanoreceptors (stretch) and chemoreceptors in the stomach wall. This stimulates short reflexes via the enteric plexuses, increasing secretory activity and motility.

Intestinal phase ('exiting of food') – Arrival of chyme from the stomach stimulates mechanoreceptors (stretch) and chemoreceptors in the duodenum triggering a reflex response to decrease activity in the stomach and increase motility and secretion within the intestine.

A more detailed explanation of the three phases will be given in Chapter 4.

Gastrointestinal motility

Gastrointestinal motility is a complex process and requires communication between many cells including smooth muscle cells of the muscularis externa, enteric neurons and interstitial cells of Cajal (ICC). Smooth muscle within the tract wall can be stimulated directly by enteric neurons or via the ICC. Absence or dysfunction of these structures may lead to motility disorders.

ICC are electrically rhythmic smooth muscle cells, derived from mesenchymal tissue. They can be found within the circular and longitudinal smooth muscle layers of the muscularis externa (intramuscular ICC) and/or as a network of branched processes around the myenteric plexus (Auerbach's) or submucosal (Meissner's) plexus (ICC of myenteric plexus and ICC of submucosal plexus).

ICCs are known as the internal gut pacemakers and are responsible for generating electrical wave activity within the gastrointestinal tract musculature. ICCs also provide mechanosensory information in response to stretch of the smooth muscle as a result of contents within the tract lumen.

- Peristalsis is the coordinated involuntary contraction of smooth muscle occurring in the oesophagus, stomach and intestines. Mechanical distention of the gastrointestinal tract wall stimulates a reflex response that stimulates alternating waves of contraction and relaxation in adjacent sections of the smooth muscle (Figure 1.7).
- Segmentation is the localised contraction of smooth muscle within the intestine. This produces a mixing action via alternating contraction and relaxation in non-adjacent sections of the digestive tract (Figure 1.7).

Table 1.1 Hormones that influence gastrointestinal tract activity

Hormone	Stimulus	Released from	Action on stomach	Action on pancreas	Action on liver	Action on small intestine	Action on large intestine	Other
Gastrin	Food in stomach, particularly proteins	G cells in stomach mucosa	Increases gastric distension Relaxes fundus Increases motility and secretion Stimulates HCl secretion Stimulates gastric emptying			Stimulates muscularis contraction	Relaxes ileocaecal valve Stimulates mass movements	
Gastric inhibitory peptide (GIP) (Glucose-dependent insulinotropic peptide)	Fatty chyme	Duodenum mucosa	Inhibits HCl production	Stimulates insulin release				
Histamine	Food in stomach	Stomach mucosa	Activate HCl production by parietal cells					
Intestinal gastrin	Acidic and partly digested food in duodenum	Duodenal mucosa	Stimulates gastric glands and motility					
Serotonin	Food in stomach	Stomach mucosa	Smooth muscle contraction					
Secretin	Acidic chyme in duodenum	Duodenal mucosa	Inhibits gastric gland secretion and gastric motility	Release of pancreatic juice rich in bicarbonate ions	Increase bile production			
Cholecystokinin (CCK)	Fatty chyme	Duodenal mucosa	Inhibits stomach secretion Inhibits stomach emptying	Release of pancreatic juice rich in enzymes	Stimulates gallbladder contraction and expulsion of stored bile	Relaxation of hepatopancreatic sphincter to release bile and pancreatic juice into duodenum		
Motilin	Fasting	Duodenal mucosa				Stimulates motility in proximal duodenum		
Somatostatin	Food in stomach Sympathetic nerve fibres	Stomach and duodenal mucosa	Inhibits gastrin, gastric secretion and motility	Inhibits secretion	Inhibits gallbladder contraction and bile release	Inhibits intestinal absorption by decreasing blood flow		
Vasoactive intestinal peptide (VIP)	Partially digested food in chyme	Enteric neurons	Inhibits acid secretion	Increases secretions		Relaxation of intestinal smooth muscle Dilates intestinal capillaries		
Glucose-like peptide (GLP-1)	Glucose in intestinal lumen	Intestinal cells of the distal ileum and colon	Inhibits acid secretion and gastric emptying	Release of insulin and suppression of glucagon		Inhibits motility		Induces satiety

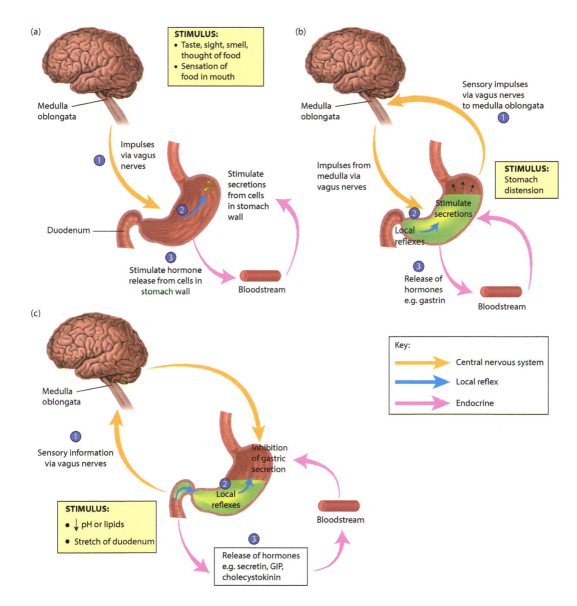

(a)

STIMULUS:
- Taste, sight, smell, thought of food
- Sensation of food in mouth

Medulla oblongata

Impulses via vagus nerves ①

②

Duodenum

Stimulate secretions from cells in stomach wall

③

Stimulate hormone release from cells in stomach wall

Bloodstream

(b)

Medulla oblongata

Sensory impulses via vagus nerves to medulla oblongata ①

Impulses from medulla via vagus nerves

② Stimulate secretions

Local reflexes

STIMULUS:
Stomach distension

③

Release of hormones e.g. gastrin

Bloodstream

(c)

Medulla oblongata

① Sensory information via vagus nerves

Inhibition of gastric secretion

② Local reflexes

STIMULUS:
- ↓ pH or lipids
- Stretch of duodenum

③

Release of hormones e.g. secretin, GIP, cholecystokinin

Bloodstream

Key:
→ Central nervous system
→ Local reflex
→ Endocrine

Figure 1.6 Phases of gastric secretion. (a) Cephalic, (b) Gastric and (c) Intestinal.

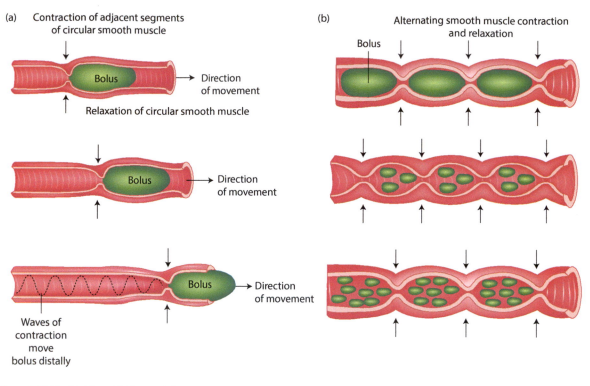

Figure 1.7 (a) Peristalsis and (b) Segmentation.

SUMMARY OF KEY POINTS

Digestive system organs are divided into

1. *Gastrointestinal tract* – oral cavity, pharynx, oesophagus, stomach, small intestine, large intestine, rectum and anus.
2. *Accessory structures* – salivary glands, teeth, gallbladder, pancreas, liver.

Gastrointestinal tract wall consists of four layers:

1. *Mucosa* – consists of three layers:
   i. *Epithelium* – composition varies according to function. Oral cavity, pharynx, oesophagus and anus consist of stratified squamous epithelium. Stomach, small intestines and colon consist of columnar epithelium.
   ii. *Lamina propria* – loose connective tissue contains blood and lymphatic vessels and sensory nerve endings.
   iii. *Muscularis mucosae* – smooth muscle tissue can contract to cause convolutions of the mucosal layer.
2. *Submucosa* – connective tissue containing blood and lymphatic vessels. Submucosal (Meissner's) nerve plexus provides sensory and motor innervation.

3. *Muscularis externa* – longitudinal and circular smooth muscle fibres to provide motility of the digestive tract. Nervous control via the myenteric (Auerbach's) nerve plexus. Propulsion is provided by *persistalsis*. Mixing is provided by *segmentation*.
4. *Serosa* – mesothelial covering of digestive organs.

Control of gastrointestinal tract function is as follows:

1. Central nervous system – long reflexes
2. Autonomic nervous system
   i. Sympathetic stimulation – inhibitory effect decreasing blood flow to the digestive tract, decreasing secretions and motility and contracting sphincters
   ii. Parasympathetic – stimulatory response, increasing motility and secretions and relaxing sphincters
3. Enteric nervous system – short or long reflexes via Auerbach's plexus and Meissner's plexus
4. Hormones – enteroendocrine cells secreting hormones into the local bloodstream to stimulate or inhibit activity within the gastrointestinal tract.

CHECK ON LEARNING

General structure

What is the relationship between the serosa and the mesentery?

Answer – The serosa, or visceral peritoneum, is a fluid-producing membrane designed to reduce friction between organs in the ventral body (abdominal cavity). It is continuous with the mesentery that supports blood vessels, lymph vessels and nerve fibres. The mesentery is continuous with the parietal peritoneum which lines the abdominal cavity helping to stabilise organs within the ventral body.

Overview of digestive system regulation

What two networks of neurons comprise the enteric nervous system?

Answer – They are the myenteric (Auerbach's) nerve plexus that is found between the circular and longitudinal muscle layers of the muscularis externa and the submucosal (Meissner's) nerve plexus which is found in the submucosa.

Increasing digestive activity is stimulated by which division of the autonomic nervous system?

Answer – The parasympathetic division stimulates smooth muscle and glandular tissue activity.

Which cranial nerve is responsible for communicating with the enteric nervous system?

Answer – The vagus nerve (cranial nerve X) is responsible.

There are two types of reflexes that regulate the digestive system and they are called short and long reflexes. Which reflex is controlled by the central nervous system and which is controlled by the enteric nervous system?

Answer – The central nervous system controls long reflexes, and the enteric nervous system controls short reflexes.

Which hormones influence digestive activity?

Answer – Gastrin, secretin, cholecystokinin and motilin influence digestive activity.

ORAL CAVITY

PRENATAL DEVELOPMENT OF THE ORAL CAVITY

The face and neck are derived from structures called *pharyngeal arches*. There are five arches (1, 2, 3, 4 and 6) that form during the fourth week of embryonic development. Only the first to fourth arches are visible externally on the developing embryo by week 5. Figure 2.1 shows the developmental anatomy of the pharyngeal arches. Pharyngeal arches are covered by ectodermal and endodermal epithelium, each arch being separated by a pharyngeal cleft. Within each arch is a pharyngeal pouch made up of endodermal tissue from the foregut tube with a mesenchymal core. Mesenchyme tissue is formed by the combination of neural crest cells that have migrated from the developing neural tube and mesoderm tissue. The pouch separates the arches internally and forms structures such as the pharyngeal, lingual and palatine *tonsils*, parathyroid glands, *middle ear cavity* and *auditory tubes*. Inside each pouch there is a basic structure that includes a nerve, muscle, cartilage and blood vessels (Figure 2.1).

- The nerve develops into a cranial nerve from the brainstem. Each arch is supplied by a specific cranial nerve. These carry motor neurons for muscle tissue innervation and sensory neurons to the skin and mucosal surfaces of the upper digestive tract (Table 2.1).

- The muscle develops into those required for *mastication*, facial expression and the *pharyngeal* and *laryngeal* muscles (Table 2.1).
- *Cartilage* develops into skeletal and *ligamentous* structures such as the inner ear bones, upper and lower jaw and laryngeal cartilages (Table 2.1).
- The *blood vessels* extend from the developing *heart* and *aorta* (Table 2.1).

Figure 2.2 shows neuromuscular derivatives of each arch.

FORMATION OF THE FACE

Embryonic development of the face commences in the fourth week of gestation. Neural crest cells combine with mesodermal cells to establish the basic structures or primordia that will form the adult face. The primordia develop around an opening or invagination of ectoderm tissues called the stomadeum, the primitive oral cavity.

The primordia are shown in Figure 2.3a:

- Frontonasal prominence – consists of tissue surrounding the developing brain
- Paired maxillary processes – derived from mesenchyme tissue from the 1st pharyngeal arch
- Paired mandibular processes – derived from mesenchyme tissue from the 1st pharyngeal arch

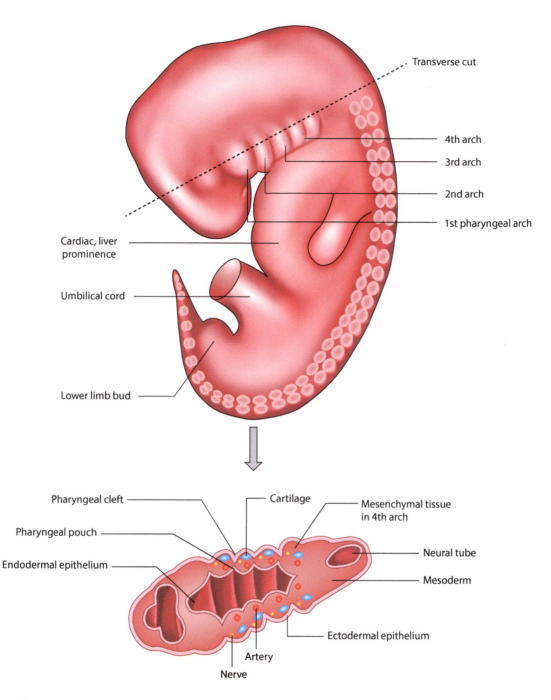

Figure 2.1 Embryology: Pharyngeal arches.

By the end of the fourth week of gestation the frontonasal prominence forms thickenings of ecto-dermal tissue or nasal placodes on each side of the developing face. Each nasal placode is divided into the larger medial and smaller lateral nasal processes. The nasal processes surround a small opening called a nasal pit (Figure 2.3b). The nasal pit gradually enlarges into a nasal sac, lined with a thick epithe-lium of olfactory tissue into which sensory nerves develop to allow the sensation of smell. The sac

Table 2.1 Embryology: Derivatives of the pharyngeal arches

Pharyngeal arch	Developmental anatomy	Cranial nerve	Muscle	Blood vessel	Cartilage/bone
I	Upper and lower jaw External ear Body of tongue (anterior 2/3)	Trigeminal (V)	*Muscles of mastication* • Tensor veli palatine • Mylohyoid • Tensor tympani	Maxillary artery	Malleus, incus, sphenoid (part)
II	External ear	Facial (VII)	*Muscles of facial expression* • Buccinators • Stylohyoid • Stapedius		Stapes, styloid process and hyoid bone
III	Palatine tonsils Root of tongue (posterior 1/3)	Glossopharyngeal (IX)	Stylopharyngeus	Common carotid arteries External carotid Internal carotid (part)	
IV	Epiglottis	Vagus (X)	Pharyngeal muscles	Subclavian artery Aortic arch	Thyroid and cricoid cartilages
VI		Recurrent laryngeal branch of Vagus (X)	Intrinsic muscles of larynx	Pulmonary arteries Ductus arteriosus Right subclavian artery	Arytenoid cartilage

is separated from the oral cavity by an oral nasal membrane.

By the end of the sixth week the medial nasal processes have enlarged and moved centrally toward the midline of the embryo's developing face and fuse together. The maxillary processes grow forward and medially below the lateral nasal processes and join with the medial nasal processes forming each side of the upper lip and primary palate (Figure 2.3c). Failure of this process results in a cleft lip. The oronasal membrane breaks down and the oral and nasal cavities merge into one oronasal space.

By week 8 the maxillary and mandibular processes have merged laterally to form the cheeks. The mandibular processes fuse centrally to form the lower jaw. The outcome of this merging will determine mouth size (Figure 2.3d).

DEVELOPMENT OF THE PALATE

Separation of the oral and nasal cavities occurs through the development of the *palate*. The palate is divided into the hard palate that forms the roof of the mouth anteriorly and the soft palate posteriorly.

Hard palate

Embryonic development of the hard palate forms as a result of fusion between the primary and secondary palates (Figure 2.3d–f).

Primary palate

The primary palate forms from the fusion of the medial nasal processes and the maxillary processes as described previously.

Secondary palate

The secondary palate forms from palatine processes or shelves during the sixth week of gestation. These arise as outgrowths from each of the maxillary processes. The shelves initially grow vertically down the side of the tongue, which sits between the two palatine shelves. At the seventh week of gestation the palatine shelves lift to sit horizontally over the tongue. Growth of the shelves continues until they meet at their midpoint. Total fusion occurs in both anterior and posterior directions. The palatine shelves fuse with the primary palate anteriorly and with each other posteriorly. The epithelial tissue covering the edges of the shelves joins forming an epithelial seam. The line gradually degenerates to allow continuity of mesenchymal tissue across the palate. Fusion of the palate relies on adhesion of epithelial tissues. Failure of closure of the palatine shelves results in a cleft palate.

The mesenchyme tissue of the palatine shelves continues to differentiate to produce the *palatine bones*, musculature and posteriorly the *soft palate*. The *nasal septum* joins the palate and the division of the nasal and oral cavities is complete. The primary and

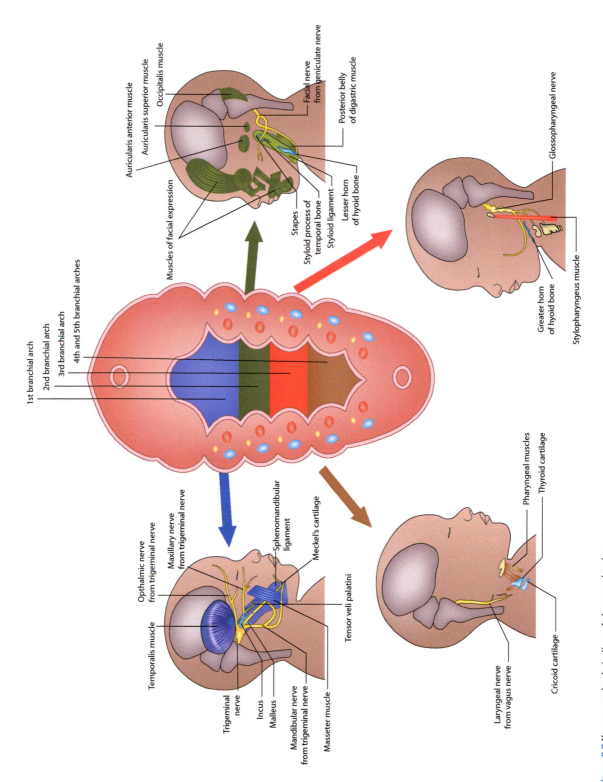

Figure 2.2 Neuromuscular derivatives of pharyngeal arches.

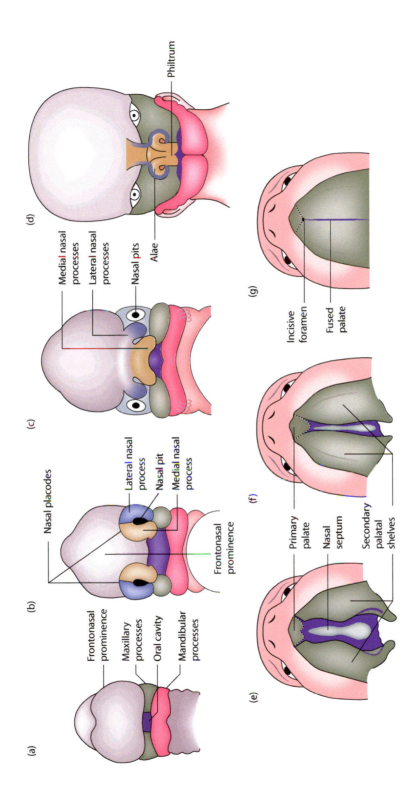

Figure 2.3 Development of the face.

secondary palates fuse to form the hard palate with closure complete by 10–12 weeks of embryogenesis. Epithelial tissue on both sides of the palate differentiates into stratified squamous keratinised epithelium on the oral side and pseudo-stratified ciliated columnar epithelium on the nasal side.

POSTNATAL DEVELOPMENT AND ADULT ORAL CAVITY

Gross anatomy

The oral or *buccal cavity* is the first point of contact for nutrients to enter the digestive tract (Figure 2.4). The main functions of the oral cavity are to

- Provide analysis of ingested nutrients
- Lubricate the oral mucosa by mucus and salivary secretions
- *Mechanically process* nutrients
- Commence the chemical digestion of carbohydrates and lipids
- Form a bolus

Nutrients are ingested into the oral cavity via the mouth. The oral cavity is lined with an oral mucosa of stratified squamous epithelium. Non-keratinised epithelium covers the inner lining of the lips, cheeks and inferior surface of the tongue. It provides a thin and delicate coating to these structures. The hard palate and tongue are covered in keratinised epithelium as a result of increased abrasion to their surfaces. The oral mucosa is continuous with the gingival or gum tissue.

The *superior* surface or roof of the oral cavity comprises the *hard palate anteriorly* and the soft palate posteriorly. The hard and soft palates provide separation of the oral cavity and *nasal cavity*. Ridges or raphe can be observed on the anterior and *lateral* surfaces of the hard palate. During mastication the tongue pushes food against the abrasive surface of the ridges to compress and mechanically break down nutrients to form a bolus.

The soft palate extends *posteriorly* to the *uvula* which can be observed suspended into the *palatoglossal arch*. The uvula prevents the premature movement of nutrients into the pharynx. Movement of the soft palate is achieved by contraction of the *levator veli palatini* and *tensor veli palatini* muscles. This is important during swallowing, as elevation of the soft palate prevents nutrients from passing into the

nasopharynx. The muscles also open the entrance to the auditory tubes. Posterior to the palatoglossal arch is the palatopharyngeal arch. The palatine tonsils sit on both sides of the oral cavity between the palatoglossal and palatopharyngeal arches. This opening between the oral cavity and oropharynx is called the *fauces*.

The floor of the oral cavity comprises the tongue. This is supported by the geniohyoid and myelohyoid muscles.

The lips constitute the anterior extent of the oral cavity. They are formed from the *obicularis oris muscle*. The outer lips are covered in *keratinised stratified squamous epithelium*. They have an extensive blood supply that provides the lips with colour. Posterior to the lips is the *vestibule* which forms a space between the lips, cheeks and teeth. The cheeks form the lateral extent of the oral cavity. They consist of the buccinators muscles and pads of adipose tissue.

DEVELOPMENTAL ABNORMALITIES OF THE ORAL CAVITY

Cleft lip and palate

Cleft lip and palate (CL/P) are the most frequently occurring congenital orofacial pathologies. They are developmentally distinct but often occur together with varying severity. They can be divided into two groups: cleft lip with or without cleft of the secondary palate and isolated cleft palate. They can be unilateral or bilateral ranging from a small notch on the upper lip to complete clefts of the lip, alveolus or palate (hard and/or soft). Minor or microforms of cleft lip and cleft palate can occur, often referred to as a submucous cleft palate. This describes a palate that initially appears normal; however, there is abnormality in the underlying mesenchymal growth with resultant bifid uvula, a notch at the posterior hard palate or misalignment of palatine muscles (Hodgkinson et al., 2005; Mosahebi and Kangesu, 2006). Figure 2.5 illustrates examples of different types of clefts.

CL/P occur in approximately 1 in 700 live births (Mossey et al., 2009; Dixon et al., 2011; Pang et al., 2013) with approximately 1,000 cases per year in the United Kingdom (Hawkes, 2012). There is a wide variation across racial and ethnic groups including highest birth prevalence rates of 1 in 500 for CL/P occurring in Asian and Native American populations. The lowest birth prevalence rates have been

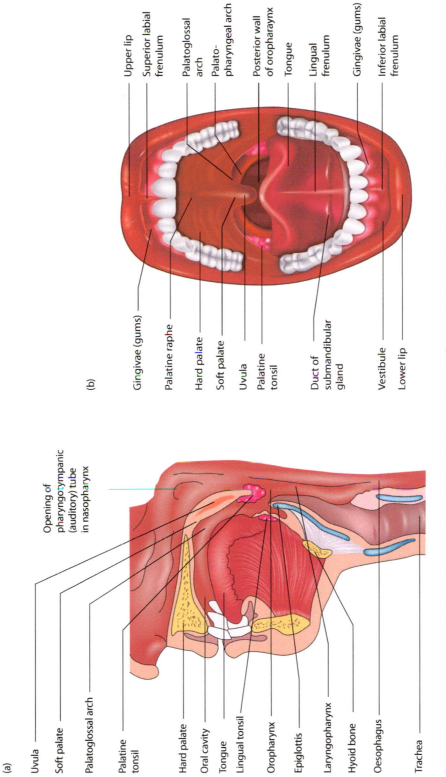

(a)

Uvula

Soft palate

Palatoglossal arch

Palatine tonsil

Hard palate

Oral cavity

Tongue

Lingual tonsil

Oropharynx

Epiglottis

Laryngopharynx

Hyoid bone

Oesophagus

Trachea

Opening of pharyngotympanic (auditory) tube in nasopharynx

(b)

Upper lip

Superior labial frenulum

Palatoglossal arch

Palato-pharyngeal arch

Posterior wall of oropharaynx

Tongue

Lingual frenulum

Gingivae (gums)

Inferior labial frenulum

Gingivae (gums)

Palatine raphe

Hard palate

Soft palate

Uvula

Palatine tonsil

Duct of submandibular gland

Vestibule

Lower lip

Figure 2.4 Anatomy of oral cavity. (a) Sagittal section through head extending to include oesophagus. (b) Open mouth showing teeth, arches, tonsils and tongue.

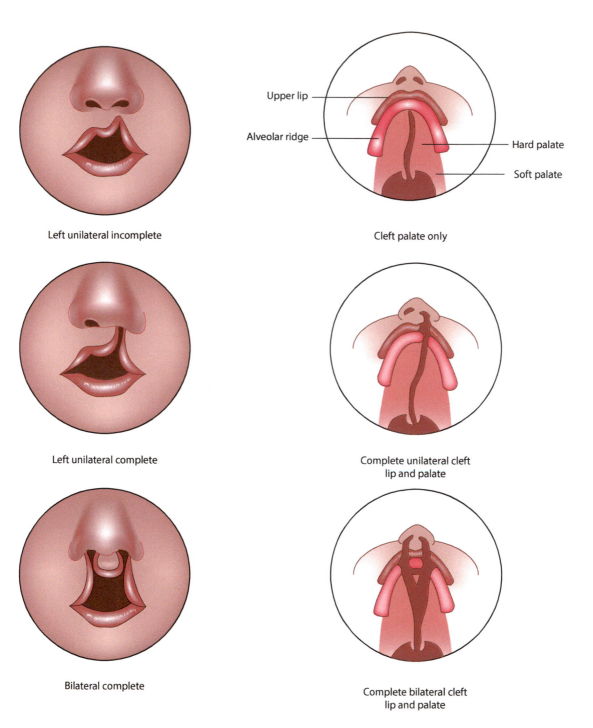

Left unilateral incomplete

Cleft palate only

Upper lip

Alveolar ridge

Hard palate

Soft palate

Left unilateral complete

Complete unilateral cleft
lip and palate

Bilateral complete

Complete bilateral cleft
lip and palate

Figure 2.5 Pathology: Types of cleft lip with or without cleft palate.

found in African-derived populations of 1 in 2500 (Dixon et al., 2011).

There are also differences in gender frequency for CL/P. Clefts involving the lip occur more frequently in males (2:1 male-to-female ratio) with clefts of the palate occurring more frequently in females (1:2 male-to-female ratio). Unilateral cases of clefts occur more frequently on the left side with a ratio of 2:1

(left to right) (Dixon et al., 2011). And, 50% of cleft lips occur with a cleft palate (Stanier and Moore, 2004).

Cleft lip with or without cleft palate and isolated cleft palate can occur with other congenital anomalies in approximately 30% of cases. This is referred to as 'syndromic CL/P'. The remaining 70% of CL/P and 50% of isolated CP present with no other apparent physical or developmental anomalies. This is classified as 'isolated non-syndromic CL/P'.

CL/P has a complex multifactorial aetiology including a combination of genetic and environmental factors. Familial aggregation includes an increased risk to a subsequent child, once a parent has an offspring with a cleft. Environmental factors associated with an increase in clefting include maternal smoking and alcohol use, pesticides for example, dioxins, anticonvulsant medications for example, phenytoin and benzodiazepines and nutrient deficiencies including zinc, vitamin B6 and folic acid. Genetic mutations for syndromic CL/P have been identified.

Cleft lip (CL) occurs as a result of failure of fusion between the medial nasal processes and the maxillary processes, during the fifth through seventh weeks of embryogenesis (Lee, 2000). Cleft palate (CP) arises from a lack of fusion of the palatine processes during weeks 6–12 of embryogenesis. Other factors implicated in CP formation are a decreased size of the palatine shelves, failure of the shelves to elevate to a horizontal position, inhibition of fusion or adhesion and failure of the tongue to drop (Abramowicz et al., 2003). Cleft palate most commonly includes the anterior, primary palate, although the posterior secondary palate can be affected with clefts becoming more severe from front to back (Hodgkinson et al., 2005). CL can be identified prenatally from ultrasound examination at 13 weeks' gestation. CP is harder to visualise but may be observed at 18–20 weeks.

CL/P can have significant effects on both a child and family. This includes complications of feeding, speech, hearing, dentition, psychological development and social integration.

Hearing

Infants with cleft palate are prone to middle ear infections (otitis media) with effusions, known as 'glue ear' (Sheahan et al., 2003; Goudy et al., 2006). This occurs as a result of functional obstruction of

the nasopharyngeal end of the auditory or Eustacian tubes. The tensor veli palatini muscle is responsible for opening and closing the auditory tubes to equalise pressure within the middle ear and assist with drainage of mucous. Loss of function due to cleft palate results in accumulation of fluid within the middle ear causing otitis media and effusion. This can lead to conductive hearing loss. Following cleft repair the majority of hearing loss is resolved; however, some infants and children are left with long-term hearing loss (Goudy et al., 2006). Hearing loss in children can have an influence on speech and language development.

Speech

Speech may be affected by lip and palate clefting. Prior to cleft repair the oral and nasal cavities are connected. This means it is difficult to create enough air pressure inside the mouth for speech, as the air exits through the nose. There is also less palate surface area for the tongue to contact to create sounds.

Speech is also affected by velopharyngeal inadequacy. This occurs when the soft palate is unable to rise during speech to cover the entrance to the nasal cavity. This is due to the altered muscle insertions of the levator and tensor veli palatini muscles which insert into the palate. Hypernasal speech, nasal emissions and nasal turbulence occur as air exits through the nose and mouth due to a lack of closure of the nasal cavity.

Following repair of the cleft some children will continue to experience velopharyngeal insufficiency. Children with clefts frequently have difficulty in speech articulation and language development. However, many continue to develop normal speech (Hodgkinson et al., 2005; Vallino et al., 2008).

Dentition

Dental malformations of size, shape, number, asymmetry and absence occur in facial clefts (Lourenço et al., 2003). The nature of dental changes depends upon the site and extent of the cleft. Commonly the upper lateral incisors are affected or completely absent or duplicate incisors may be present. Disruption by the cleft can cause teeth to erupt at abnormal sites or *Hypodontia*, where teeth are missing.

Feeding

Feeding also causes difficulties in infants with CL/P. Due to the connection between the nasal and oral cavities the infant is unable to generate the negative pressure required to create suction on the nipple or teat. The cleft also provides an opening via which fluid may pass into the nasal cavity. This can occur directly or through the cleft. This also interferes with the compression of the nipple onto the hard palate to express milk. Cleft lips also prevent an adequate seal between the lips and nipple or teat and difficulties arise in maintaining the correct nipple or teat position.

THE TONGUE

Prenatal development of the tongue

Development of the tongue commences during week 4 of gestation. The pharyngeal arches contribute to the embryological development of the tongue. Swellings of mesenchyme tissue form on the floor of the pharynx, in the pharyngeal arches I–IV.

- First pharyngeal arch (I)
  - Three swellings form at the distal extent of the pharynx: Two lateral lingual swellings and a central swelling called the *tuberculum impar*. The swellings merge to form the anterior two thirds of the tongue.
- Second pharyngeal arch (II)
  - The second arch contribution diminishes as the tongue develops and is not visible in the mature tongue.
- Third pharyngeal arch (III)
  - The hypobrachial eminence is derived from the third arch. It forms the posterior one third of the tongue. A demarcation line at the point of fusion of the anterior and posterior sections of the tongue is called the *sulcus terminalis*.
- Fourth pharyngeal arch (IV)
  - The epiglottis is derived from the epiglottal swelling at the posterior aspect of the tongue.

During weeks 8–9 of embryogenesis muscle tissue migrates into the tongue. This is innervated by the hypoglossal nerve (*cranial nerve* XII). Sensory innervation of the anterior two thirds of the tongue develops from the trigeminal (*cranial nerve* V) and facial (*cranial nerve* VII) nerves. Posterior sensory innervation develops from the glossopharyngeal (*cranial nerve* IX) and vagus nerves (*cranial nerve* X). The tongue epithelium proliferates to produce *papillae* and *taste buds* appear. By week 9 the tongue is functional. It

has matured, and recognisable adult tongue structures are evident.

Postnatal development and adult tongue
Gross anatomy and function

At birth the tongue has a rounder shape than the adult tongue and fills a large proportion of the mouth in relation to the size of the oral cavity. By the age of 5 years the tongue descends further towards the *larynx* and occupies less space in the oral cavity.

The tongue forms the base of the oral cavity. It is covered by oral mucosa and is divided into the root or pharyngeal portion and the body or oral portion. It is a large striated, skeletal muscle which is attached at its base to the *hyoid bone*. It is also tethered to the floor of the oral cavity by the centrally placed *lingual frenulum*. The skeletal muscle tissue which forms the bulk of the tongue is made up of two muscle groups:

- The *intrinsic muscles* have their origin and insertion within the tongue. They are responsible for changes in shape and size of the tongue and are essential to assist in manipulation of food during chewing. There are four groups of muscles: inferior longitudinal muscle, superior longitudinal muscle, transverse muscle and vertical muscle. Each group represents a different orientation of muscle fibres. Together they create up and down movements, flattening, narrowing and lengthening of the tongue. They are innervated by the *hypoglossal nerve (cranial nerve XII)*.
- The *extrinsic muscles* arise outside of the tongue. They include four muscles: genioglossus, styloglossus, palatoglossus and hyoglossus muscles. They provide movement for retraction and protrusion of the tongue. They are also important to raise the *bolus* toward the pharynx in preparation for swallowing. They are innervated by the *hypoglossal nerve (cranial nerve XII)*.

The tongue also provides sensory information regarding taste. The superior surface of the tongue is covered in tiny projections called papillae. The papillae are divided into four groups: *filiform, fungiform, foliate* and *circumvallate* papillae (Figure 2.6).

- Filiform papillae occur as elongated projections over the anterior two thirds of the tongue. They provide an abrasive surface for mastication. The filiform papillae do not contain taste buds.

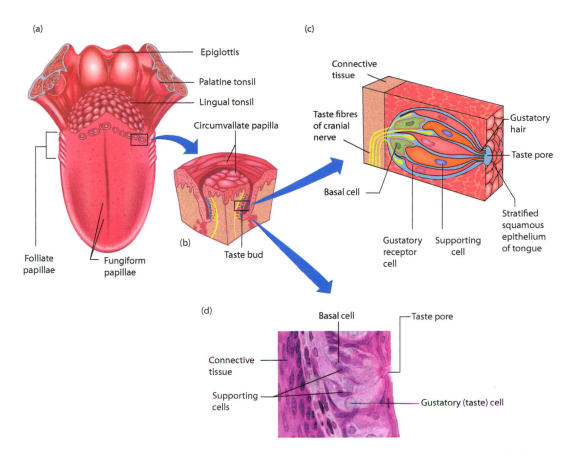

Figure 2.6 Tongue and taste buds. (a) Gross anatomy of the tongue, (b) enlarged section of circumvallate papilla, (c) cross section through a taste bud and (d) histological section through a taste bud.

- Fungiform papillae are distributed towards the tip and sides of the tongue, dispersed between the filiform papillae. They are mushroom shaped and provide taste sensation via the cranial nerves.
- Foliate papillae are found bilaterally on the posterior-lateral sides of the tongue. They form furrows which lie near to the molar teeth.
- The circumvallate papillae form a 'V' shape just anterior to the root of the tongue and the *sulcus terminalis*. There are between 8 and 12 papillae which form a demarcation line between the oral and pharyngeal components of the tongue. Like the fungiform papillae, they provide taste sensation via the cranial nerves.

As nutrients enter the oral cavity they are mixed with saliva. The saliva and food mixture flows around and between the papillae. Taste buds distributed along the sides of the papillae utilise sensory gustatory hairs protruding from within the taste bud pore to stimulate sensory impulses. Gustatory receptor cells are chemoreceptors from which impulses are directed to the central nervous system for recognition and distinguishing different taste sensations (Figure 2.6). These include bitter, sweet, salt, sour, *umami* and water. As a person ages there may be a decline in discrimination of these taste sensations.

The pharyngeal component of the tongue does not contain taste buds. It does however contain the lingual tonsils which are part of the lymphoid system.

Developmental abnormalities of the tongue
Ankyloglossia

Ankyloglossia or 'tongue tie' is a congenital abnormality associated with a short, tight or thickened lingual frenulum which 'ties' the tongue to the floor of the mouth. The prevalence is approximately 2%–5%

and occurs with greater frequency in males (Hong, 2013; Power and Murphy, 2015). There are no specific known causes for ankyloglossia; however, it can occur with other congenital abnormalities such as cleft lip and palate.

There is no consensus on a reliable definition for ankyloglossia. Diagnosis is variable in relation to appearance and function of the tongue. Current opinion suggests that emphasis should be placed on functional assessment of the tongue and feeding as part of the diagnosis of the condition (Edmunds et al., 2012; Emond et al., 2014; Power and Murphy, 2015).

There is considerable inconsistency in the amount of tongue restriction, with variable effects on tongue function. Many infants are asymptomatic and continue to be able to breastfeed successfully. However, for those with severe tightness of the frenulum, this can result in a restricted range of motion of the tongue in forward protrusion and/or lateral mobility. In some cases, the frenulum may extend to the tip of the tongue causing an indentation at the anterior edge. Ankyloglossia may cause difficulties with infant feeding, such as prolonged or frequent feeding times, inadequate milk intake and poor latching. For the mother, nipple soreness, breast pain, mastitis and low milk supply can occur (Edmunds et al., 2012; Kotlow, 2013). In older children and adults, ankyloglossia may result in difficulties in articulation of speech, maintaining oral hygiene, licking the lips or food, kissing and discomfort beneath the tongue.

Movement of the tongue is an important element of breastfeeding. Ankyloglossia prevents the tongue being extended over the lower gum line. In order to compensate and keep the mother's nipple in its mouth, the infant has to use its jaw. Maintenance of an effective seal to the breast is compromised as the tongue moves back to the floor of the mouth more quickly. Infants bite or latch strongly to the breast to suckle, and may compress the tip of the nipple, rather than areaolar tissue. This leads to ineffective milk release. Lactation advice is essential, and the recognition of the benefits of breastfeeding has encouraged mothers to persevere; however, some mothers cease breastfeeding in favour of bottle feeding. These problems do not occur for all infants with ankyloglossia. Most are still able to feed adequately from breastfeeding, as residual elasticity of the frenulum is able to compensate.

Most ankyloglossia is managed conservatively; however, where there is significant functional restriction, frenotomy or frenectomy may be performed by the surgical division of the lingual frenulum. This is usually undertaken in the first few weeks following birth without analgesia. The effectiveness of frenotomy has been shown to provide improvement to those with difficulty breastfeeding or with difficulties in speech articulation in older children and adults. There is however some controversy as to the effectiveness and timing of frenotomy.

THE TEETH

Prenatal development of the teeth

Odontogenesis is the process of tooth formation and development. It commences in week 6 gestation. Figure 2.7 shows the basic tooth structures. Teeth and their associated structures are derived from a combination of *stomadeal* ectoderm/epithelium and neural crest-derived mesenchyme.

- The ectoderm forms the enamel portion of the teeth from cells called *ameloblasts*.
- The mesenchyme forms the dentine, pulp, cementum and periodontal structures. Dentine derives from cells called *odontoblasts* and cementum from *cementoblasts*.

Odontogenesis is a highly coordinated and complex process, involving over 200 genes. It necessitates coordinated cell communication between the ectodermal and mesenchyme tissues involved. The process can be divided into the following stages: bud, cap, and bell stages (Figure 2.8).

Bud stage

Primary thickening of the oral ectoderm in week 6 of gestation forms an epithelial band. The epithelial band forms a continuous 'horseshoe'-shaped ridge around the margins of the developing oral cavity. This is called the *dental lamina*. It is from here that the tooth buds arise. The formation of the dental lamina in the lower jaw precedes that of the upper jaw.

At intervals along the dental lamina, in both the upper and lower jaws, swellings of the dental lamina occur. These swellings are epidermal cells

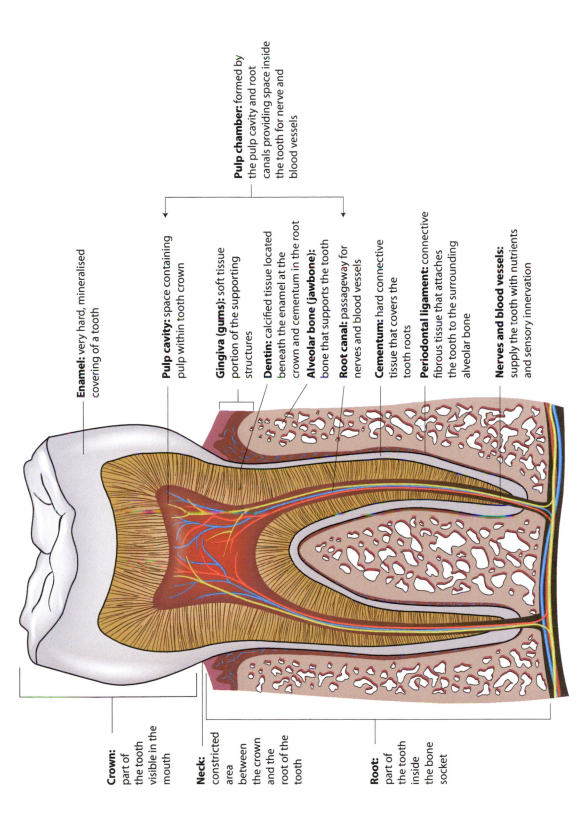

Enamel: very hard, mineralised covering of a tooth

Pulp cavity: space containing pulp within tooth crown

Pulp chamber: formed by the pulp cavity and root canals providing space inside the tooth for nerve and blood vessels

Gingiva (gums): soft tissue portion of the supporting structures

Dentin: calcified tissue located beneath the enamel at the crown and cementum in the root

Alveolar bone (jawbone): bone that supports the tooth

Root canal: passageway for nerves and blood vessels

Cementum: hard connective tissue that covers the tooth roots

Periodontal ligament: connective fibrous tissue that attaches the tooth to the surrounding alveolar bone

Nerves and blood vessels: supply the tooth with nutrients and sensory innervation

Crown: part of the tooth visible in the mouth

Neck: constricted area between the crown and the root of the tooth

Root: part of the tooth inside the bone socket

Figure 2.7 Section through an adult tooth.

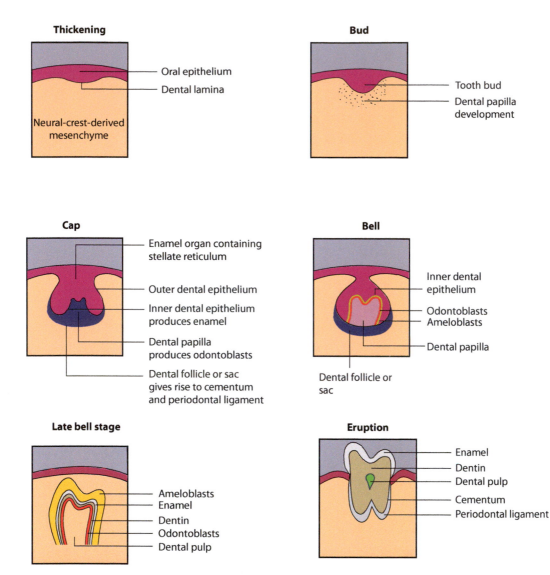

Thickening

Oral epithelium
Dental lamina

Neural-crest-derived mesenchyme

Bud

Tooth bud
Dental papilla development

Cap

Enamel organ containing stellate reticulum

Outer dental epithelium

Inner dental epithelium produces enamel

Dental papilla produces odontoblasts

Dental follicle or sac gives rise to cementum and periodontal ligament

Bell

Inner dental epithelium

Odontoblasts
Ameloblasts

Dental papilla

Dental follicle or sac

Late bell stage

Ameloblasts
Enamel
Dentin
Odontoblasts
Dental pulp

Eruption

Enamel
Dentin
Dental pulp
Cementum
Periodontal ligament

Figure 2.8 Embryology: Stages of tooth development.

proliferating into the subjacent mesenchyme tissue. The swellings indicate the eventual positions of individual teeth. Each swelling is called an epithelial bud. At week 7 epithelial buds are evident for two incisors, one canine and two premolar teeth in both the upper and lower jaws.

At weeks 8–9 the epithelial tissue of the dental lamina protrudes further into the mesenchyme. This is the first stage in the development of the primary tooth germ.

Cap stage

The cap stage commences around week 10 gestation. The epithelial tissue continues to grow into the underlying mesenchyme and takes on the appearance of a cap. The structure is now called the *enamel organ*. It contains a group of star-shaped cells and aminoglycans called the *stellate reticulum*. These attract water and swell inside the enamel organ. The enamel organ, as the name suggests, is responsible for the production of enamel that covers the external surface of the tooth.

As the cap enlarges, mesenchyme tissue is caught between the developing folds of the enamel organ. This forms the dental papilla which will develop into the dentin and the tooth pulp.

The enamel organ and dental papilla become enclosed together by a dental follicle. This limits the spread of the developing dental papilla and produces the supporting structures of the tooth.

Bell stage

The bell stage commences in week 14 as the enamel organ takes on a bell shape. As this structure develops there are changes in the epithelium associated with the tooth development. The epithelial tissue that surrounds the dental papilla differentiates into ameloblasts that will form the tooth enamel. Mesenchymal cells of the dental papilla differentiate into dentin producing odontoblasts.

The dental papilla becomes further enclosed by the enamel organ and development of the tooth crown starts. During the bell stage the dental lamina separates from the developing tooth.

Development of the crown always starts with the laying down of dentin.

- *Dentin* is formed from the dental papilla. *Odontoblasts* form a layer of dentin next to the inner dental epithelium. Dentin production continues towards the inside of the tooth.
- Enamel is formed from *ameloblasts*. The cells secrete enamel onto the surface of the dentin initially and then gradually build up the layer of enamel on top of the developing tooth.
- *Cementum* is formed by cementoblasts that form from the dental follicle. The cementum is laid down at the tooth root to assist in securing the tooth to the adjacent tissues.
- The *periodontal ligament* develops as a connection between cementum and the bone socket into which the tooth sits.

By week 30 gestation layers of *dentin* and enamel are evident within the tooth structure.

Branches of nerves and blood vessels form in the mesenchyme tissue surrounding the tooth during its early development. As the tooth enlarges the nerves and blood vessels grow into the dental papilla. They provide vascular supply and drainage and nervous innervation to the dental papilla. This eventually differentiates into the *dental pulp*. By week 40 gestation the crown is three quarters developed and the neurovascular bundle is maturing into the *dental papilla*.

Alveolar bone develops from the dental follicle. This forms the sockets in which the teeth will sit. This can occur independently from the development of the tooth; however, to ensure that the tooth develops in the correct position the two processes must be coordinated. The tooth remains in the alveolar bone until eruption occurs. The *gingival tissues* (gum tissues) develop at this stage.

Postnatal development and adult teeth

Gross anatomy and function

Infant and child tooth development

At birth the primary or deciduous teeth are embedded within the gum or gingival tissues of the oral cavity. The primary or 'milk' teeth remain here until tooth eruption occurs, usually between the ages of 6 and 24 months. During this time enamel deposition continues at the crown of the tooth. Once complete the epithelium overlying the tooth fuses with the overlying oral mucosa. This forms a pathway for tooth eruption. The crown of the tooth pushes apically to erupt from within the gingiva, a process commonly known as 'teething'. This occurs as a result of growth of the root, dentin and pulp beneath. Secondary or permanent teeth lie in the gingival tissue behind the deciduous teeth. *Osteoclastic* activity reabsorbs the roots of the deciduous teeth, to be replaced by 32 permanent teeth. This occurs from the age of 6 years (Figure 2.9).

Adult teeth

The digestive process is started by the teeth in the oral cavity, grinding the food mechanically to start breaking it down. This is called *mastication*. Teeth cut and grind the nutrients in order to mix them with salivary secretions. This is assisted by the tongue and enables the food to be mixed with digestive enzymes such as *salivary amylase* and *lingual lipase*. These enzymes start the first stages of *starch* and lipid digestion, respectively.

The *crown* is the exposed portion of the tooth which sits above the gingiva or gums. It is covered by enamel, a hard, translucent crystalline substance that covers the underlying dentin. It provides a hard protective covering for the exposed tooth surface and is the most mineralised and resilient tissue of the

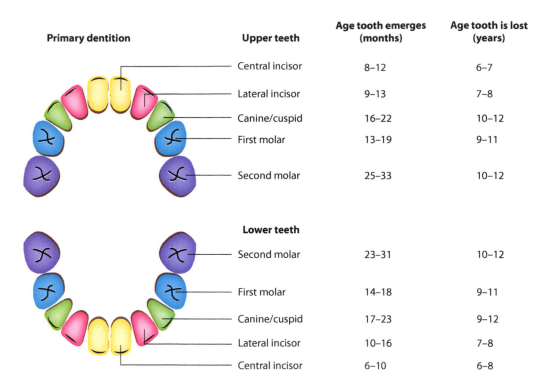

Primary dentition	Upper teeth	Age tooth emerges (months)	Age tooth is lost (years)
	Central incisor	8–12	6–7
	Lateral incisor	9–13	7–8
	Canine/cuspid	16–22	10–12
	First molar	13–19	9–11
	Second molar	25–33	10–12
Lower teeth			
	Second molar	23–31	10–12
	First molar	14–18	9–11
	Canine/cuspid	17–23	9–12
	Lateral incisor	10–16	7–8
	Central incisor	6–10	6–8

Figure 2.9 Child dentition.

human body. It consists mainly of a combination of organic calcified salts and water.

Dentin is a hard mineralised substance similar to bone, consisting of water, collagen and crystalline hydroxyapatite. The majority of the tooth consists of dentin.

Within the dentin is the dental pulp. This is a cavity within the tooth composed of loose connective tissue. Nerves and blood vessels follow the *root canal* into the dental pulp. The *apical foramen* provides an opening to the root canal at the base of the tooth. Innervation of the teeth is via the maxillary and mandibular branches of the trigeminal nerve (*cranial nerve* V). Blood vessels are the superior and inferior alveolar arteries and branches of the maxillary artery.

The neck of the tooth is the area between the crown and root. It is at this point that the gingival tissues approach the tooth forming a groove called the *gingival sulcus*. Epithelial tissue at the base of the sulcus attaches the gingiva to the tooth.

The root sits below the gingiva into the bone socket or alveolus of the upper and lower jaw. The structure and shape of the root vary according to

tooth type. The tooth is held into the alveolus by the *periodontal ligament* and cementum. The periodontal ligament forms a fibrous connection with the tooth, called a *gomphosis*.

An adult has 32 permanent teeth (Figure 2.10). In adults the last teeth to appear are the third molars or wisdom teeth; however, in some people they fail to descend.

There are four main types of teeth classified according to their shape and function:

- *Incisors* are utilised for cutting and biting due to their sharp apices. They have a single root.
- *Canine* or *cuspid* teeth have a pointed, conical shape ideal for tearing and piercing food. Canines have a single root.
- *Premolars* or bicuspids have a more flattened, broad crown ideal for crushing and grinding. They have one or two roots.
- *Molars* also have flat, broad crowns for crushing and grinding. When the upper and lower jaws are closed the premolars and molars fit together to facilitate the process.

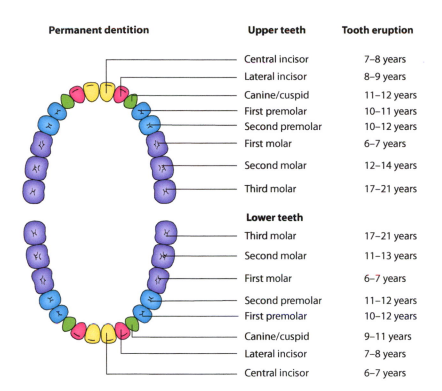

Permanent dentition	Upper teeth	Tooth eruption
	Central incisor	7–8 years
	Lateral incisor	8–9 years
	Canine/cuspid	11–12 years
	First premolar	10–11 years
	Second premolar	10–12 years
	First molar	6–7 years
	Second molar	12–14 years
	Third molar	17–21 years
	Lower teeth	
	Third molar	17–21 years
	Second molar	11–13 years
	First molar	6–7 years
	Second premolar	11–12 years
	First premolar	10–12 years
	Canine/cuspid	9–11 years
	Lateral incisor	7–8 years
	Central incisor	6–7 years

Figure 2.10 Adult dentition.

SALIVARY GLANDS

Prenatal development of the salivary glands

There are three pairs of major salivary glands: the *parotid, submandibular* and *sublingual* glands. Each secretes saliva into the oral cavity. In addition to the major glands there are approximately 600–1000 minor *buccal* glands distributed throughout the oral cavity and upper digestive tract. The major salivary glands are derived from *ectomesenchymal* tissue between the sixth and eighth weeks of gestation. A solid cord of epithelial cells, derived from the *stomadeum*, forms into the surrounding mesenchyme tissue. The cells branch to form the basic *acinar* and *ductal* structures of the mature salivary gland. The central cells of the branches disintegrate to form the lumen of the ducts and the end secretory portion of the gland.

The parotid gland enlarges first and grows posteriorly. At the same time the *facial nerve (cranial nerve VII)* grows anteriorly, until complete development of the parotid gland encloses the facial nerve. The submandibular and sublingual glands form at 6 and 8 weeks, respectively. The minor buccal glands arise from oral ectoderm and nasopharyngeal endoderm. They develop at 3 months' gestation.

The secretion of saliva is controlled by the autonomic nervous system. The *postganglionic fibres* of the sympathetic and parasympathetic nerves synapse with *myoepithelial* and acinar cells in the developing gland. The myoepithelial cells provide contraction of the gland epithelium during secretion. The acinar cells produce saliva.

Continued stimulation of the salivary glands by autonomic stimulation promotes their maturation. Sympathetic nerve stimulation causes the acinar cells to mature, and parasympathetic stimulation provides overall gland growth. The salivary glands start secreting saliva from week 16 of embryological development.

By 4–6 months of age saliva secretion increases. During this time it is not inactivated by gastric acid and thus can contribute to the digestion of starches in the stomach and small intestine.

Postnatal development and adult salivary glands

Gross anatomy and function

The parotid, submandibular and sublingual salivary glands are the major *tubuloalveolar glands* responsible for the production of saliva within the oral cavity.

• The *parotid gland* is the largest of the major salivary glands. It is situated anterior and inferior to the ear, lying between the *masseter muscle* and overlying

skin. It occupies a triangular space containing gland tissue. Saliva drains from the gland via the *parotid duct (Stensen's duct)*. The duct is 4–6 cm in length and 0.5 cm in diameter. It runs from the anterior border of the parotid gland penetrating the buccinator muscle of the cheek. It enters the oral cavity at the level of the second maxillary molar (Figure 2.11).

• The submandibular gland lies between the *digastric* and *mylohyoid* muscles of the cheek and jaw. Saliva

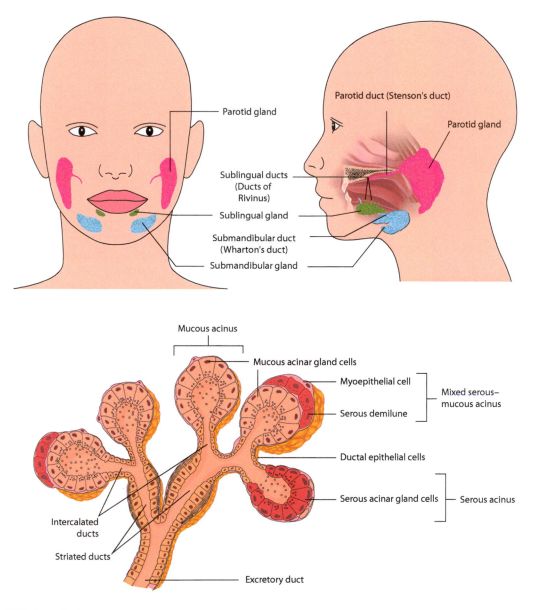

Figure 2.11 Salivary glands.

from the submandibular gland drains into the oral cavity via the *submandibular* or *Wharton's duct*. The duct exits on the medial side of the gland to drain into the oral cavity, just lateral to the lingual frenulum (Figure 2.11).

- The sublingual gland is the smallest of the three major salivary glands. It lies deep to the floor of the oral mucosa. It has no dominant duct; however, there are 10 small ducts called the *Ducts of Rivinus*. They exit the superior surface of the gland, beneath the tongue (Figure 2.11).

Saliva production

Saliva has an important role to play in the maintenance of oral health and the preparation of nutrients for swallowing and digestion. Table 2.2 shows the functions of saliva.

Salivary glands can produce saliva at a rate of 0.5–1 mL/min/g of gland. This is equivalent to 1–1.5 L of saliva per day. Saliva is cleared from the mouth by reflex swallowing. The glands are composed of three cell types; acinar epithelial cells, ductal epithelial cells and myoepithelial cells which are embedded within a supporting connective tissue (Figure 2.11):

- *Acinar epithelial cells* are responsible for the primary production of saliva that is secreted into the ducts of the gland. Acinar cells are packed with secretory granules that release their products via *exocytosis* into the lumen of the duct. There are two types of acinar cells:

Table 2.2 Functions of saliva

Mucin moistens the oral mucosa and nutrients as they enter the oral cavity to facilitate bolus formation

Initiation of digestive processes in the oral cavity by the production of *amylase* to digest starch and *lingual lipase* to digest fats

High content of calcium and phosphate ions important for the mineralisation of the enamel of new teeth

Provides antimicrobial protection of the oral cavity via
- Secretory IgA
- Lysozyme
- Salivary peroxidase
- Lactoferrin

Medium for dissolved foods to stimulate taste buds

Bicarbonate provides a buffer to maintain pH range 5.6–7

Provides a *mucin* coat over the teeth and oral cavity important in the prevention of dental caries and oral infection, respectively

- *Serous acinar gland cells* produce saliva rich in proteins such as amylase, an enzyme involved in the initial digestion of starch in the oral cavity.
- *Mucus acinar gland cells* produce saliva rich in mucin. This is a *glycoprotein* that moistens, lubricates and coats the surface of the oral mucosa.
- *Ductal epithelial cells* line the lumen of the gland ducts and modify the saliva as it moves along the lumen towards the excretory ducts.
- *Myoepithelial cells* sit between the acinar and ductal cells and assist in the movement of secretions along the lumen of the duct.

Formation of saliva

Saliva is formed by the passive and active transportation of *electrolytes* and proteins from the surrounding *interstitial fluid* into the acinar cells. The solutes are then transported to the lumen of the salivary gland ducts (Figure 2.11). Acinar cells have a high *plasma membrane* permeability due to the presence of *aquaporins*. These are membrane proteins that act as selective water channels. They are responsible for facilitating the *osmotic* movement of water across the acinar cells, in response to electrolyte concentrations. The saliva end product reflects a plasma-like, *isotonic* fluid, containing water, electrolytes and proteins.

Once inside the duct, the saliva is subject to modification by reabsorption and secretion. The duct of the salivary glands is divided into three anatomical areas: the *intercalated duct*, the *striated duct* and the *excretory duct*.

- The intercalated duct secretes bicarbonate into the lumen of the duct and absorbs *chloride ions* (Cl^-).
- The striated duct absorbs *sodium ions* and secretes *potassium ions* (K^+) into the saliva.
- The excretory duct makes no modifications.

The saliva secreted from the salivary glands is always *hypotonic* to plasma. The main components of saliva are 99% water, mucin, enzymes, K^+, Ca^{2+}, phosphate, Cl^-, *carbonic anhydrase*, *urea* and bicarbonate. However the composition is variable depending upon the gland producing it and the stimulus for production.

- The parotid glands produce the majority of saliva during ingestion of nutrients. This accounts for approximately 69% of saliva production; however, this reduces significantly during periods of rest to approximately 26%. This reflects the fact that parotid gland acinar cells are serous and thus their main function is to produce a thin, serous saliva rich in antibacterial proteins and enzymes. These are able to facilitate digestive processes in the mouth.

- The submandibular glands are more active during periods of rest. They produce approximately 69% of saliva volume at rest; however, during nutrient ingestion this decreases to 26%. These glands are mixed and contain both mucus and serous acinar gland cells; however, the serous cells predominate.
- The sublingual glands produce a constant smaller volume of viscous saliva, approximately 5% of the total saliva volume. This does not change with the ingestion of nutrients. The saliva is mucin based, due to the presence of mainly mucus acinar gland cells. This contributes to the viscosity of the saliva produced and lubrication of the oral mucosa.

Control of salivary secretions

The production of saliva is controlled by behavioural, neural, physical and chemical stimuli. Chemoreceptors in the mucosa of the oral cavity are stimulated by irritants, acids, spices and chemicals from food. The physical presence of nutrients or the mechanical movement of chewing stimulates mechano-receptors. Sensory neurons transmit impulses from these receptors to the *cerebral cortex* and salivary *nuclei* in the *medulla* of the *brainstem*. Conscious recognition of the thought, sight or smell of food also stimulates the salivary nuclei. Even chewing with an empty mouth can stimulate a response. Motor responses are coordinated via the autonomic nervous system. Parasympathetic innervation is via the glossopharyngeal nerve (cranial nerve IX) to the parotid glands and the facial nerve (cranial nerve VII) to the submandibular and sublingual glands. This stimulates the production of copious amounts of thin, watery saliva. Sympathetic innervation stimulates smaller volumes of viscous, mucin-based saliva.

Ageing and the salivary glands

As a person ages the composition of his or her saliva changes. The amount of amylase and mucin decreases producing a thicker, more viscous saliva. In older people common changes in saliva production are related to drug therapy. This can lead to difficulties in swallowing, chewing, oral dryness and difficulty with dentures.

Changes associated with different stages of the lifespan

Sjögrens syndrome

Sjögrens syndrome (SS) is a progressive autoimmune inflammatory disorder of the lacrimal and salivary glands. It causes dryness of mucosal surfaces leading to xerophthalmia (dry eyes) and xerostomia (dry mouth), together with non-specific symptoms including malaise and fatigue.

SS predominantly affects women (9:1 female-to-male ratio) with onset in middle age, but can affect children, men and older people, with an increased prevalence rate occurring with increasing age (Ramos-Casals et al., 2012; Mavragani and Moutsopoulos, 2014).

SS can be categorised as either primary or secondary. Primary SS (pSS) is classified as occurring in a healthy individual with no other associated disease. Secondary SS (sSS) occurs with other systemic auto-immune diseases such as rheumatoid arthritis and systemic lupus erythematosus. It accounts for 60% of all SS cases (Kassan and Moutsopoulos, 2004). The cause of SS is considered to be multifactorial including a combination of genetic, immune and environmental factors (e.g. retroviruses, hormones).

SS occurs as a result of inflammation in the salivary and lacrimal glands. Inflammation of the epithelial cells may be triggered by a virus in those who are genetically predisposed. The infection and inflammation cause epithelial cell death or apoptosis (Larché, 2006). Chemical mediators are released from the damaged cells and promote the movement of lymphocytes into the gland. The continued inflammation results in atrophy and fibrosis of the acinar cells and destruction of ductal cells (Fox, 2005). Lymphocytes also interfere with the normal nervous stimulation and response of salivary glands. It has also been suggested that aquaporins in the epithelial acinar cells may be decreased which results in a decrease in production and flow of saliva.

SS can significantly affect a person's quality of life. Clinical manifestations include the glandular effects of xerostomia and xerophthalmia occurring in 90%–95% of people with pSS (Mavragani and Moutsopoulos, 2014).

- *Xerophthalmia* (95%) results in dry eyes and decreased tear production. Symptoms include itching, grittiness and soreness of the eyes, with ocular fatigue, photosensitivity and a decrease in visual acuity. This can lead to corneal ulcers, eyelid infection and destruction of the conjunctival epithelium (kerato-conjunctivitis sicca).

- *Xerostomia* (90%) relates to dryness of the oral mucosa. Reduced saliva volume leads to difficulties in speech, eating, retaining and controlling dentures, dysphagia and may lead to tooth decay and periodontal disease. *Angular cheilitis* is a common feature.

  In the advanced stages of SS the oral mucosa becomes dry and glazed with fine wrinkles across its surface.

- Increases in *oral infections* such as candidiasis are associated with SS. The antibacterial properties of saliva such as IgA are lost which allows the colonisation of bacterial and fungal infections.

- Saliva is important in maintaining a stable oral pH. Increases in the colonisation of bacteria such as *Streptococcus mutans* occur in SS, and small decreases in pH may lead to demineralisation of teeth and contribute to the development of *dental caries* of people with SS.

- Lack of saliva causes the tongue to become dry. It can stick to the hard palate generating a 'clicking' sound when released. This can interfere with speech and swallowing. The tongue appears red with the formation of lobules across its surface. Tongue papilla may be partially or completely lost, affecting taste.

- Parotid gland swelling and inflammation occur in approximately 50% of cases of pSS (Skopouli et al., 2000). This is usually asymptomatic, occurring bilaterally and can be a predictor of lymphoma. There is a 10–50 times higher risk of developing lymphoma, occurring in 5%–10% of people with pSS (Ramos-Casals et al., 2012; Bootsma et al., 2013).

- Nasal and throat symptoms, extending to the larynx, can develop, which may present as a persistent dry cough and shortness of breath (xerotrachea/bronchitis sicca). *Dysphagia* occurs frequently as a result of decreased saliva production and often necessitates the need to drink liquids to assist swallowing. Decreased saliva production also prevents the neutralisation of gastric acid reflux into the oesophagus and trachea.

People with pSS may also develop extraglandular features such as arthritis (15%–30%), vasculitis (purpura 10%), Raynaud's phenomenon (18%–37%), fatigue (70%), nephritis (2.5%), thyroid disease (14%–33%), peripheral neuropathies (2%–10%) and central nervous system (3%–20%) effects, such as headache, migraine, mood disorders and cognitive dysfunction (Ramos-Casals et al., 2012; Bootsma et al., 2013; Mavragani and Moutsopoulos, 2014; Morreale et al., 2014).

PHARYNX

Prenatal development of the pharynx

The pharynx is a passageway for nutrients and air to pass to the oesophagus and trachea, respectively. The *pharynx* is formed as part of the foregut of the developing embryo. It develops from

- Endoderm which forms the mucosal epithelial lining of the pharynx
- Ectoderm which forms the epithelial covering of the pharynx
- Neural crest cells which form skeletal and muscle tissue
- Mesoderm cells which form the pharyngeal musculature

These structures develop from the individual pharyngeal arches. It is a process that must be carefully coordinated to ensure structures develop at the right time and in the right place.

During foetal life the pharynx increases in width and length. It is divided into the nasopharynx, oropharynx and laryngopharynx. During foetal life the pharynx is more compliant or collapsible than in its adult form. This decreases in the first year of life but can still be a cause of *apnea* in children.

Postnatal development and adult pharynx

Gross anatomy and function

The pharynx is a muscular tube extending from the posterior aspect of the oral and nasal cavities to the *cervical* end of the oesophagus, at the *cricopharyngeus muscle* and *upper oesophageal sphincter*. It allows the passage of air and nutrients to either the *trachea* or oesophagus, respectively. The powerful skeletal muscle structure of the pharynx facilitates swallowing or *deglutition*. This moves the bolus from the oral cavity to the oesophagus.

The pharynx is divided into three parts: the nasopharynx, the oropharynx and the *laryngopharynx*.

The pharynx is lined with non-keratinised stratified squamous epithelium. It has a well-developed muscularis externa to facilitate swallowing. The longitudinal muscle group is made up of the *palatopharyngeus*, *stylopharyngeus* and *salpingopharyngeus* muscles. These elevate and shorten the pharynx during swallowing. The circular muscle group consists of the superior, middle and inferior constrictors, which contract from superior to inferior to clear the bolus from the pharynx.

Neuromuscular control of the pharynx is via the *pons* and medulla of the brainstem. Sensory and motor innervation is via the trigeminal (*cranial nerve* V), glossopharyngeal (*cranial nerve* IX), vagus (*cranial nerve* X) and hypoglossal (*cranial nerve* XII) nerves.

SUMMARY OF KEY POINTS

1. Mouth – a cavity lined with stratified squamous (keratinised on gums, hard palate and dorsum of tongue).
2. Vestibule – area bounded by lips, cheeks, teeth and gums.
3. Palate – the roof of the mouth that can be divided into hard palate – formed by the palatine processes of maxillary bones and the palatine bones; soft palate – soft fold containing skeletal muscles which terminates posteriorly in the uvula.
4. Tongue – a muscular organ anchored in the floor of the mouth. Consists of bundles of skeletal muscle fibres which run in longitudinal, transverse and vertical planes. These muscles change the shape of the tongue for speech and swallowing. The median septum divides the tongue into bilaterally symmetrical halves. The lingual frenulum secures the tongue to the floor of the mouth. A very short frenulum produces the condition 'tongue-tied'.
5. Extrinsic muscles – gross movements of the tongue are produced by the three extrinsic muscles which insert on the tongue and have their origins on portions of skull bones and the hyoid bone:
   i. Genioglossus – protrudes the tongue (origin is mandible)
   ii. Hyoglossus – depresses the tongue (origin is hyoid bone)
   iii. Styloglossus – retracts and elevates the tongue (origin is the styloid process of temporal bone).
6. Lingual papillae – projections of the lamina propria on the dorsum of tongue. There are four types of these projections:
   i. Filiform papillae – the most numerous, they cover the anterior two thirds of the dorsum. They give the tongue a roughness needed in licking semisolid foods. Heavily keratinised, they give the tongue a 'coated' appearance.
   ii. Fungiform papillae – located on the sides of tongue interspersed among the filiform papillae. Taste buds are found around these papillae.
   iii. Folliate papillae
   iv. Circumvallate papillae – form a V-shaped formation near the posterior margin of the tongue. The largest numbers of taste buds are associated with these papillae.
7. Salivary glands – ducted exocrine glands producing saliva. Two types of acinar secretory cells are found in the glandular tissue:
   i. Serous cells producing a watery secretion containing amylase
   ii. Mucous cells producing a viscous liquid containing the glycoprotein mucin
8. Submandibular glands – are bilaterally located at the median aspect of the mandibular angle. Their ducts bring saliva to the oral cavity at the base of the frenulum. They are mixed glands, containing approximately equal numbers of serous and mucous cells.
9. Sublingual glands – are anterior to the submandibular glands under the tongue. Cells of these glands are mostly mucous producing. Very little amylase is found in this saliva.
10. Parotid glands – are anterior and inferior to the external ears lying in a connective tissue capsule. Parotid ducts bring saliva into the vestibule alongside of the second upper molar. The glandular cells are mostly serous.
11. Fauces – are the passageway from the mouth to the pharynx. This short corridor is guarded by four pillars; the two palatoglossal arches are more anterior followed by the two palatopharyngeal arches. In between the two sets of arches on either side are the palatine tonsils. During swallowing, contraction of the muscles in these arches constricts the pillars preventing food from reentering the mouth.
12. Pharynx – receives food from the oral cavity via the fauces as the tongue moves up and back. The food enters the oropharynx first. Contractions of muscles in the soft palate raise this structure to prevent food from entering the nasopharynx. The oropharynx and the more inferior laryngopharynx are common passageways for food and air. These regions are lined with stratified squamous epithelium and well supplied with mucous glands.

CHECK ON LEARNING

Oral cavity

A limited amount of digestion takes place in the mouth: Which enzymes are involved and what do they do?

Answer – Amylase breaks down starches (polysaccharides to disaccharides); lipase breaks down fats.

Name the three salivary glands.

Answer – They are the parotid, submandibular and sublingual glands.

What is the name of the membrane that secures the tongue to the floor of the mouth?

Answer – This is the frenulum.

List three functions of the tongue important for digestion.

Answer – Three functions are mechanical breakup of food material, formation of a bolus and sensory analysis of food material (taste buds).

What type of epithelial cells line the mouth, pharynx and oesophagus?

Answer – Stratified squamous epithelial cells line the mouth, pharynx and oesophagus.

Taste buds are found at the base of papillae on the tongue. Name the four types of papillae.

Answer – They are circumvallate, filiform, foliate and fungiform.

What are the five different taste sensations?

Answer – They are sweet, sour, salty, bitter and umami.

Explain the pathway for taste.

Answer – Saliva dissolves nutrients, nutrients drain down into the base of the papillae, the chemicals stimulate the sensory receptors of the taste buds and taste sensations are translated into a nervous impulse which travels to the sensory cortex of the brain where the different taste sensations are interpreted.

What is the function of mucin?

Answer – Mucin is a glycoprotein that helps to bind the bolus together.

CASE STUDY

Cleft lip and palate

Stanley is 6 years old. He was born with a cleft lip and palate. He underwent surgical repair of the cleft lip and palate but has developed gradual conductive hearing loss. He has also had speech therapy due to slow language development and difficulties in articulation of words. Due to the extent of clefting Stanley has absent incisors at the site of the original cleft. Stanley's mother has smoked during all her pregnancies and Stanley's sister Poppy also has a cleft lip.

Stanley attended a follow-up appointment with his paediatrician. He presented with a sore throat and pain in his right ear. On examination the eardrum is bulging, inflamed and red. An otitis media with effusion was diagnosed.

Explanation of normal and altered physiology

The following table sets out the normal and altered anatomy and physiology which explains the person's problems.

Normal physiology	Altered anatomy/physiology and related problems
Explain the process of embryological development of the face. Embryological development of the face commences in week 4 gestation from five facial primordia: • One frontonasal prominence • Two maxillary processes • Two mandibular processes The processes enlarge and grow towards one another, fusing to create the oral cavity, upper and lower jaws and primary and secondary palates.	*Cleft lip and cleft palate are common craniofacial malformations. They often occur together and can form a significant cleft extending from the palate to the upper lip and nasal cavity.* *What is the process of embryological development of a cleft lip?* Cleft lip is the incomplete fusion of the maxillary processes and the medial frontonasal processes. Fusion of the midline to form the upper lip and philtrum should be complete between 7 and 8 weeks' gestation. Cleft lip is associated with primary palate development. *What is the process of embryological development of a cleft palate?* Cleft palate occurs as a result of failure of fusion of the maxillary palatine shelves during the formation of the secondary palate. The nasal and oral cavities are connected.

(Continued)

During embryological development the embryo may be exposed to environmental factors or teratogens which may affect the normal developmental processes.

What is a teratogen?
Any agent that causes an abnormality following foetal exposure during pregnancy.

Cleft lip with cleft palate has been associated with a number of environmental or teratogenic factors.

What factors may be associated with the development of cleft lip and palate?

- Smoking
- Alcohol
- Anticonvulsants
- Benzodiazepines
- Folate insufficiency
- Zinc insufficiency

Feeding and nutrition

At full term an infant has developed the ability to suckle and maintain a vacuum within the oral cavity to be able to feed from the breast or bottle.

Explain the physiological process occurring during sucking.

1. An intact palate is required to initiate the sucking reflex. The palate is stimulated by the presence of the nipple or teat in the infant's mouth.
2. The presence of pressure from the tongue onto the nipple or teat facilitates the process. A closed seal created by the infant's mouth around the nipple creates a negative pressure inside the mouth. The infant uses the resistance of the palate to press the nipple or teat against. A wave of pressure is created by the movement of the infant's tongue to express fluid directly into the pharynx.
3. The tongue lowers to allow expansion of the nipple or teat. They fill with fluid and the process repeats.

Infants with cleft lip and palate often have difficulty in feeding.

Explain the reasons for this in terms of altered anatomy and physiology.

- Infant has difficulty in creating a seal around the nipple or teat due to the cleft lip.
- Infant is unable to generate negative pressure and create suction.
- Infant has decreased ability to suck.
- Cleft palate provides a connection between the oral and nasal cavity. Fluid may enter into nasal cavity and escape through the nose.
- The cleft palate interferes with the compression of the nipple onto the hard palate to express milk.

Speech

What is the role of tensor veli and levator veli palatini muscles in speech?
The tensor and levator veli palatini muscles insert into the hard and soft palate. The muscles raise the palate during speech to prevent air from entering the nasal cavity.

Cleft lip and palate may result in speech and language difficulties. These may be resolved in childhood but some children and adolescents retain speech difficulties into adulthood.

Speech in those with cleft lip and palate can be referred to as 'hypernasal speech'.

Explain why hypernasal speech occurs:

1. Pre-cleft repair
Prior to repair the oral and nasal cavities are connected.
There is less palate surface area for the tongue to contact to make sounds.
It is difficult for the child to create enough air pressure inside the oral cavity for speech.
There is altered attachments of the tensor and levator veli palatini muscles.
Velopharyngeal inadequacy occurs when the soft palate is unable to rise during speech to cover the entrance to the nasal cavity.
Hypernasal speech occurs as a result of air escaping through the nose.

(Continued)

2. Post-cleft repair

Velopharyngeal function is not always restored by cleft repair. If attachment is still insufficient then hypernasal speech will continue.

What other factors can influence speech?

- Hearing loss. Difficulty in interpreting sounds
- Insufficient palate function
- Cleft interferes with speech sounds in the mouth – normally made through interaction of throat and palatine muscles
- Poor dentition
- Timing of cleft repair

Hearing

What is the role of the auditory/eustachian (pharyngotympanic) tubes?

Drainage of the middle ear by the auditory tubes is important in the prevention of middle ear infections (otitis media) and effusion. The tubes open to equalise pressure between the middle ear cavity and external pressure.

Children with cleft lip and palate have an increased risk of otitis media and effusion.

Explain the anatomical and physiological reason for this condition in cleft lip and palate.

- Poor drainage of the middle ear due to inefficient functioning of the auditory/eustachian (pharyngotympanic) tubes
- Obstruction of the nasopharyngeal end of the tubes
- Poor *tensor veli palatini* function
- Increased pressure of fluid in the middle ear
- Otitis media

What are the long-term effects?

- Conductive hearing loss
- Tympanic membrane scarring

Dentition

What role does the primary palate have in the development of teeth?

Development of the primary palate results in the development of the alveolar ridge at the intermaxillary segment. This contains the four front incisor teeth.

Children with cleft lip and palate often require dental and orthodontic treatment.

How might the development of a cleft lip and palate affect normal tooth development?

- Malformations of the size, shape, number and symmetry of teeth
- Malpositioned teeth
- Missing teeth
- Upper lateral incisor – missing or malpositioned
- Alterations in pattern of tooth eruption
- Hypodontia can occur outside of the cleft site
- Cross bite

These can depend upon the severity of the cleft.

CLINICAL CHALLENGES

1. Infants and children may be admitted to hospital for repair of a cleft palate. At what stage in a child's development is this most likely to occur? What does the repair involve?
2. Consider the long-term problems associated with cleft lip and palate in adults that may present in the clinical area.
3. Consider what the ongoing role of the multidisciplinary team is in the management of cleft lip and palate.
4. How is otitis media managed in children?

OESOPHAGUS

PRENATAL DEVELOPMENT OF THE OESOPHAGUS

The oesophagus is a muscular tube that provides a connection between the pharynx and stomach. It is of endoderm origin and is derived from the *caudal* portion of the primitive foregut tube. The oesophagus and trachea develop from this single structure. During the fourth week of gestation a lung bud grows from the ventral surface of the foregut where the trachea and bronchial tree develop as tubes. The oesophagus elongates and commences development of the oesophageal wall. The muscle layer of the wall starts its development in week 6 from mesenchyme tissue. This will form the circular and longitudinal muscle layers of the adult oesophagus. At this stage the trachea and oesophagus are joined. Separation of the oesophagus and trachea commences with the development of tracheo-oesophageal folds between the ventral trachea and dorsal oesophagus. These fuse to form a tracheo-oesophageal septum/groove that separates the two structures in a rostro-caudal direction. Failure of this process can lead to the development of oesophageal atresia or tracheo-oesophageal fistula.

The epithelial tissue lining the oesophagus is of ectoderm origin, developing as ciliated epithelial cells in week 10 and maturing to stratified squamous epithelium by week 25. Any remaining ciliated cells develop into oesophageal glands.

At each end of the oesophagus a sphincter develops to control the movement of food into and out of the oesophagus. The upper oesophageal sphincter forms from the lower pharyngeal arches, while the lower oesophageal sphincter is derived from mesenchyme tissue that surrounds the oesophagus as it enters the stomach. In infants the tone of the *lower oesophageal sphincter* is reduced and peristalsis is immature. This is associated with increased *reflux* and *regurgitation* in infants. At birth the oesophagus is approximately 10 cm long and 0.5 cm in diameter.

POSTNATAL DEVELOPMENT AND ADULT OESOPHAGUS

Gross anatomy and function

The oesophagus is a muscular tube providing a conduit for nutrients to pass from the pharynx to the stomach. At rest the oesophagus is collapsed into folds; however, these disappear when the oesophagus is distended by a bolus. The adult oesophagus ranges between 25 and 30 cm in length and lies posterior to the trachea. It lies within the thoracic cavity and pierces the *diaphragm* to enter the abdominal cavity, at the *oesophageal hiatus* (Figure 3.1). Like most parts of the digestive tract, the oesophageal wall is composed of a mucosa, submucosa, muscularis externa and adventitia.

- The mucosa is composed of non-keratinised squamous epithelium, which appears a smooth,

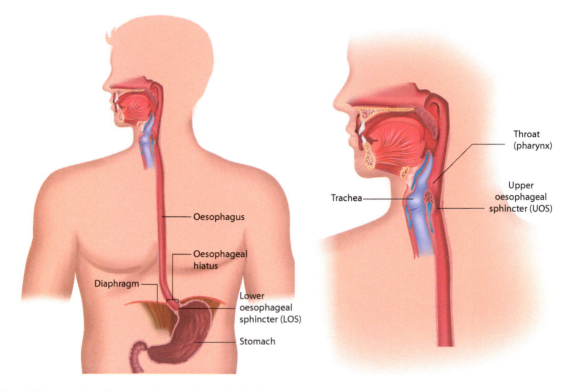

Figure 3.1 Anatomical position of oesophagus and associated sphincters.

pale pink at endoscopy. The 'gastro-oesophageal junction' or 'oesophago-gastric junction' is the point at which the oesophagus meets the stomach. This forms the point of transition between the oesophageal mucosa and the columnar epithelium of the gastric cardia mucosa. This is known as the 'squamocolumnar junction' (SCJ) or 'Z' line.

This is a short transition meaning that the distal part of the oesophagus may be inadvertently exposed to acid-secreting mucosa. This is prevented by the presence of the lower oesophageal sphincter that directs acid back towards the stomach. The oesophageal mucosa is protected if refluxate enters the oesophagus by peristaltic waves which push the acidic contents back into the stomach. Bicarbonate (pH 7.8–8) from saliva also assists in neutralising the acid refluxate.

- The submucosa is scattered with oesophageal glands, particularly in the lower third, which produce mucus. This aids the smooth passage of the bolus through the oesophagus.

The oesophageal submucosa also contains a network of capillaries. Branches of the inferior thyroid artery, aortic oesophageal artery and left gastric artery supply the oesophageal tissues. Venous drainage is from submucosal veins to the *vena cava* and left *gastric vein* which is a branch of the *hepatic portal vein*. Submucosal veins are significant in the formation and haemorrhaging of *oesophageal varices*.

As food passes through the oesophagus it stimulates sensory chemo-, mechano-, thermo- and noci-receptors in the oesophageal mucosa and submucosa. Responses to these stimuli are made through the parasympathetic and sympathetic branches of the autonomic nervous system. Parasympathetic stimulation increases oesophageal muscle contraction and peristalsis and increases secretions from oesophageal glands. Sympathetic stimulation decreases blood supply and increases oesophageal sphincter contractions.

- The muscularis contains both circular and longitudinal layers of muscle tissue. The muscle type is variable along the oesophageal length. The upper third consists of *striated skeletal muscle*, the middle third a combination of striated and smooth muscle and the lower third smooth visceral involuntary muscle only.

- The adventitia consists of a thin layer of *connective tissue* which differentiates into serosa (peritoneum) as the oesophagus enters the abdominal cavity.

Movement of food into and out of the oesophagus is controlled by two distinct sphincters; the upper-oesophageal (crico-pharyngeal sphincter) and the lower oesophageal (cardiac) sphincters.

- The *upper oesophageal sphincter* (UOS) sits approximately 1 cm below the vocal cords, adjacent to the vertebral bodies of cervical vertebrae C5 and C6. It corresponds to the 'C' shaped *cricopharyngeus muscle* which provides a barrier to the efflux of oesophageal and gastric contents when the muscle is contracted. The UOS sphincter usually remains closed when a bolus is not being transported. Speech and emotion can however influence the pressure exerted by the UOS and full closure may not be maintained. Pressure in the UOS falls during sleep and anaesthesia.

- The *lower oesophageal sphincter* (LOS) or *cardiac sphincter* is a complex structure (Figure 3.2). It is an area of distal oesophagus approximately 4 cm long, lying within an area referred to as the 'gastro-oesophageal junction'. The intrinsic component of the LOS is formed from a combination of circular smooth muscle of the oesophageal wall and proximal stomach. Extrinsically, the skeletal muscle of the diaphragm acts as an external sphincter applying pressure to the LOS. The LOS is also supported by the presence of a *phreno-oesophageal membrane or ligament* which runs around the edge of the crural diaphragm as it meets the oesophagus. It extends upwards, penetrating into the submucosa of the oesophagus. This assists in controlling the upward and lateral movement of the LOS.

- One third of the LOS lies proximal to the diaphragm and two thirds of the LOS lies below the diaphragm within the abdomen. An anatomical flap is created at the gastro-oesophageal junction which assists in keeping the distal part of the LOS within the abdomen.

- These structures exert control of the movement of food into the stomach and prevent reflux of stomach contents back into the oesophagus. In order to provide an effective barrier to the movement of food out of the stomach, the LOS must maintain enough pressure to keep the sphincter closed. It has to overcome the tendency of reflux from increased stomach pressure that arises from peristaltic contractions following a meal or during inspiration. It acts as a one-way valve to allow ingested materials to enter the stomach and at the same time prevent stomach contents from refluxing into the oesophagus. The combination of smooth intrinsic muscle and diaphragm contraction enables the sphincter to remain closed.

- The intrinsic muscular structure of the oesophageal wall also assists LOS function. The inner muscularis layer of the oesophagus forms semicircular 'clasp' muscles towards the gastro-oesophageal junction. These 'C' shaped structures arise from the left and right sides of the oesophageal wall, 'clasping' one another from either side. The oblique gastric 'sling' muscles run around the left side of the gastro-oesophageal junction and extend over the anterior and posterior side of the stomach following the lesser curvature. They form the additional oblique muscle layer of the stomach and assist in maintaining what is called the angle of His (Figure 3.2). Contraction of the 'clasp' and 'sling' muscles assists in maintaining the integrity of the LOS.

- The muscles of the LOS maintain a basal tone to create a higher pressure than that inside the stomach to prevent reflux of the stomach contents into the oesophagus. This is aided by contraction of the diaphragm and the unidirectional peristaltic waves, assisted by gravity, directing ingested food towards the stomach. Saliva also assists in neutralising any refluxed stomach contents. Failure of these processes can lead to gastro-oesophageal reflux.

- During swallowing the LOS and diaphragm must relax to allow food to enter the stomach. At the same time the distal oesophagus and LOS are pulled upwards as a result of muscle contraction. Control of the LOS is via the vagus nerve which stimulates excitatory and inhibitory neurons in the myenteric plexus within the oesophageal sphincter wall to contract and relax. Tone of the LOS is also under neurohormonal influences. Substances such as nicotine, secretin, cholecystokinin and prostaglandin decrease LOS tone while gastrin and *substance P* increase LOS tone.

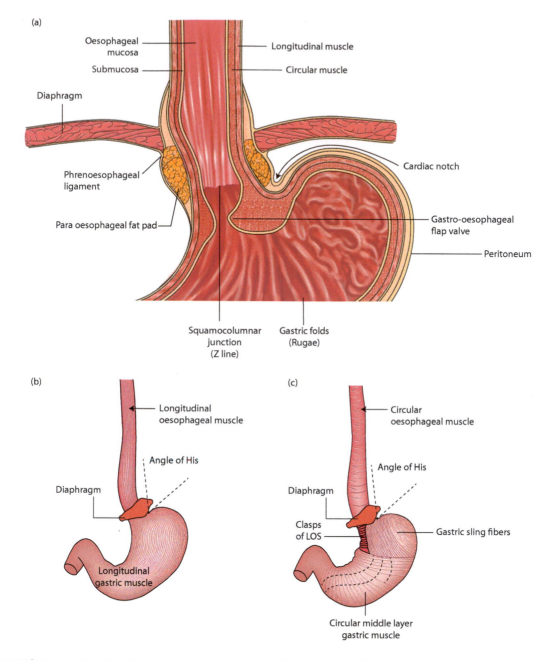

Figure 3.2 Gastro-oesophageal junction and associated musculature. (a) Gastro-oesophageal junction, (b) longitudinal muscle structure and (c) circular muscle structure.

- Transient lower oesophageal sphincter relaxations (TLOSRs) also occur independent of swallowing. They are mediated by the vagus nerve and allow gaseous exit from the stomach, for example during belching. They occur more frequently following meals or if the stomach is distended. The duration of TLOSRs is longer than relaxation of the LOS during swallowing and therefore has the potential for reflux to occur.

- Oesophageal transit is approximately 6–8 seconds, at a rate of 1–4 cm/s depending upon the size and consistency of the bolus.

OROPHARYNGEAL FUNCTION AND AGEING

Oropharyngeal motility may be affected in the older person but it does not correlate with symptoms or have significant effect on the older person unless associated with a disease process. The effects of ageing occur within the muscularis of the pharynx and oesophagus, including effects on the upper and lower oesophageal sphincters.

In an older person there is a low resting UOS pressure and during the pharyngeal phase of swallowing there is delayed and incomplete UOS relaxation. Ageing prolongs the oropharyngeal transit and clearance time during swallowing and may lead to pharyngeal residues.

As the oesophagus ages there is a decrease in the amplitude and velocity of peristaltic contractions. This may be associated with a reduction in myenteric ganglion cells. There is also thickening of the muscularis and evidence of a decrease in striated muscle fibres in the proximal oesophagus, with these being replaced with smooth muscle cells.

There is a decrease in LOS pressure and reduced relaxation at the lower oesophageal sphincter. This leads to decreased oesophageal emptying. There is also movement of the LOS into the chest. Decreased hypersensitivity in the proximal oesophagus may lead to a delay in oesophageal swallowing.

DEVELOPMENTAL ABNORMALITIES OF THE OESOPHAGUS

Oesophageal atresia and tracheo-oesphageal fistula

Oesophageal atresia is a congenital malformation where the oesophagus fails to unite into a continuous tube during embryological development. Oesophageal atresia can occur with or without *tracheo-oesophageal fistula* (TOF), where a connection develops between the trachea and oesophagus.

Oesophageal atresia accounts for 1 in 2500–3000 live births (Shaw-Smith, 2006; Spitz, 2007) with one third of infants with oesophageal atresia being premature (Hosie and Gavens, 2013).

Oesophageal atresia and TOF can be classified according to anatomical configuration (Figure 3.3).

The most common type is oesophageal atresia with a distal tracheo-oesophageal fistula (Hosie and Gaverns, 2013; Smith, 2014; Slater and Rothenberg, 2016).

OA/TOF occurs as an isolated anomaly in the majority of cases but in less than 1% of cases occurs in association with other familial disorders or syndromes (Spitz, 2007). These include VACTERL association, CHARGE association, cardiac anomalies and Trisomy 18 (Edward's syndrome) (Bradshaw et al., 2016; Spitz, 2007). VACTERL is a group of pathologies including vertebral, anorectal, cardiac anomolies, tracheo-oesophageal fistula, and renal and limb pathologies. CHARGE association includes coloboma (developmental defect of the eye), heart anomaly, choanal atresia, retardation, and genital and ear anomalies. OA and TOF have also been associated with duodenal atresia and intestinal malrotation (Smith, 2014). Approximately 50% of all infants with oesophageal atresia have additional defects including cardiac, anorectal, genitourinary, digestive, vertebral, skeletal, respiratory, genetic or other disorders such as cleft lip and palate.

Oesophageal atresia and TOF arise during the first 6 weeks of embryonic development. During the fourth week the respiratory bud develops from the foregut tube. After rapid growth the oesophagus and trachea separate by a process of apoptosis. A TOF may form due to failure of the trachea and oesophagus to separate completely.

Oesophageal atresia is difficult to detect but may be predicted prenatally by ultrasound scan. Increased accuracy of diagnosis can be seen when there is an absent or small foetal stomach 'bubble' and polyhydramnios. Polyhydramnios is an excess accumulation of amniotic fluid during pregnancy and has a predictive value for oesophageal atresia of 55%–56% (Spitz, 2007; Smith, 2014). It is seen in approximately 33% of cases of OA/TOF (Bradshaw, 2016), although it is not specific to OA/TOF and can occur in association with other pathologies. In oesophageal atresia it occurs as a result of the inability of the foetus to swallow amniotic fluid.

Initial diagnosis may be made by attempting to pass a nasogastric tube. This is usually unsuccessful and resistance can be felt as the tube meets the end of the oesophageal pouch. Diagnosis is confirmed by chest X-ray and will assist in the diagnosis of an associated TOF. A nasogastric tube is inserted into the oesophagus until it meets resistance and the patency

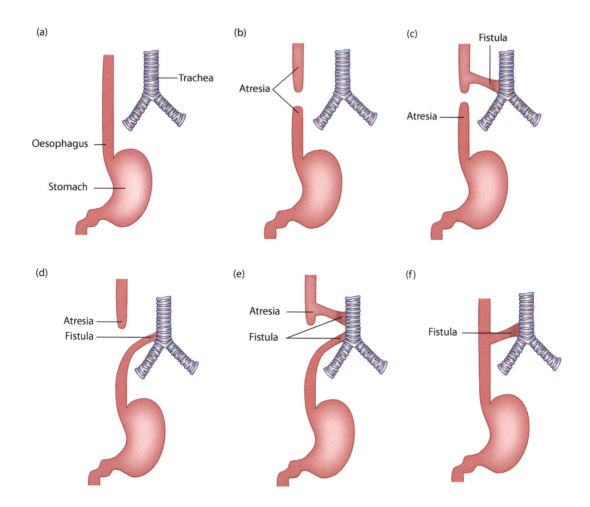

Figure 3.3 Types of oesophageal atresia and trachea-oesophageal fistula. (a) Normal anatomy, (b) Type A: oesophageal atresia without fistula (10%), (c) Type B: oesophageal atresia with proximal TEF (<1%), (d) Type C: oesophageal atresia with distal TEF (85%), (e) Type D: oesophageal atresia with proximal and distal TEF (<1%), and (f) Type E: TEF without oesophageal atresia (H-type fistula) (4%).

of the oesophagus can be ascertained from the position of the catheter, which shows curling of the tube at the oesophageal pouch. Presence of a TOF will show air in the stomach and distal bowel.

Infants with OA are unable to feed successfully. Any fluid may be swallowed normally but the infant may immediately cough or gag, regurgitating the liquid through the mouth and nose. If a TOF is present the fistula may allow fluid into the trachea or air into the stomach. Excess air may result in a distended abdomen. Clinical features in the newborn include excessive salivation, drooling, coughing, sneezing and choking which can lead to aspiration, cyanosis and respiratory distress (Hosie and Gravens, 2013;

Slater and Rothenberg, 2016). Long-term complications may include tracheomalacia (weakness of the tracheal wall), dysmotility of the oesophagus and gastro-oesophageal reflux disease.

CHANGES ASSOCIATED WITH DIFFERENT STAGES OF THE LIFESPAN

Gastro-oesophageal reflux disease in infants

Gastro-oesophageal reflux (GOR) is the effortless return of gastric content into the oesophagus with or without regurgitation or vomiting. It is a normal physiological occurrence in many infants during the first year of life with 70%–85% of infants having frequent daily episodes of regurgitation within the first 2 months of life (Czinn and Blanchard, 2013). Regurgitation is the effortless movement of refluxate into the throat and mouth. GOR decreases with increasing age and in 65%–95% of infants reflux is self-limiting and resolution is often spontaneous by age 2 (Fike and Mortellaro, 2011; Hassan and Ng, 2012). These infants are often known as 'happy spitters'.

Gastro-oesophageal reflux disease (GORD) occurs in infants when gastric reflux leads to adverse symptoms that affect the well-being of infants (Martigne et al., 2012; Czinn and Blanchard, 2013). GORD affects up to 6.2%–8% of infants and children (Fike and Mortellaro, 2011; Martigne et al., 2012). Regurgitation is often associated with meal size and the type of feed.

Paediatric GORD has been associated with cow's milk allergy, respiratory disease, neurological disorders such as cerebral palsy, oesophageal atresia and hiatus hernia (Hassan and Ng, 2012). Infants of low birth weight with chronic lung disease also have an increased risk.

GORD is associated with TLOSRs not associated with swallowing, which allow the stomach contents to reflux into the lower oesophagus (Fike and Mortellaro, 2011). The TLSORs can be caused by stomach distention and increased intra-abdominal pressure caused by straining, coughing, increased respiratory effort and postprandial (after a meal) seating postures (Czinn and Blanchard, 2013). This may be made worse by slow gastric emptying. Clearance of the refluxed material is impeded by insufficient peristalsis.

Refluxate containing acid, pepsin and bile from gastric secretions contacts the oesophageal mucosa. This results in an increase in regional blood flow and the production of local chemical mediators, such as prostaglandins. This increases the permeability of the oesophageal mucosa to acid, resulting in inflammation. The inflammatory response impairs function at the lower oesophageal sphincter resulting in poor motility. This favours reflux of gastric contents into the oesophagus and the development of oesophagitis.

Clinical features of GORD include recurrent regurgitation and vomiting, feeding refusal, arching of the back, especially during feeds, poor weight gain, irritability, oesophagitis and dysphagia or painful swallowing (Hassan and Ng, 2012; Czinn and Blanchard, 2013; Papachrisanthou and Davis, 2015). Respiratory symptoms include hoarseness, wheezing, recurrent and chronic cough, recurrent pneumonias and aspiration (Fike and Mortellaro, 2011; Hassan and Ng, 2012). All of these can lead to failure to thrive. Excess crying and irritability occur in response to pain associated with the burning sensation of refluxed gastric acid into the oesophagus. Sudden infant death syndrome (SIDS) may occur as a result of impaired swallowing and the decreased ability for the infant to rouse himself or herself (Page and Jeffery, 2000).

Gastro-oesophageal reflux disease in adults (GORD)

Gastro-oesophageal reflux disease (GORD) refers to the entry of refluxate from the stomach into the oesophagus, pharynx, trachea or *bronchial tree* that causes symptoms or damage to the oesophageal mucosa (Kahrilas, 2008). The potential to cause inflammatory damage to all of these structures is possible, but particularly the oesophageal mucosa leading to *oesophagitis,* ulceration, bleeding, *fibrosis* and *stricture* (Watson and Bowling, 2004).

GORD can be classified in two ways; *erosive oesophagitis* where gross abnormality of the mucosa is evident, with breaks and erosions of the oesophageal mucosa or *non-erosive reflux disease* where symptoms occur without abnormality of the oesophageal mucosa. According to Talley and Ford (2005) 40%–60% of patients with heartburn do not have oesophageal erosions.

Symptoms of GORD include *dyspepsia*, heart burn, regurgitation, *epigastric pain* and an acid taste in the mouth (Watson and Bowling, 2004; Talley and Ford 2005; Bredenoord et al., 2013; Noble, 2013). These symptoms frequently occur postprandially (after eating) but can occur during sleep. Sleep disturbance is associated with severe oesophagitis or Barrett's oesophagus and has shown to be a risk factor for adenocarcinoma (Orr, 2010).

Mild reflux disease occurs when refluxate enters the oesophagus during transient LOS relaxations (TLOSRs) postprandially (after eating), resulting in mild oesophagitis (Lee and McColl, 2013). Symptoms can be induced or exacerbated by lying flat, bending, straining or wearing tight clothing. Obesity and pregnancy can cause reflux by increasing the intra-abdominal pressure forcing stomach contents upwards towards the oesophagus, while smoking causes relaxation of the lower oesophageal sphincter (Watson and Bowling, 2004; Lee and McColl, 2013). Hiatus hernia is associated with disruption of LOS pressure and sphincter function.

Severe reflux is associated with erosive oesophagitis and is a risk factor for *Barrett's oesophagus*, with 10%–15% of those with oesophagitis going on to develop Barrett's oesophagus, a precursor to oesophageal *adenocarcinoma* (Jankowski et al., 2000; Patti and Waxman, 2010).

The development of GORD has been associated with a number of factors.

Prevention of reflux into the oesophagus is a result of contraction of the LOS. It prevents ingested food and gastric juice from entering the oesophagus, which can lead to damage of the oesophageal mucosa. Loss of LOS tension results in refluxate containing stomach acid, pepsin, duodenal juice and *bile acids* entering the distal oesophagus. Defects in peristalsis have also been observed with erosive oesophagitis, where clearance of acid toward the stomach is impaired, leading to oesophagitis and mucosal lesions (Roman and Kahrilias, 2015). Delayed gastric emptying, increased intra-gastric pressure, oesophageal hypersensitivity to acid, presence of an acid pocket nearer to the squamocolumnar junction (SCJ), loss of gastro-oesophageal flap valve function and increased frequency of transient lower oesophageal sphincter relaxations (TLOSRs) have been implicated in GORD (Reider et al., 2010; Bredenoord et al., 2013).

Mucosal damage arises from the diffusion of high concentrations of *hydrogen ions* from the lumen of the oesophagus into the mucosal tissue, down a concentration gradient. These changes are sensed by afferent sensory nerves containing acid sensing *ion channels*. These activate the nerve fibres and produce heartburn (Orlando, 2006). At the same time, acid is allowed to penetrate into the basal layer of the squamous cell epithelium of the oesophagus through gaps in the damaged epithelium. Acid entering the cells initiates the process of mucosal destruction, causing erosion and ulceration. *Pro-inflammatory cytokines* produced during this inflammatory process affect the *neuromuscular* control of the lower oesophageal

sphincter causing weakness and decreased peristalsis (Orlando, 2006; Reider et al., 2010). This increases the probability of reflux and continued acid injury.

Barrett's oesophagus

Barrett's oesophagus, also known as Barrett's *metaplasia* or columnar lined oesophagus (CLO), is associated with long-standing reflux disease and oesphagitis (Watson and Bowling, 2004; Salmon, 2007). It is defined as 'an oesophagus in which any portion of the normal distal squamous epithelial lining has been replaced by metaplastic columnar epithelium, which is clearly visible endoscopically (greater than or equal to 1 cm) above the gastro-oesophageal junction and confirmed histopathologically from oesophageal biopsies' (Fitzgerald et al., 2014). The oesophageal mucosa may appear as red, velvety mucosa extending in a circular fashion around the gastro-oesophageal junction or as 'tongues' of tissue extending into the oesophagus (Flejou, 2005). During endoscopy *segmental change* of the oesophageal mucosa to columnar epithelium around the gastro-oesophageal junction is measured. Barrett's oesophagus is difficult to recognise as it occurs in an area of *transitional* epithelium at the gastro-oesophageal junction (Spechler and Souza, 2014). Most cases of Barrett's oesophagus show no symptoms and therefore may go undiagnosed (Spechler and Souza, 2014; De Silva and Fitzgerald, 2015). Prevalence is estimated at 1.6%–6.8% (Gilbert et al., 2011) with the global rate of diagnosis increasing yearly.

Barrett's oesophagus is a premalignant condition with a risk of progression to oesophageal adenocarcinoma of 0.2%–0.4% per year (Watson and Bowling, 2004; Jankowski et al., 2010; De Silva and Fitzgerald, 2015). Resolution of Barrett's oesophagus rarely occurs with many cases showing no change, neither showing progression nor regression (Jankowski et al., 2010). Risk factors for Barrett's oesophagus include males over the age of 45 years, a long history of GORD, obesity associated with an increased waist circumference, smoking, an absence of *Helicobacter pylori* and a positive family history, supporting a genetic predisposition (Fitzgerald et al., 2014; Schneider and Corley, 2015). Of those with GORD, 10%–15% develop Barrett's oesophagus (Patti and Waxman, 2010).

Damage to the stratified squamous epithelium of the oesophageal mucosa, often due to chronic oesophageal reflux, results in metaplasia. This is the replacement of the normal stratified squamous epithelial cells of the oesophagus with columnar epithelium at the gastro-oesophageal junction (Nakagawa et al., 2015). The columnar epithelium is 'intestine-like' containing abundant goblet cells and mucus cells. It may rarely contain mature enterocytes, Paneth cells and enteroendocrine cells (Flejou, 2005). It is thought that the change arises from *stem cells* in the oesophagus or adjacent glandular tissues that are induced to undergo altered differentiation into columnar epithelium; however, the specific stem cell of origin has not yet been identified (Nakagawa et al., 2015). Damage to the oesophageal epithelium by chronic GORD leads to mucosal irritation and eventually the normal process of a stem cell division and cell differentiation is disrupted. Multiple stem cells can be produced at each division (Jankowski et al., 2000) and once initiated, colonisation of the mucosa with columnar cells occurs quickly. Metaplasia that occurs in Barrett's oesophagus can develop into dysplasia (abnormal appearance of cells). The presence and type (high or low grade) of dysplasia in Barrett's oesophagus are an indicator of an increased risk of carcinoma. In addition there may also be associated cellular chromosomal changes, abnormalities of gene expression and abnormalities in the regulation of cell cycles (Flejou, 2005; Almond et al., 2014).

Oesophageal adenocarcinoma

Oesophageal cancer is the 13th most common cancer in the United Kingdom with 8750 new cases diagnosed each year (Cancer Research UK, 2016). There are two types of oesophageal cancer; squamous cell carcinoma and adenocarcinoma, the latter being more prevalent. Oesophageal adenocarcinoma is a malignant tumour of oesophageal glandular epithelium. Rates of oesophageal adenocarcinoma are increasing across the Western world (Schneider and Corley, 2015) and this has become the most common cancer arising in the oesophagus (De Silva and Fitzgerald, 2015). The UK annual incidence is 13.2 per 100,000. It is the sixth most common cause of death related to cancer (Pennathur et al., 2013; De Silva and Fitzgerald, 2015).

Risk factors associated with oesophageal adenocarcinoma are increasing age, white males, GORD, smoking, abdominal obesity (particularly increased body mass index and waist circumference) and absence of *Helicobacter pylori* (Jankowski et al., 2010; Lepage et al., 2013; Almond et al., 2014; Schneider and Corley, 2015). The progression from Barrett's metaplasia to dysplasia and cancer is increased in smokers (De Silva and Fitzgerald, 2015). A diagnosis of Barrett's oesophagus is an indicator of the potential to develop oesophageal adenocarcinoma but not all cases of Barrett's oesophagus progress to adenocarcinoma (Lepage et al., 2013). Disease progression is from normal oesophageal squamous mucosa to metaplasia, dysplasia and cancer. The extent and type (high or low grade) of dysplasia will determine progression to adenocarcinoma.

Oesophageal adenocarcinoma is often asymptomatic, with symptoms only occurring late in the disease progression. Symptoms include dysphagia (difficulty swallowing), progressing from solids to liquids. There is associated weight loss, anaemia and symptoms of disease spread (metastasis). Common sites of metastasis are the liver, lungs, adrenal glands and peritoneum.

Staging of the cancer is based upon the depth of penetration through the oesophageal wall structures, lymph node involvement and presence or absence of metastases. The staging of cancer at diagnosis is an important indicator in the prognosis of the disease (Lepage et al., 2013).

Achalasia in adults

Achalasia is a rare motility disorder of the oesophagus. It affects approximately between 0.3 and 1.63 of adults per 100,000 of the population, occurring equally in men and women (Boeckxstaens et al., 2014). The precise etiology is unknown but it is likely to be associated with a combination of genetic, immune and environmental factors. Antibodies to the myenteric plexus, inflammatory infiltrates containing T lymphocytes in the myenteric plexus and the association with autoimmune connective tissue disease, point towards an autoimmune etiology. Infectious agents such as poliomyelitis, *varicella zoster*, herpes simplex virus and Guillain-Barre syndrome have all preceded achalasia and may suggest a viral etiology. There is no clear hereditary or genetic pattern.

Achalasia occurs as a result of impaired or absent relaxation of the lower oesophageal sphincter (LOS) and the absence of oesophageal peristalsis following swallowing. Failure of relaxation and opening of the LOS results in obstruction, stasis and fermentation of food within the lower oesophagus. The oesophageal mucosa becomes inflamed, followed by hyperplasia of the epithelium and subsequent dysplasia in some cases. The pathogenesis of achalasia is associated with the loss of inhibitory innervation of the oesophageal myenteric plexus. The myenteric neurons are less numerous or absent (Boeckxstaens et al., 2014). Inhibitory neurotransmitters such as nitric oxide and vasoinhibitory peptide are lost as a result of inflammation and fibrosis of the myenteric plexus. Loss of oesophageal sensitivity and compliance has also been shown to occur (Brackbill et al., 2003). Nitric oxide and vasoinhibitory peptide are essential for the relaxation of the lower oesophageal sphincter and relaxation of smooth muscle cells in the muscularis externa of the oesophageal wall during peristalsis. Their absence results in a tight lower oesophageal sphincter and a lack of peristalsis (Mittal and Balaban, 1997; Richter, 2013). Histological examination has shown thickening of the muscularis at the LOS and distal oesophagus, particularly within the circular muscle, and inflammation and collagen deposition within the myenteric plexus (Richter, 2013).

Achalasia is considered a premalignant condition although the risks are variable. Barrett's oesophagus and squamous cell carcinoma of the oesophagus have been linked with achalasia. This is a more prevalent outcome following treatment, where relaxation of the lower oesophageal sphincter predisposes to gastro-oesophageal reflux and subsequent oesophagitis.

Clinical features of achalasia include dysphagia (>90%), chest pain (25%–64%), heartburn (18%–52%), regurgitation of undigested food (76%–91%), respiratory pathologies such as nocturnal cough and aspiration and weight loss (35%–91%) due to a lack of peristalsis and impaired oesophageal emptying (Mittal and Balaban, 1997; Brackbill et al., 2003; The Society for Surgery of the Digestive Tract, 2004; Boeckxstaens et al., 2014).

DEGLUTITION

Prenatal deglutition

The process of infant feeding is complex and not only relies on anatomical and physiological development but is also influenced by environmental, social and cultural factors. *Deglutition* is the process of swallowing, the method of moving ingested nutrients from the oral cavity to the stomach, via the pharynx and oesophagus. *In utero* the developing embryo and foetus relies upon a nutrient supply from the mother via the placenta (*passive nutrition*); therefore, the act of swallowing is not required to deliver nutrients. However a foetus of 10–14 weeks' gestation is capable of swallowing amniotic fluid. It does this to assist in the regulation of amniotic fluid volume and composition, to recycle solutes and to assist in the maturation of the digestive tract. Co-ordinated *sucking* and swallowing is vital to the infant in gaining nutrients. Sucking is visible at 18–24 weeks by the movement of the tongue backwards and forwards. Stability in the rhythm of sucking and swallowing is achieved between 32 and 40 weeks.

It is not until birth that the process of sucking and swallowing is required as a nutritive process. The effectiveness of this process depends upon the age of the infant at birth. Sucking and swallowing in premature babies is less efficient than in full-term infants due to the lack of necessary *sensorimotor* development. The following section explores the mechanisms of obtaining nutrients during the postnatal period.

Postnatal deglutition

After birth it is essential that the developing infant receives adequate nutrition to sustain growth and development. The effectiveness of this depends upon the age of the infant, and the ability to co-ordinate the processes of sucking, swallowing and breathing.

At birth feeding is dependent on reflexive processes which are controlled by the brainstem. These include *rooting*, *gagging*, sucking and swallowing (Figure 3.4). *Pre-term* infants have less well-developed reflexes; however, by full term the necessary sensorimotor developmental changes are maturing, as the brain itself matures, a process called *encephalisation*.

The *rooting reflex* is associated with the sensory stimulation of skin around the mouth which causes the infant to turn the head toward the feeding stimulus, usually the breast or teat of a bottle. The infant's mouth gapes to accept the breast or teat. With increasing age this becomes a visual response to the sight of food rather than a physical stimulus.

The *sucking reflex* occurs once the mouth is 'attached' to the breast or teat. The palate is stimulated by the presence of the nipple or teat in the

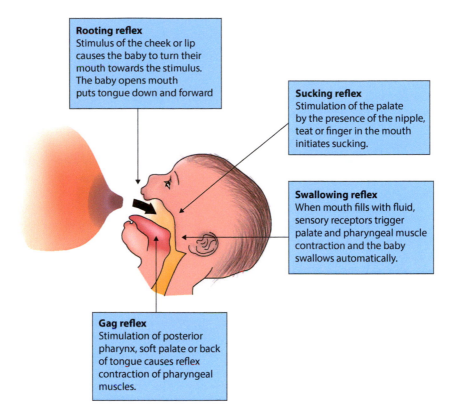

Rooting reflex
Stimulus of the cheek or lip causes the baby to turn their mouth towards the stimulus. The baby opens mouth puts tongue down and forward

Sucking reflex
Stimulation of the palate by the presence of the nipple, teat or finger in the mouth initiates sucking.

Swallowing reflex
When mouth fills with fluid, sensory receptors trigger palate and pharyngeal muscle contraction and the baby swallows automatically.

Gag reflex
Stimulation of posterior pharynx, soft palate or back of tongue causes reflex contraction of pharyngeal muscles.

Figure 3.4 Feeding reflexes in the infant.

infant's mouth and initiates the sucking reflex. This is important as inadequate stimulation of the palate may lead to feeding difficulties. This is enhanced by the closing of the lower jaw and pressure of the tongue on the lower surface of the teat or nipple. A seal is then created with the lips, gums and tongue onto the nipple or teat, allowing a negative pressure inside the oral cavity and pharynx to develop. Initially the seal is weaker and allows leakage of fluid from the mouth during feeding. By 4 months a tighter seal is developed. Once in position, the infant rolls the tongue from anterior to posterior, creating a wave of pressure onto the nipple or teat, to express milk or fluid directly into the pharynx. The tongue then lowers to allow for expansion of the nipple and teat, which refill and the process continues.

There are two types of sucking in *post-term* infants; '*non-nutritive*' and '*nutritive*'. Non-nutritive occurs in the absence of food or when little or no fluid is available. It occurs in short, fast bursts and is often associated with preterm infants. 'Nutritive' sucking occurs in the presence of adequate fluid, in longer bursts of sucking. Initially sucking and swallowing occur in a 1:1 ratio. As the infant matures the runs of sucking and swallowing become more rapid and organised. Infants gradually adjust feeding patterns to improve the efficiency of obtaining nutrients.

Swallowing commences as the tongue propels the liquid bolus onto the pharynx. Sensory receptors in the oral cavity and pharynx mucosa trigger the contraction of muscles in the palate and pharynx, which move upwards to prevent oral contents from entering the nasopharynx and nasal cavity. This occurs as long as the bolus volume is enough to stimulate the sensory receptors. At the same time inhibition of *inspiratory neurons* occurs to prevent the aspiration of the bolus. Reflexive coughing or swallowing occurs as a response to the presence of bolus contents in the upper airway, sensed by chemoreceptors.

As liquid enters the pharynx, the pharyngeal muscles contract and propel the bolus into the oesophagus.

The laryngeal opening closes and the upper oesophageal sphincter relaxes. This allows the passage of the bolus down the oesophagus. Mechanoreceptors in the oesophageal wall sense the presence of the bolus and stimulate peristalsis. Distention of the oesophageal wall causes relaxation of the lower oesophageal sphincter, via the vagus nerve (X) and the bolus proceeds into the stomach. Air is also swallowed with the bolus and thus there are periods of transient lower oesophageal sphincter relaxations (TLOSRs) to allow the air to escape. This may allow some reflux of stomach contents.

During feeding it is important that the infant maintains *respiration.* In preterm infants this is difficult as the neurological control mechanisms are immature and thus deprivation of respiration occurs in favour of feeding. As a result *hypoxia* and *hypercapnia* may ensue, where there is a lack of *oxygen* and increase in *carbon dioxide* levels, respectively, during feeding. The co-ordination of the neural processes of swallowing and respiration improves at full term and by 2–3 months of age alternation of swallowing and respiration occurs. This is significant for infants with lung disease or brain injury who may not be able to respond to changes in blood oxygen and carbon dioxide levels, giving rise to extended periods of *apnea.*

As infants get older the anatomical and physiological processes involved in feeding continue to mature, and infants are able to accept different consistencies of nutrients. 'Weaning' is the process of changing from a purely fluid diet to one that contains solid food. This usually takes place at 6 months of age. Infants are able to chew from 5 months and gradually continue to develop more co-ordination of movements of the tongue, lip and jaw to facilitate the movement of food within the oral cavity and to accommodate the changes in consistency of nutrients. By the age of 4–5 years, the more mature adult tongue movements and swallowing are present.

Deglutition in adults

Deglutition is the process of swallowing which involves the transportation of a bolus from the oral cavity through the pharynx and into the stomach via the oesophagus. There are two types of swallowing, *volitional* and *reflexive.* Volitional swallowing involves the voluntary initiation and regulation of swallowing via brain centres outside of the brainstem. Reflexive swallowing occurs as a result of stimulation of the pharynx directly from, for example, saliva. These processes only differ in how swallowing is initiated. The physical process of swallowing is the same in each from the pharynx down.

Deglutition is controlled by the co-ordination of sensory and motor neurons, the *cerebral cortex,* the paired brainstem swallowing centres, the *insula* and the *parietal* and *occipital lobes* of the brain. These are responsible for the sensory and motor integration of swallowing, control of pharyngeal muscles, the mechanical and chemical stimulation of the oesophagus and the voluntary decision to swallow. This demonstrates the extensive involvement of many anatomical regions of the brain during swallowing. This may be clinically relevant to pathologies such as *cerebrovascular accidents,* more commonly known as strokes, where regional vascular damage of the brain results in dysphagia or difficulty in swallowing.

Deglutition occurs in three phases: the *buccal, pharyngeal* and *oesophageal* phases (Figure 3.5). These phases are similar to those seen in the infant.

The buccal or oral phase of swallowing

The buccal phase of swallowing involves the voluntary preparation of food in the oral cavity. *Mastication* is the process of chewing where nutrients are moved around the oral cavity by the tongue and movements of the mandible (lower jaw). The movement of the tongue pushes nutrients against the *raphe* and hard palate to crush the oral cavity contents and to push the nutrients between the molars and premolars for grinding and crushing. The combination of these movements and the mixing of nutrients with saliva forms a bolus. During the buccal phase of swallowing, the tongue is initially elevated against the hard palate posteriorly to prevent the bolus from entering the oropharynx too early. The bolus, once formed, is pushed up against the palate as the tongue rises and in a rolling motion pushes the bolus towards the oropharynx. At the same time palatine and pharyngeal muscles contract to raise the palate and to close off access to the nasopharynx. The tongue remains elevated to prevent movement of the bolus back into the oral cavity, until the bolus reaches the laryngopharynx.

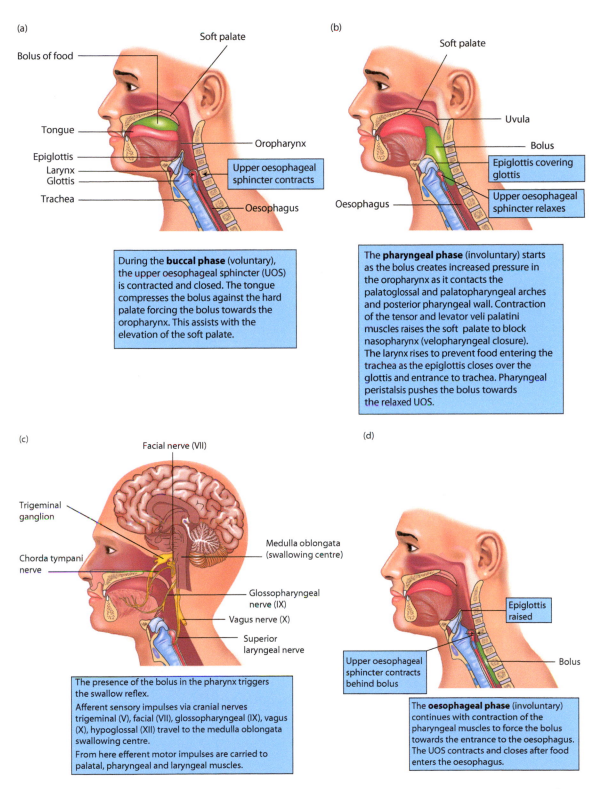

(a)

Bolus of food

Soft palate

Tongue

Epiglottis
Larynx
Glottis

Trachea

Oropharynx

Upper oesophageal
sphincter contracts

Oesophagus

During the **buccal phase** (voluntary),
the upper oesophageal sphincter (UOS)
is contracted and closed. The tongue
compresses the bolus against the hard
palate forcing the bolus towards the
oropharynx. This assists with the
elevation of the soft palate.

(b)

Soft palate

Uvula

Bolus

Epiglottis covering
glottis

Upper oesophageal
sphincter relaxes

Oesophagus

The **pharyngeal phase** (involuntary) starts
as the bolus creates increased pressure in
the oropharynx as it contacts the
palatoglossal and palatopharyngeal arches
and posterior pharyngeal wall. Contraction
of the tensor and levator veli palatini
muscles raises the soft palate to block
nasopharynx (velopharyngeal closure).
The larynx rises to prevent food entering the
trachea as the epiglottis closes over the
glottis and entrance to trachea. Pharyngeal
peristalsis pushes the bolus towards
the relaxed UOS.

(c)

Facial nerve (VII)

Trigeminal
ganglion

Chorda tympani
nerve

Medulla oblongata
(swallowing centre)

Glossopharyngeal
nerve (IX)

Vagus nerve (X)

Superior
laryngeal nerve

The presence of the bolus in the pharynx triggers
the swallow reflex.

Afferent sensory impulses via cranial nerves
trigeminal (V), facial (VII), glossopharyngeal (IX), vagus
(X), hypoglossal (XII) travel to the medulla oblongata
swallowing centre.

From here efferent motor impulses are carried to
palatal, pharyngeal and laryngeal muscles.

(d)

Epiglottis
raised

Bolus

Upper oesophageal
sphincter contracts
behind bolus

The **oesophageal phase** (involuntary)
continues with contraction of the
pharyngeal muscles to force the bolus
towards the entrance to the oesophagus.
The UOS contracts and closes after food
enters the oesophagus.

Figure 3.5 Phases of adult deglutition (swallowing). (a) Buccal phase, (b and c) pharyngeal phase, (d and e) oesophageal phase.   (*Continued*)

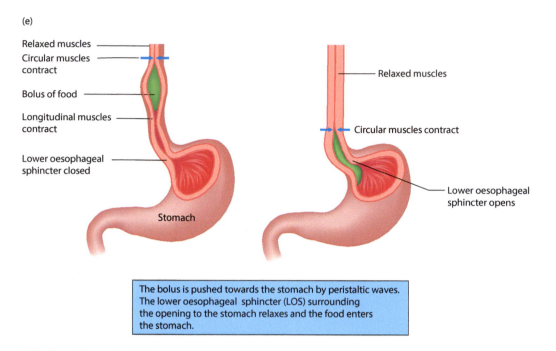

(e)

The bolus is pushed towards the stomach by peristaltic waves. The lower oesophageal sphincter (LOS) surrounding the opening to the stomach relaxes and the food enters the stomach.

Figure 3.5 (Continued) Phases of adult deglutition (swallowing). (a) Buccal phase, (b and c) pharyngeal phase, (d and e) oesophageal phase.

Pharyngeal phase

The pharyngeal component of swallowing is an involuntary process, initiated by stimulation of sensory receptors in the mucosa of the pharynx. The bolus moves through the pharynx due to reflex contractions of pharyngeal muscles, stimulated by the presence of the bolus in the oropharynx. The pharyngeal phase takes approximately 1 second but is dependent on the size and consistency of the bolus. As the bolus approaches the larynx, the larynx contracts and elevates anteriorly, in order that the *epiglottis* can close over the entrance to the *trachea* as the bolus passes. This is also assisted by pressure from the bolus on the epiglottis itself as it passes to the laryngopharynx. The pharyngeal phase of swallowing is also enhanced by the stimulation of sensory taste nerve fibres of the glossopharyngeal and facial nerves that supply the taste buds in the tongue. These synapse with the brainstem swallowing centres to stimulate pharyngeal muscle contraction.

Oesophageal phase

As the bolus reaches the laryngopharynx, the pressure of the bolus causes relaxation of the upper oesophageal sphincter. Once inside the oesophagus the bolus is moved by involuntary peristalsis and the influence of gravity to the stomach. The circular and longitudinal muscles contract together to increase the force generated. Oesophageal peristalsis is induced by *cholinergic fibres*.

AGEING AND DEGLUTITION

Changes in deglutition can be observed in the healthy older person. Overall tongue movement during the early part of swallowing is reduced and pharyngeal stimulation is delayed. The duration of movement of the bolus through the pharynx is reduced. The delays in swallowing can also be associated with a decrease in taste sensitivity.

The Oesophagus

1. Muscular tube that extends from the laryngopharynx to the stomach.
2. Receives food from the pharynx as a result of swallowing.
3. Passes through the mediastinum and penetrates the diaphragm at the oesophageal hiatus.

The wall of the oesophagus shows a number of variations from the rest of the digestive tract:

1. The main aim of the oesophagus is to transport food from the mouth to the stomach so the mucosa is made up of stratified squamous epithelium with mucous-producing cells to make the surface of the epithelium smooth and slippery.
2. The submucosa has numerous mucus-secreting glands to aid transport.
3. The myenteric plexus in the muscularis externa generates waves of contraction, initiated by the vagus nerve.
   i. Food passes through the oesophagus by muscular contractions of the wall called *peristalsis*. The food enters the stomach through the gastro-oesophageal junction. This opening is guarded by a sling of muscle from the diaphragm called the lower oesophageal or cardiac sphincter (skeletal muscle).
4. Deglutition (swallowing) – deglutition occurs in three phases:
   i. Buccal phase
   ii. Pharyngeal phase
   iii. Oesophageal phase

CHECK ON LEARNING

Oesophagus

How does the structure of the oesophageal epithelium aid the function of the oesophagus?
Answer – The epithelium of the oesophagus is made up of multiple layers of stratified squamous epithelial cells. As these cells move towards the lumen of the oesophagus they become more flattened in shape. The flattened shape together with the mucus from the goblet cells aids the smooth transition of the bolus to the stomach.

There is a transition in the oesophagus from one type of muscle to another. What are these two types of muscle?
Answer – The types are striated (skeletal) and smooth muscle.

What is the function of the upper and lower oesophageal sphincters?
Answer – The upper oesophageal sphincter is made up of circular skeletal muscle and prevents air from entering the oesophagus, and the lower oesophageal sphincter prevents reflux of acid into the oesophagus.

What type of contraction propels the bolus through the oesophagus?
Answer – Peristalsis propels the bolus.

What are the three phases of deglutition?
Answer – The three phases are as follows: buccal phase, pharyngeal phase and oesophageal phase.

Describe the sequence of events that takes place with deglutition.
Answer – The bolus is generated, the mouth closes, the tongue pushes against the hard palate, the tongue contracts and arches back forcing the bolus to the oropharynx, the soft palate closes off so that no food or fluid can enter the nasal cavity, when the bolus touches the pharyngeal wall a reflex contraction of the pharyngeal muscles forces the bolus down past the laryngopharynx and the epiglottis closes preventing entry of food and fluid into the larynx and trachea. The bolus passes through the upper oesophageal sphincter and moves via peristalsis and gravity down the oesophagus to the stomach.

Which nerve initiates peristalsis?
Answer – The vagus nerve initiates peristalsis.

CASE STUDY

Upper GI physiology from the patient's perspective

Mrs. Ann Hughes (58), a married woman working part time as a PA, has a 2-year history of chest pain and acid reflux. She occasionally has trouble swallowing and has a sore throat most of the time. She has lost 3 kg in weight over 6 months. She has been prescribed 20 mg of omeprazole once daily for 4 weeks but her symptoms have persisted. She is referred by her general practitioner for an oesophago-gastro-duodenoscopy (OGD). The upper digestive tract is examined and biopsies of the oesophagus and duodenum taken. There is mild oesophagitis and the biopsy confirms Barrett's oesophagus.

Explanation of normal and abnormal physiology

The following table sets out the normal and altered anatomy and physiology which explains the person's problems.

(*Continued*)

Normal anatomy/physiology	Altered anatomy/physiology and related problems

The main function of the oesophagus is to transport food from the mouth to the stomach.

The lower oesophageal sphincter prevents reflux of acid from the stomach into the oesophagus.

In the stomach hydrogen (H+) ions and chloride ions (Cl−) are secreted from the parietal cells in the gastric mucosa. H+ ions combine immediately with Cl− ions to make hydrochloric acid (HCl) in the stomach.

What is the function of hydrochloric acid in the stomach?
This is for converting pepsinogen into pepsin so that proteins can be digested into peptides. HCl also 'sterilises' the stomach contents to reduce the incidence of gastroenteritis.

The gastric mucosa is not damaged by acid secretion because the mucus it secretes provides protection from HCl and pepsin action.

Describe the histology of the oesophageal mucosa.
The mucosa is composed of non-keratinised squamous epithelium. This becomes darker at the distal end of the oesophagus at the gastro-oesophageal junction. This forms the point of transition between the oesophageal mucosa and gastric mucosa.

How is the histology of the oesophagus related to its function?
The epithelium consists of multiple layers of stratified squamous epithelial cells. As these cells move towards the lumen of the oesophagus they become more flattened in shape. The flattened shape together with the mucus from the goblet cells aids the smooth transition of the bolus to the stomach.

The muscularis externa contractions result in peristalsis which facilitates the movement of the bolus towards the stomach.

The oesophageal submucosa has numerous mucus-secreting glands to aid transport.

The myenteric plexus in the muscularis externa of the oesophagus generates waves of contraction (peristalsis). The presence of food in the oesophagus stimulates mechano- and chemo-receptors which generates a short reflex to the myenteric plexus bringing about contraction.

Describe a second pathway that initiates contraction of the myenteric plexus bringing about waves of contraction in the oesophagus?

Peristalsis is also initiated by stimulation from the vagus nerve (involuntary nervous system).

The junction of the oesophagus with the stomach is just below the diaphragm and is marked by the lower oesophageal sphincter (LOS). The combination of the LOS muscle itself, and the diaphragm encircling the LOS (oesophageal hiatus), keep gastric secretions and contents in the stomach until they are expelled into the duodenum.

What is gastro-oesophageal reflux disease (GORD)?
It refers to the entry of refluxate from the stomach into the oesophagus, pharynx and in some cases trachea. The refluxate causes inflammation to the mucosa.

How does the refluxate cause inflammation?
High concentrations of hydrogen ions move by diffusion (down a concentration gradient) from the oesophageal lumen into the mucosal tissue causing cell destruction.

List the constituents of refluxate.
It contains stomach acid, pepsin, duodenal juice and bile acids.

What is the long-term danger of exposing the oesophageal mucosa to HCl?
The normal cell structure of the oesophageal mucosa cells is altered in the inflammatory response. The 'damage' to cell structure and development by inflammation can lead to their permanent alteration (metaplasia) and the development of cancer of the oesophagus. The pre-malignant phase of damage is known as Barrett's oesophagus. In Barrett's oesophagus the stratified squamous epithelial cells that line the oesophagus are replaced by columnar epithelial cells.

Mrs. Hughes' tissues biopsy confirmed Barrett's.

Why might the patient have trouble swallowing intermittently?
The presence of refluxate in the oesophagus causes an inflammatory response (oesophagitis). Cytokines produced during this inflammatory process affect the neuromuscular control of the lower oesophageal sphincter causing weakness and decreased peristalsis.

Why is the patient complaining of a sore throat?
HCl and stomach secretions are refluxing back up the oesophagus to the upper respiratory tract and spilling over into the larynx causing inflammation (swelling, redness and pain). This is more likely to happen at night when the person is lying down and there is less 'help' from gravity afforded by being upright.

Why does this patient have chest pain?
The presence of refluxate in the oesophagus mucosa is sensed by afferent sensory nerves containing acid-sensing ion channels. These activate the nerve fibres and produce heartburn.

Why might the patient be losing weight?
The discomfort in the chest will be exacerbated on eating as will the sensation of reflux, for several hours after eating. In addition if there is some difficulty swallowing, the patient will probably be eating and drinking less in order to lessen the discomfort and thus will be losing weight.

What are causes of GORD?
Weak lower oesophageal sphincter (LOS) can cause GORD. Smoking can cause relaxation of the LOS.

An oesophageal hiatus may be too large. Obesity and pregnancy can increase abdominal pressure forcing gastric content into the oesophagus. A hiatus hernia can cause GORD.

(Continued)

Background – initial investigations

The table below provides the rationale behind the investigations that may be used to diagnose Mrs. Hughes' condition.

Investigation	Result	Rationale
Biopsy of the oesophageal mucosa via OGD	Presence of columnar epithelium confirming Barrett's oesophagus	Altered histology (metaplasia) observed. Caused by acid inflammation. Replacement in the oesophagus of stratified squamous epithelium with columnar epithelium.
Barium or gastrograffin swallow	Negative for hiatus hernia	Contrast x-ray used to look for movement of substances through the oesophagus and any abnormality. Could be used to rule out motility disorders or other causes of dysphagia.
Ambulatory pH monitoring pH test via probe transnasally inserted into the oesophagus for 24 hours	Low (<2) pH in the oesophagus some or most of the time	To indicate the degree and duration of reflux of acid into the oesophagus which gives an indication of the exposure of the oesophageal mucosa to acid.
Pharyngo-laryngoscopy	Inflamed pharynx and larynx	To check for damage to the upper respiratory tract which would be due to exposure to acid flowing from the lower oesophagus up the oesophagus and over into the upper respiratory tract.

CLINICAL CHALLENGES

1. How is gastro-oesophageal reflux managed with medication?

2. Barrett's metaplasia is considered to be a precancerous condition. How may this progress clinically in the oesophagus? What types of carcinoma may develop?

Chapter 4

THE STOMACH AND GASTRIC FUNCTION

Specific learning outcomes

- Describe the embryonic development of the stomach.
- Describe the gross anatomy, histology and physiological function of the stomach.
- Discuss the physiological processes involved in gastric mechanical and chemical digestion.
- Explain the mechanism and regulation of gastric secretions.
- Discuss the physiological effects of ageing on the structure and function of the stomach.
- Discuss common developmental abnormalities of the stomach.
- Discuss common disorders of the stomach.
- Explain the pathogenesis of common gastric disorders.
- Compare and contrast the normal physiology of the stomach with the altered physiology seen with dysfunction of the stomach.

PRENATAL DEVELOPMENT OF THE STOMACH

The gastrointestinal tract is formed from endodermal tissue, initially divided into the foregut and hindgut. These are endodermal tubes, surrounded by mesoderm. The stomach develops from the foregut diverticulum. The mesodermal tissue develops cavities within it called *coelom* on either side of the developing stomach. As the coelom increase in size, the stomach becomes suspended by a dorsal (back) and ventral (front) mesogastrium. The stomach is surrounded by visceral peritoneum, and the two mesenteries attach it to the parietal peritoneum, lining the developing cavity (Figure 4.1a and b).

The stomach begins as a simple hollow tube and then dilates, generating an enlarged lumen in the fourth week of gestation. The dorsal border of the stomach grows more rapidly than the ventral border and this causes the generation of a curve in the stomach called the greater curve. During the seventh week the stomach rotates 90° clockwise about a longitudinal axis (Figure 4.1c–e). The rotation generates a space behind the stomach called the lesser sac, also called the omental bursa.

During the eighth week the stomach and duodenum rotate about a ventro-dorsal (antero-posterior) axis. The cranial end of the stomach moves left and downwards and the caudal end moves right and upwards. This has the effect of drawing up the stomach, pulling the duodenum into the C-shaped position identified in adults (Figure 4.1f). The rotation of the stomach helps to move the dorsal mesentery into place forming the various folds known as the greater and lesser omentum. The dorsal mesentery hangs from the greater curvature and becomes the greater omentum. The ventral mesentery extends from the lesser curvature and is attached to the liver and forms the lesser omentum. The rotations serve to position the stomach towards the epigastric region.

The rotations of the stomach and the development of the omenta generate the spaces found in the peritoneal cavity. The space behind the stomach is termed the lesser sac or omental bursa, and the space in front of the stomach is termed the greater sac. The rotation of the stomach also serves to position the nerve supply, with the right vagus nerve supplying the posterior wall of the stomach and the left vagus nerve supplying the anterior wall (Figure 4.1).

The cells in the stomach mucosa responsible for gastric secretions emerge between weeks 10 and 12.

(a) Transverse view

Lumen of
developing
stomach

Dorsal
mesogastrium

Coelom
(developing
peritoneal cavity)

Ventral
mesogastrium

Coelom

(b) Transverse view

Lumen of
developing
stomach

Dorsal
mesogastrium

Left vagal branch

Right vagal
branch

Ventral
mesogastrium

(c) Oblique view

Dorsal
mesentery
(posterior)

Left vagal
branches

Right vagal
branches

Ventral
mesentry
(anterior)

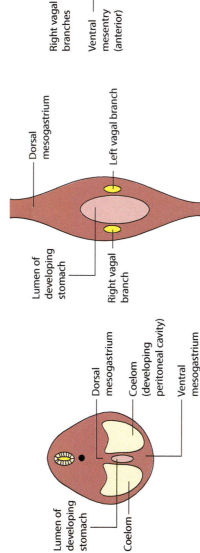

(d) Oblique view: The dorsal (posterior)
wall of the stomach expands during
the 4th and 5th weeks to form the
greater curvature.

(e) Oblique view: During the 7th week, the
stomach rotates clockwise on its longitudinal
axis. The dorsal mesentery (greater curvature)
sits on the left side. The ventral mesentery
(lesser curvature) sits on the right side.

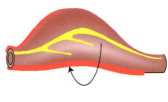

(f) Frontal view: During the 8th week, the stomach rotates
about an anterior : posterior axis

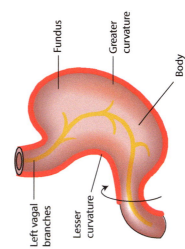

Fundus

Greater
curvature

Body

Left vagal
branches

Lesser
curvature

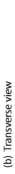

Figure 4.1 Rotations of the stomach.

By the end of week 12 parietal cells are producing hydrogen and chloride ions which come together to form hydrochloric acid in the gastric pits. Exocrine cells that line the gastric epithelium are secreting the enzymes pepsin, lipase, intrinsic factor and rennin and gastric enteroendocrine cells are releasing the hormone gastrin.

The stomach can be seen on ultrasound scan by the ninth week of gestation. By week 14 the characteristic structures such as the greater and lesser curvature, fundus, body and pylorus can be distinguished.

POSTNATAL DEVELOPMENT AND ADULT STOMACH

Gross anatomy and function

Prior to birth it is the function of the placenta to ensure that there is adequate exchange of nutrients and waste products which will enable the embryo to grow. This is called passive nutrition. After birth the neonate needs to adapt to active nutrition involving the processes of ingestion, digestion and absorption. Following birth the mechanical functioning of the gastrointestinal tract and digestion are still quite immature. The infant has to go through a number of stages before it can ingest, process and absorb all the dietary nutrients required to sustain growth and development. The mechanisms of sucking and swallowing exist before birth but do not become fully functional until after birth. Sucking and swallowing are complex physiological processes that require neurological and muscular coordination and take time to fully develop following birth. For the first 3 months after birth swallowing is an involuntary action and is governed by an automatic reflex action. Once the connections between the striated skeletal muscles in the pharynx and the associated neural pathways to sensory and motor pathways in the brain are fully established voluntary control can commence. This is normally established by the age of 6 weeks.

Food material entering the stomach will have been through the processes of mechanical and chemical digestion. Mastication together with the injection of saliva will have taken place in the mouth so food material that enters the stomach has already experienced limited mechanical and chemical digestion. The process of mastication and mixing with saliva will have started breaking down complex food materials. There are five general functions of the stomach:

1. Temporary storage of food
2. Chemical processing of food through the action of acids and enzymes
3. Mechanical processing of food through the action of gastric smooth muscles
4. Release of intrinsic factor required for the absorption of vitamin B_{12}
5. Limited absorption

The stomach of a child is round until the child reaches 2 years old. The stomach then elongates and at the age of approximately 7 it assumes the J-shape structure found in adults. The stomach lies between the oesophagus and duodenum in the superior part of the abdominal cavity under the diaphragm (see Chapter 1; Figure 1.1). The left side of the stomach is called the greater curvature and the right is the lesser curvature. The size and shape of the stomach are continually changing and are dependent upon two factors: the size of the individual and the size of the meal. In adults it is approximately 15–25 cm long and in neonates is the size of a hen's egg. The stomach's ability to store large volumes of food is attributed to rugae and a third oblique muscle layer. Generally adult stomachs have a volume of approximately 1.5 L but this can be distended up to 4 L. At rest an empty adult stomach contains approximately 50 mL.

Anatomically, the stomach can be divided into four sections (Figure 4.2):

1. *Cardia* – The cardia surrounds the superior opening of the stomach and connects to the oesophagus. It contains an abundance of mucus-secreting glands that help protect the stratified squamous epithelial cells of the distal oesophagus.
2. *Fundus* – The dome-shaped section of the stomach to the left of the abdominal oesophagus is the fundus.
3. *Body* – Inferior (below) to the fundus is the largest region of the stomach, called the body, and it is here that the bulk of the gastric glands are found that secrete the enzymes and acids.
4. *Pylorus* – The region that connects the stomach to the duodenum inferiorly at the gastro-duodenal junction is the pylorus. It has two major parts: the pyloric antrum that connects to the body of the stomach and the pyloric canal that joins the duodenum. The pathway of chyme from the pyloric canal to the duodenum is controlled by a thick

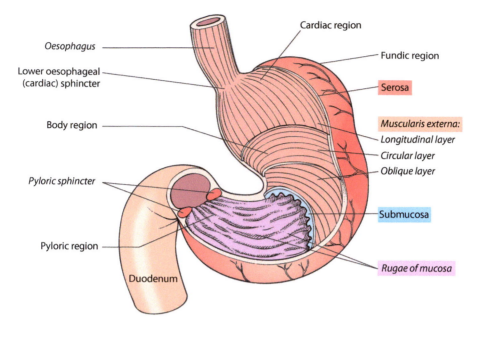

Figure 4.2 Gross anatomy of stomach.

band of circular muscle called the pyloric sphincter. Glands embedded in the mucosa of the pylorus secrete mucous and digestive hormones that regulate mechanical and chemical digestion.

The stomach has a rich blood supply from the coeliac artery which gives rise to three branches: left gastric artery, common hepatic artery and splenic artery. There are two arterial arcades that sit along the lesser and greater curvatures of the stomach that provide a large proportion of the circulation. Venous drainage is by corresponding veins from which blood drains into the portal vein and the superior mesenteric vein.

FUNCTIONAL HISTOLOGY OF THE STOMACH

The stomach wall, like the rest of the gastrointestinal tract, is made up of four layers: mucosa, submucosa, muscularis and serosa (Figure 4.3); however, there are some modifications. Unlike the rest of the gastrointestinal tract the stomach has an additional muscle layer. On the inside of the circular layer of the muscularis externa there is an oblique smooth muscle layer. This additional muscle layer has two functions: the first is to provide support as the gastric volume

expands. The second is to help with mechanical digestion by assisting the churning process, breaking up food material and increasing the surface area for the acids and enzymes to function.

When the stomach is empty the mucosa and submucosa are thrown up into folds called *rugae*. As the stomach receives food and expands these folds flatten out.

At the junction where the oesophagus joins the stomach there is a clear transition from stratified squamous epithelium that provides protection for the oesophagus, to columnar epithelium which specialises in secretion. This is called the Z line or squamocolumnar junction (SCJ). The stomach epithelium covers the surface of the stomach and has many small openings that extend down into the lamina propria. These are called gastric pits and lead onto gastric glands which are lined with a number of secretory cells. There are four major types of secretory epithelial cells that cover the surface of the stomach: mucous cells, parietal cells, chief cells and G cells (Figure 4.3):

1. *Mucous cells* – These are the most abundant secretory cells of the gastric epithelium. They cover the whole of the surface of the stomach and extend down into the gastric glands where 'neck cells' also produce mucous. They are particularly

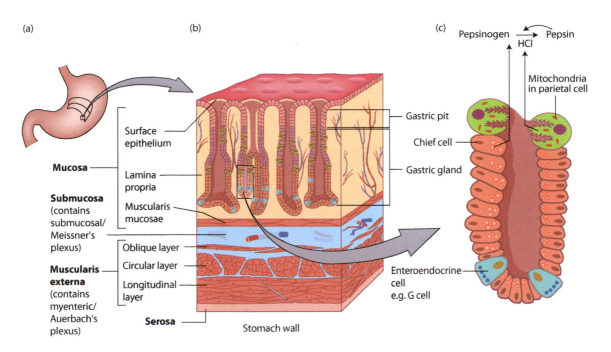

(a)

(b)

(c)

Pepsinogen → Pepsin
HCl

Mitochondria
in parietal cell

Gastric pit

Chief cell

Gastric gland

Mucosa

Surface
epithelium

Lamina
propria

Submucosa
(contains
submucosal/
Meissner's
plexus)

Muscularis
mucosae

**Muscularis
externa**
(contains
myenteric/
Auerbach's
plexus)

Oblique layer

Circular layer

Longitudinal
layer

Serosa

Enteroendocrine
cell
e.g. G cell

Stomach wall

Figure 4.3 Histology of stomach. (a) Stomach wall, (b) gastric pit and gland and (c) HCl and pepsin production.

abundant in gastric glands of the cardia and pylorus. They produce a bicarbonate-rich mucus that lubricates and protects the epithelium from acids and enzymes and other noxious substances. Mucous is made up of mucin (protein) and glycoproteins which adheres to the gastric mucosa.

2. *Parietal cells* – The most abundant secretory cells within the gastric glands are parietal cells and chief cells. Parietal cells secrete hydrochloric acid and intrinsic factor. The acid is vital for the activation of pepsinogen and destruction of ingested microorganisms such as bacteria. The acid also denatures (alters the chemical structure) proteins and inactivates enzymes in food.

Hydrochloric acid keeps the contents of the stomach at a pH of between 1.5 and 2. Hydrochloric acid is not produced within the parietal cell because it would destroy the cell. The hydrogen and chloride ions that make up hydrochloric acid are transported separately by different mechanisms and come together in the gastric lumen outside of the cell. Hydrogen ions are created inside the cell as the enzyme carbonic anhydrase converts carbon dioxide and water to carbonic acid. The carbonic acid dissociates into hydrogen ions and bicarbonate ions. The hydrogen ions

are transported via one pathway to the lumen of the gastric gland via active transport. Bicarbonate ions are transported out of the cell in exchange for chloride ions. The outflow of bicarbonate into the blood results in a slight elevation of blood pH known as the 'alkaline tide'. Via the process of diffusion the chloride ions then move through the cell to the gastric gland lumen (Figure 4.4).

Intrinsic factor is also produced by the parietal cells. It is a glycoprotein that binds to vitamin B_{12} in the terminal ileum of the small intestine. This binding forms a complex that binds with receptors on the wall of the ileum (small intestine) allowing transfer of vitamin B_{12} across the ileal wall into the blood. Dietary vitamin B_{12} is released from ingested proteins in the stomach through the action of pepsin and acid. This vitamin is required for the maturation of erythrocytes and deficiency leads to anaemia. It is also required for the healthy functioning of nerve fibres. The rate of secretion of intrinsic factor increases during the first 2 weeks after birth. Concentrations of intrinsic factor reach adult levels by 3 months of age.

3. *Chief cells* – Chief cells secrete pepsinogen which is an inactive proenzyme. When pepsinogen comes into contact with hydrochloric acid, in the gastric

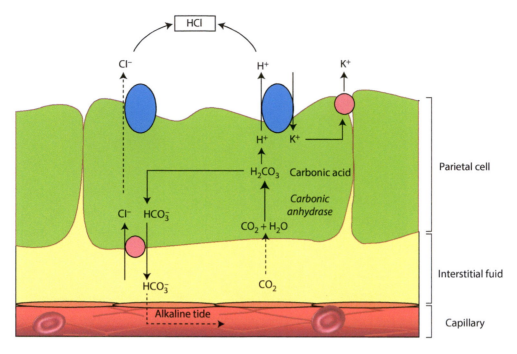

Figure 4.4 Formation of HCl.

lumen, the acid converts pepsinogen into pepsin. Pepsin is an active proteolytic enzyme which breaks down proteins.

The chief cells of neonates produce chymosin, also known as rennin (not produced in adults). Chymosin coagulates milk proteins and then gastric lipase starts the process of digestion of the fats in the milk. The production of chymosin is maximal during the first few days after birth. After this, production will decline and be replaced by pepsin, the main protein-digesting enzyme. The secretion of pepsinogen in infancy (prior to weaning) is lower than that for adults. This is believed to be attributed to breastfeeding where there is reduced protein in the diet in comparison to what is present following weaning.

4. *G cells* – Different types of enteroendocrine cells are found within the stomach mucosa. These cells produce more than seven different hormones which diffuse into nearby blood vessels. The principal hormone secreted from the gastric epithelium is gastrin. This is important for acid secretion and gastric motility. Gastrin is produced by the G cells which are found predominantly in the gastric pits of the pyloric antrum. The primary stimulus for the secretion of gastrin into the bloodstream is the presence in the stomach of food that contains peptides and amino acids (from protein digestion). Gastrin has three major effects on gastric function: stimulation of gastric acid from parietal cells, pepsinogen from chief cells and contraction of the muscles of the stomach to aid mechanical digestion. Up until the age of 4 months infants have much higher concentrations of gastrin than adults. This is because during infancy gastrin plays an important role in maturation of gut function.

REGULATION OF GASTRIC ACTIVITY

During infancy the digestive system can be described as immature. Relative to an adult, ingested food moves rapidly through the gastrointestinal tract. The rate of peristalsis is much greater and this affects the frequency, consistency and colour of stools. Gastric emptying in the newborn is approximately 2–3 hours and between 3 and 6 hours in the older infant and child.

Hydrochloric acid production by the parietal cells in the gastric mucosa starts by week 12. During infancy gastric acidity is believed to be low but there is a lack of agreement about acidity levels during infancy. Hydrochloric acid secretion is high during the first 10 days after birth. The rate of secretion then decreases until day 30. After 3 months the rate of secretion is at the level of adults. An acid environment in the stomach is necessary for enzyme action and therefore this has an impact upon the efficiency of digestive enzymes and hormones. Gastric activity increases steadily to 10 years of age where it then plateaus. During the time of adolescence (10–15 years) the rate of hydrochloric acid production by the parietal cells increases, which seems to correspond with the increased ingestion of food during this time.

Effective digestion of complex foods requires participation from both the nervous and endocrine systems (see Chapter 1; 'Overview of control and regulation of the digestive system'). The secretory cells of the stomach mucosa and the muscles of the muscularis externa are regulated by direct stimulation from the central nervous system, short reflexes distributed throughout the stomach wall and from hormones released along the gastrointestinal tract (see Chapter 1; Table 1.1).

The way the nervous and endocrine systems interact to regulate gastric activity can be summarised into three phases: cephalic, gastric and intestinal (Figure 4.5).

(a)   **Cephalic phase**

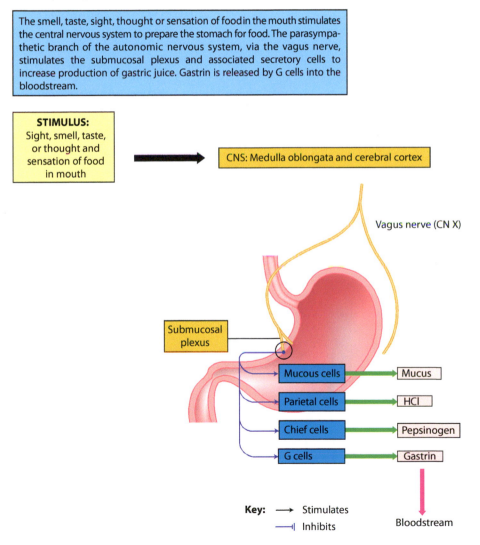

The smell, taste, sight, thought or sensation of food in the mouth stimulates the central nervous system to prepare the stomach for food. The parasympathetic branch of the autonomic nervous system, via the vagus nerve, stimulates the submucosal plexus and associated secretory cells to increase production of gastric juice. Gastrin is released by G cells into the bloodstream.

STIMULUS:
Sight, smell, taste, or thought and sensation of food in mouth

CNS: Medulla oblongata and cerebral cortex

Vagus nerve (CN X)

Submucosal plexus

Mucous cells → Mucus
Parietal cells → HCl
Chief cells → Pepsinogen
G cells → Gastrin

Bloodstream

Key: → Stimulates
⊣ Inhibits

Figure 4.5 The three phases of gastric secretion.

(Continued)

(b) **Gastric phase**

The arrival of food in the stomach stimulates neural and endocrine responses to initiate the **gastric phase**. The gastric phase is stimulated specifically by:

1. Stomach distension activating stretch receptors
2. Increased pH of stomach contents activating chemoreceptors
3. Presence of undigested food, e.g. proteins and peptides stimulating gastrin production

Stretch receptors and chemoreceptors stimulate secretory cells via the submucosal and myenteric plexuses. Entero-endocrine G cells produce the hormone gastrin which is released into the bloodstream. Secretory activity from mucous, parietal and chief cells occurs into the stomach lumen. The muscularis externa is stimulated via the myenteric plexus to produce mixing waves. During the gastric phase ingested food is mixed and churned with gastric juices and is referred to as chyme. The gastric phase may last for 3–4 hours.

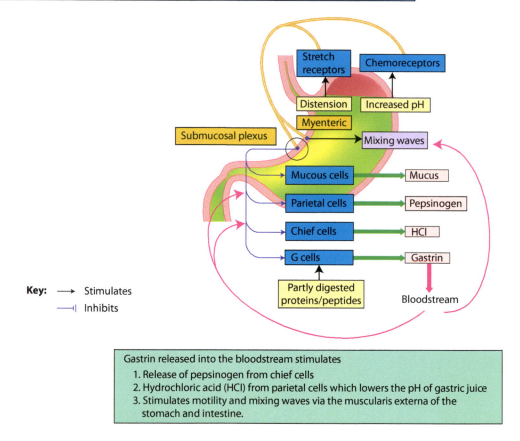

Key: → Stimulates
      ⊣ Inhibits

Gastrin released into the bloodstream stimulates

1. Release of pepsinogen from chief cells
2. Hydrochloric acid (HCl) from parietal cells which lowers the pH of gastric juice
3. Stimulates motility and mixing waves via the muscularis externa of the stomach and intestine.

Figure 4.5 (Continued) The three phases of gastric secretion.

Cephalic phase ('getting ready for food') – The CNS receives sensory information from the olfactory nerve (smell), the gustatory nerve (taste) and the optic nerve (sight). Interpretation by the CNS of this information, and the anticipation of food, leads to nerve impulses being sent from the CNS informing the stomach that it needs to prepare for the imminent arrival of food. Nerve impulses through the parasympathetic nervous system travel via the vagus nerve (*cranial nerve* X) stimulating the submucosal plexus within the stomach submucosa to release mucus from the mucous cells, pepsinogen from the chief cells and hydrochloric acid from the parietal cells. The G cells are also induced to release gastrin which, via the circulatory system, stimulates the parietal cells to release hydrochloric acid and stimulates a low level of gastric motility.

(c)   **Intestinal phase**

The entry of chyme into the duodenum signals the start of the **intestinal phase**, after several hours of mixing in the stomach. The presence of chyme containing H^+, fats and part digested proteins in the duodenum inhibits gastric neural and entero-endocrine activity. The inhibition of gastric activity carefully controls gastric emptying and ensures secretory, digestive and absorptive functions of the duodenum are maximised.

Enterogastrones, e.g. CCK, secretin and GIP are also stimulated by the presence of the above substances in chyme and act to reduce gastric activity.

The arrival of chyme in the duodenum stimulates stretch and chemoreceptors triggering the **enterogastric reflex**. The entero gastric reflex

1. Inhibits activity of vagal nuclei in the medulla oblongata decreasing central stimulation of the stomach
2. Inhibits local reflex activity leading to a decrease in gastric secretory and motor activity
3. Activates the sympathetic nervous system to trigger contraction of the pyloric sphincter to prevent further movement of chyme into the duodenum

The reflex results in decreased gastric activity with inhibition of gastrin production and decreased motility which protects the duodenum from excess amounts of chyme and acidity.

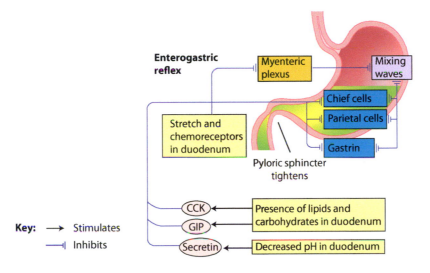

Figure 4.5 (Continued) The three phases of gastric secretion.

Gastric phase ('arrival of food') – When food arrives at the stomach it triggers a number of additional changes and these can be summarised as distension and a change in pH.

The distension and change in pH caused by the arriving food stimulate the stretch receptors (also termed *baroreceptors*) and chemoreceptors in the stomach mucosa. These changes are detected by short reflexes coordinated by the submucosal and myenteric plexus. Impulses from the submucosal plexus stimulate the parietal and chief cells to increase gastric

secretion of acid and pepsinogen. Impulses from the myenteric plexus stimulate contraction of the gastric muscles causing vigorous smooth muscle contractions. Contractions of smooth gastric muscle have two main functions: to mix food and gastric secretions to create a liquid called *chyme*. At the end of the gastric phase chyme will then be ejected through the pyloric sphincter into the small intestine, a process called *gastric emptying*. Impulses from the gastric neurons also stimulate gastrin release from the G cells, which enhances the release of gastric secretions and smooth muscle contraction, further contributing to the volume of gastric juice and the mixing waves. The goal of the gastric phase is to generate enough acids, enzyme and mixing waves to create the right environment for the effective chemical and mechanical breakdown of food. The trigger for eventually stopping acid and enzyme secretion and digestive movement is when the pH drops to less than 2.

Intestinal phase ('exiting of food') – Once food has reached the right 'soup'-like consistency and pH (less than 2) it is ready to enter the duodenum. It is important that gastric emptying of chyme through the pyloric sphincter is controlled so that acids that arrive in the duodenum can be neutralised and nutrients can be absorbed more efficiently in the small intestine. Pancreatic enzymes and enzymes from the small intestine epithelial cells (enterocytes) cannot function in an acid environment. The arrival of chyme in the small intestine triggers a neural and endocrine response. The stimulation of short reflexes and the release of hormones work together to inhibit the release of gastric acids and pepsinogen and slow gastric motility.

As chyme enters the duodenum it stimulates stretch and chemoreceptors that trigger gastric inhibitory impulses called the enterogastric reflex. The enterogastric reflex inhibits neural stimulation via the myenteric plexus thus slowing gastric motility. It also has the effect of stimulating contraction of the pyloric sphincter. The enterogastric reflex plays a vital role in controlling the rate at which chyme enters the duodenum.

The presence of certain nutrients in the small intestines triggers the release of hormones from enteroendocrine cells directly into the lamina propria which are then absorbed into the blood circulation and further contribute to suppression of gastric activity. Lipids and carbohydrates stimulate the release of cholecystokinin (CCK) and gastric inhibitory peptide (GIP). CCK and GIP inhibit the release of acids and enzymes and GIP also slows down gastric motility. As chyme enters the duodenum it will bring with it acid which will lower the pH in the duodenum. This stimulates enteroendocrine cells to release secretin which has the effect of inhibiting the release of acid from the parietal cells and pepsinogen from the chief cells. Secretin also triggers the release of a bicarbonate-rich secretion from epithelial duct cells lining pancreatic and biliary ducts. This bicarbonate-rich secretion has a pH of 7.5–8.8 which travels along the pancreatic

and biliary ducts and enters into the duodenum via the hepatopancreatic ampulla. It serves to dilute and buffer the acids within the chyme that enter into the duodenum. This provides the right pH for enzyme activity in the small intestine.

The main function of the intestinal phase is to control the rate at which chyme enters into the duodenum. Collectively hormones from enteroendocrine cells and stimulation via the enterogastric reflex suspend gastric secretion and motility. As the chyme in the duodenum is processed and moves on, stimulation of enteroendocrine cells and stretch and chemoreceptors will diminish and secretory and motor activity in the stomach will resume until the next cephalic phase.

Gastric emptying in infants is affected by the composition of feeds. Among healthy adults there is considerable variability concerning transit time through the stomach. Also the length of time food stays in the stomach will be dependent upon the composition of food material ingested. The transit time of breast milk through the stomach is much faster than formula feed. This is believed to be associated with the lower fat content, greater emulsification and reduced ratio of casein to whey found in breast milk. What this research suggests is that the rate of gastric emptying in infants is governed by the level of long-chain triglycerides (fat content). Gastric emptying in the newborn is approximately 2–3 hours and between 3 and 6 hours in the older infant and child.

The gastric phase is likely to end after approximately 4–5 hours when the stomach is completely empty. If the meal is substantial the gastric phase might be even longer because with a large meal the gastric phase will be intermittent as it is suppressed by neural and hormonal messages from the duodenum as chyme is ejected from the pylorus into the duodenum.

GASTRIC DIGESTION IN INFANTS

In the neonate birth initiates the transition from a passive mechanism for the acquisition of nutrients (i.e. placenta) to a system whereby the infant must ingest, digest and absorb nutrients from an external source. Although gastric hormone and gastric gland secretion is active at birth their activity is relatively low. This means that compared to the adult stomach (pH 2) the pH of the neonate stomach is only mildly acidic (close to neutral). The lack of acidity in the stomach means that salivary amylase remains active and therefore starch digestion continues. It also means that protein digestion in the stomach is limited because without an acid environment activation of pepsinogen to pepsin will be limited.

There are three important digestive enzymes in the stomach. The chief cells of the gastric mucosa release pepsin and gastric lipase. The third enzyme present is salivary amylase.

Protein digestion begins in the stomach. The chief cells of the gastric mucosa produce different types of pepsinogens: pepsinogen A and pepsinogen C. The gastric mucosa of the neonate also produces chymosin, also called rennin which is essential for the breakdown of milk proteins. These enzymes are secreted in an inactive form and become active when exposed to the acid environment of the stomach of a pH less than 4. Pepsin activity can be detected after 16 weeks in foetal development. Pepsin activity in the stomach of a newborn is low; however, compensation for this is provided by intestinal enteropeptidases and pancreatic trypsins and chymotrypsins which have a higher activity in the newborn. Intestinal protein digestion through the action of pepsin activity is fully developed in infants at 3–8 months of age. As a consequence of this it is believed that the stomach of a neonate does not contribute significantly to overall protein digestion.

Fat digestion begins in the stomach. Gastric fat digestion is also much more significant in infants than it is in adults. The enzymes responsible for catalysing (breaking down) fats in the stomach originate from two sources: lingual lipase comes from the lingual serous glands in the mouth and gastric lipase from the gastric mucosa. Gastric lipase breaks down fats to free fatty acids and diglycerol and is important for releasing fatty acids from milk. Gastric lipase is active in the relatively low pH environment of the infants. By the age of 3 months the pH is even lower and this inactivates much of the gastric lipase. Fatty acids are essential for infant development, particularly brain, retinal and growth development. Triglyceride is the main energy source of the neonate. Other lipases such as pancreatic lipase and bile salt-dependent lipase are active in the small intestine and convert the triglyceride to monoglyceride which can then be absorbed. The activity of lingual and gastric lipase is essential because, unlike pancreatic and bile salt-dependent lipase, they are able to penetrate the phospholipid component of the milk fat globule membrane and hydrolyse triglycerides. Therefore the partial hydrolysis of fat in the stomach is a prerequisite for the completion of digestion and absorption of fatty acids and monoglycerol in the small intestine. Bile salts also contribute to the breaking down of the milk fat globule membrane.

Gastric lipase breaks down triglycerides to diglyceride and pancreatic lipase breaks down diglyceride to monoglyceride. Breast milk lipase is an important lipase for the infant because it is able to completely hydrolyse triglyceride (Lonnerdal, 2003). It is therefore possible for the combined action of gastric and milk lipase to complete milk fat digestion without the need for pancreatic lipase. The free fatty acids released by the hydrolysis of triglycerides by milk lipase are more easily absorbed than monoglyceride at the low bile salt concentration present in the newborn (Lonnerdal, 2003).

Amylase activity in the neonate is low when compared to that of an adult. However, the amylase in breast milk (milk amylase) is able to hydrolyse starches given, as supplements, to partially breastfed infants. Lonnerdal (2003) explains that it is the milk amylase that enables breastfed as opposed to formula-fed infants to be better able to tolerate starch supplements. The low activity of amylase in newborns is compensated for by the high activity of brush border enzymes – glucoamylase, sucrose-isomaltase and lactase – which are able to break down lactose and short-chain glucose polymers.

At birth the digestive system is still relatively immature. However it is clear from the explanations above that the newborn has a number of active compensatory mechanisms that enable adequate nutrition to be achieved.

AGEING AND GASTRIC DIGESTION

Adult requirements for nutrients, vitamins and minerals do not change significantly as a consequence of ageing. However, the ageing process can affect an individual's ability to digest and absorb nutrients.

In an older person there is a decrease in gastric compliance, particularly in the fundus and antrum. The antrum fills more quickly which leads to early satiety or feeling full. There is delayed emptying of the stomach, particularly solid foods, but liquids are emptied more quickly. This may predispose to reflux.

Age-related reductions in the production of digestive enzymes by the stomach and small intestine have an impact upon nutrient absorption. Age-related reductions in the production of hydrochloric acid (hypochlorhydria) in the stomach can limit protein digestion in the older person. Hydrochloric acid is needed to convert pepsinogen to the active enzyme pepsin required to break down proteins to peptides. An increased prevalence of hypochlorhydria has been seen in people with *Helicobacter pylori*. Age-related reductions in the production of intrinsic factor, required for the absorption of vitamin B_{12}, have also been identified which affect digestion. Age-related gastric reductions in bicarbonate-rich mucous from goblet cells make the gastric mucosa more vulnerable to the action of acids and pepsin.

DEVELOPMENTAL ABNORMALITIES OF THE STOMACH

Pyloric stenosis

Infantile hypertrophic pyloric stenosis (IHPS) is the most common cause of gastric outlet obstruction in infancy. It affects 2–5 per 1000 live births (Sørensen et al., 2002; Hernanz-Schulman, 2003; Georgoula and Gardiner, 2012). Aetiology (causes) is unclear but is believed to be multifactorial including both genetic (hereditary) and environmental factors. There is a positive family history in 17% of cases (Taylor et al., 2013). IHPS has been associated with postnatal erythromycin (antibiotic) and infant sleeping position. IHPS is most commonly seen in infants aged between 2 and 8 weeks, however approximately 10% of cases occur in premature infants (Schechter et al., 1997; Feenstra et al., 2012; Hsu et al., 2014). It occurs more frequently in males (Feenstra et al., 2012; Hsu et al., 2014) and with declining risk with subsequent births within a family, showing highest prevalence in firstborns (Ranells et al., 2011; Georgoula and Gardiner, 2012; Taylor et al., 2013). Infants with IHPS are clinically normal at birth but during the first weeks of life parents report increasing episodes of vomiting. This vomiting is termed *non-bilious projectile vomiting* which can lead to dehydration, weight loss and electrolyte imbalance. Diagnosis is made through clinical examination and ultrasound scan. Clinical signs include a palpable pyloric tumour or 'olive' and visible peristaltic waves. Ultrasound features include a pyloric muscle mass, little or no gastric emptying, decreased relaxation of the pyloric muscle and increased pyloric thickness and increased pyloric muscle length (Hsu et al., 2014).

The stenosis or obstruction in the pylorus is caused by hypertrophy and hyperplasia of the longitudinal and circular muscle layers that make up the muscularis externa. This causes narrowing of the pyloric antrum, the pyloric canal becomes lengthened and the pylorus becomes thickened. This causes partial or complete obstruction leading to delayed gastric emptying, dilation of the stomach and the resultant vomiting.

Congenital diaphragmatic hernia

Congenital diaphragmatic hernia (CDH) is caused by the failure of the diaphragm to fuse properly during foetal development. Normal development sees the diaphragm develop as a septum between the heart and the liver. It then projects posterolaterally and closes at the Bochdalek foramen at approximately 8–10 weeks' gestation. This provides separation of the thoracic and abdominal cavities. Failure of the diaphragm to fuse allows abdominal organs to move up into the thoracic cavity and occupy the space for the lungs (Figure 4.6). The most common type of hernias are Bochdalek hernias. The incidence of congenital diaphragmatic hernia is 1 in 2500–3000 live births (Kline-Fath, 2012; McHoney, 2014) with a prevalence of 2.3 per 10,000 births (McGivern et al., 2015). It occurs with more frequency on the left side (McHoney, 2014).

CDH is associated with significant morbidity and mortality and variable survival rates (Edmonds et al., 2013). Approximately 50%–85% of cases are diagnosed prenatally during routine ultrasound scan (McHoney, 2014). Undiagnosed cases normally present at or very soon after birth depending upon the severity of the hernia. Smaller hernias may go unnoticed until adult life.

CDH may occur as an isolated pathology or associated with other co-existing anomalies. Infants with CDH often present with lung hypoplasia, pulmonary hypertension and co-existing anomalies associated commonly with the heart and nervous system. It is also often associated with other genetic and chromosomal syndromes such as trisomy 18 (Edwards syndrome) (McGivern et al., 2015). Gastro-oesophageal reflux is common in later life and neurodevelopmental delay, including motor and cognitive deficits, is common (Losty, 2014).

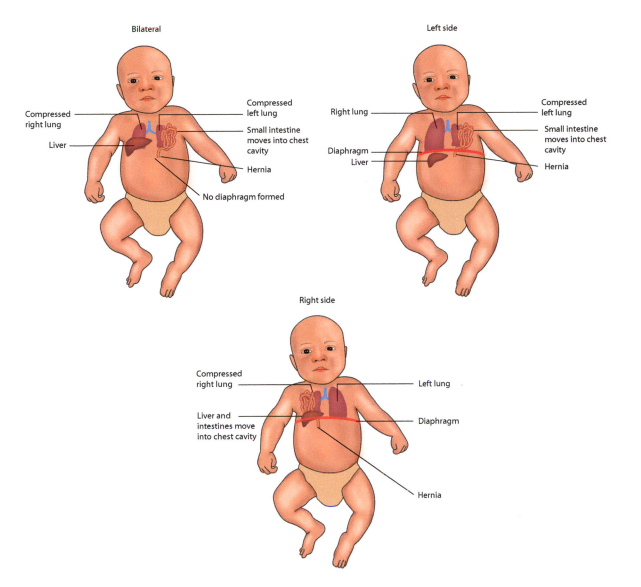

Figure 4.6 Congenital diaphragmatic hernia.

The aetiology (cause) of CDH is not clear but associations with specific genes and teratogenic factors, such as vitamin A have been implicated (Kline-Fath, 2012).

CHANGES ASSOCIATED WITH DIFFERENT STAGES OF LIFESPAN

Functional dyspepsia

Functional dyspepsia or 'non-ulcer' dyspepsia is a relapsing and remitting disorder occurring in the gastroduodenal region of the gastrointestinal tract.

It refers to a group of digestive symptoms including sensation of pain in the upper abdomen, bloating, fullness during or after a meal, early satiety, regurgitation, nausea, vomiting and chest pain (Feinle-Bisset et al., 2003; Talley and Ford, 2015). The diagnostic criteria include the presence of chronic symptoms that occur at least weekly, over a period of 6 months in the absence of other structural or functional disorders (Talley et al., 1999; Talley and Ford, 2015). Global prevalence is between <2% and 57% depending upon geographical population (Ford et al., 2015). And, 80% of individuals with dyspepsia state that their symptoms are aggravated by ingesting a meal (Bisschops et al., 2008).

Functional dyspepsia is divided into two subcategories: epigastric pain syndrome where intermittent pain and burning are experienced at least once per week in the epigastric region which may or may not be meal related; and postprandial distress syndrome where fullness is experienced a number of times per week following a normal-sized meal or early satiety occurs which prevents a person from finishing a meal (Talley and Ford, 2015).

A proposed disease model for functional dyspepsia is of activation of immune cells in the duodenum by allergens and pathogens in a genetically predisposed individual. Release of inflammatory mediators and cytokines can lead to tissue injury and meal-related symptoms. These include increased gastric acid secretion, visceral hypersensitivity, disordered gastric motility and delayed gastric emptying (Wallander et al., 2007; Walker et al., 2014). Other factors implicated in the development of functional dyspepsia include female gender, smoking, obesity, alcohol, medications such as NSAIDs (non-steroidal anti-inflammatory drugs) and *H. pylori* (Ford et al., 2015). Psychological factors such as stress, anxiety, anger and depression have been implicated (Banning, 2004; Mahadera and Goh, 2006; Wallander et al., 2007). There is also an association between dyspepsia and subsequent irritable bowel syndrome.

Hiatus hernia

A hiatus hernia is the upward escape of the stomach through the hiatus of the diaphragm to lie within the chest. There are two main types of hiatus hernia: sliding and para-oesophageal or rolling. Sliding hiatus hernia is the most common of the two occurring in almost 95% of cases (Fofaria and Morris, 2015) and is associated with reflux. In this situation the top of the stomach protrudes through the hole in the diaphragm called the oesophageal hiatus. This hiatus, or hole, is what allows the oesophagus to enter the thoracic cavity and join the stomach in the abdominal cavity at the gastro-oesophageal junction (GOJ). The hernia may slide up and down, disrupting the GOJ (Figure 4.7). The oesophageal hiatus may dilate, with laxity of the phreno-oesphageal ligament.

The rolling or para-oesophageal hiatus hernia is less common and occurs when part of the stomach protrudes up through the hiatus into the thoracic cavity and lies parallel to the oesophagus. It is not associated with GORD (Figure 4.7).

Diagnosis of the hiatus hernia is usually made by endoscopic examination of the gastric mucosa and the gastro-oeophageal junction. Hiatus hernia affects the anti-reflux barrier at the gastroesophageal junction and is now regarded as one of the major causative factors of GOR (Kasapidis et al., 1995). According to Kawanishi (2006), 31.9% of patients who underwent endoscopy investigations for symptomatic gastroesophageal reflux disease (SGERD) had a hiatus hernia. Failure of oesophageal clearance, impaired acid emptying, reduced sphincter pressure during straining and increases in transient LOS relaxations (TLOSRs) have been implicated in hiatus hernia associated GOR (Lee and McColl, 2013). The hiatus hernia can act as a trap for stomach acid which may escape into the oesophagus during transient LOS relaxation (TLOSR) or if the pressure of the LOS is low. This is particularly the case in large hiatus hernias where there is disruption of the LOS and diaphragm (Boeckxstaens, 2005).

The prevalence of hiatus hernia increases with age (Collen et al., 1995; Amano et al., 2001; Loffeld and Van Der Putten, 2002; Roman and Kahrilas, 2015) and is associated with increased body mass index. It is well known that the majority of patients with active reflux oesophagitis (inflammation of the oesophagus caused by reflux of acid) have a hiatus hernia. However the presence of a hiatus hernia is not a prerequisite in developing reflux disease, although it is a risk factor (Amano et al., 2001; Fofaria and Morris, 2015). Hiatus hernia has also been associated with an increased risk of developing Barrett's oesophagus but links to oesophageal adenocarcinoma are not clear (Roman and Kahrilas, 2015).

Aetiology (causes) is unclear but is believed to include both genetic (hereditary) and environmental factors. Weakness or rupture of the phreno-oesophageal ligament which surrounds the diaphragm and oesophageal hiatus is thought to occur, particularly with ageing where loss of elastic fibres and replacement with adipose tissue has been observed (Lee and McColl, 2013). The progressive weakening of LOS muscles associated with ageing may be a

(a)

(b)

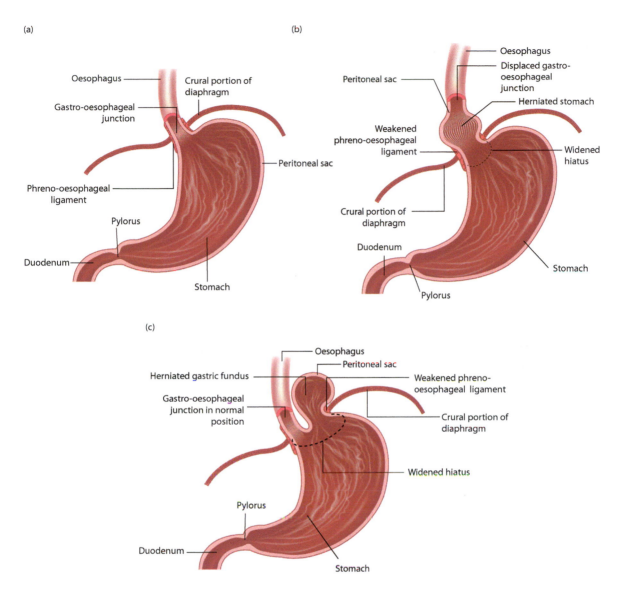

Oesophagus

Crural portion of diaphragm

Gastro-oesophageal junction

Peritoneal sac

Phreno-oesophageal ligament

Pylorus

Duodenum

Stomach

Oesophagus

Displaced gastro-oesophageal junction

Peritoneal sac

Herniated stomach

Weakened phreno-oesophageal ligament

Widened hiatus

Crural portion of diaphragm

Duodenum

Stomach

Pylorus

(c)

Oesophagus

Peritoneal sac

Herniated gastric fundus

Gastro-oesophageal junction in normal position

Weakened phreno-oesophageal ligament

Crural portion of diaphragm

Widened hiatus

Pylorus

Duodenum

Stomach

Figure 4.7 Hiatus hernia. (a) Normal anatomy, (b) sliding hiatus hernia and (c) para-oesophageal hernia.

contributory factor. Any factor that increases intra-abdominal pressure can also increase the risk of hiatus hernia, factors such as obesity, persistant cough and pregnancy.

Helicobactor pylori infection

Helicobactor pylori infection (*H. pylori*) is a gram–negative microaerophilic spiral–shaped bacterium which colonises the stomach mucosa. It is one of the most common bacterial infections and is linked to a number of digestive diseases in both children and adults.

Most people with *H. pylori* are asymptomatic but all of them will have a level of inflammation of the gastric mucosa called gastritis. *H. pylori* is recognised as a major risk factor for the development of gastritis, with 10%–15% developing peptic ulcer disease, 0.1% gastric mucosa–associated lymphoid tissue (MALT) lymphoma and 1%–3% gastric cancer

(Peek and Crabtree, 2006; Ertem, 2013; Oppong et al., 2015).

Prevalence of infection is much higher in developing than developed countries. It varies from 80% in developing countries to 6%–25% in developed countries (Wang and Peura, 2011; Oppong et al., 2015). *H. pylori* affects over half of the adult population worldwide. Acquisition of *H. pylori* is believed to occur in early childhood (Rothenbacher et al., 2000) and the infection usually persists throughout life (Oppong et al., 2015). *H. pylori* is associated with increased prevalence of gastritis and intestinal metaplasia with increasing age. Overcrowding in childhood and poor hygiene have been associated with increases in *H. pylori* in some countries.

The progression of *H. pylori* to peptic ulceration is influenced by a number of factors that include strain of *H. pylori*; host factors, such as genetic susceptibility; environment for example smoking; and diet (i.e. the presence or absence of certain vitamins and nutrients) (Noto and Peek, 2012). Factors such as these have all been implicated as playing a role in the pathogenesis of atrophic gastritis. *H. pylori* causes disease by the production of a variety of virulence factors which may affect the cells signalling processes and facilitate the formation of neoplastic changes (Wang et al., 2014). These allow it to evade the powerful gastric juices of the stomach. It also produces a urease enzyme that catalyses hydrolysis of urea into ammonia which is used to detect its presence in a urea breath test.

H. pylori causes acute and chronic inflammation in gastric epithelial cells and stimulates a wider inflammatory response, recruiting immune cells to the site of infection. It also stimulates pro-inflammatory cytokines which mediate the inflammatory response and results in inflammation and ulceration (Wang et al., 2014). *H. pylori* can cause ulceration in both the stomach and duodenum.

In the stomach, acute and chronic inflammation of the gastric mucosa is as a direct result of colonisation of *H. pylori* in the gastric mucosa. Gastritis may develop from a chronic superficial gastritis to atrophic gastritis (Noto and Peek, 2012).

Gastritis can occur anywhere in the stomach but is most commonly seen in the antrum and corpus of the stomach (Siurala et al., 1985; Sherman, 1994). Gastritis in the corpus or body of the stomach causes hyposecretion of acid and predisposes to an increased risk of gastric cancer. Duodenal ulceration is thought to result from gastritis in the stomach antrum. This has a negative feedback effect on the production of the hormone gastrin, which increases acid production in the stomach. This increases the acidic load within the duodenum which causes damage to the duodenal mucosa. Metaplasia of the duodenal cells can occur which allows *H. pylori* to colonise the duodenum, causing duodenal inflammation and ulceration (Oppong et al., 2015). It is associated with a decreased risk of gastric cancer (Atherton, 2006). A study carried out by Kato et al. (2004) showed that *H. pylori* is the most important causal factor for the development of duodenal ulcers in children. The ulcers are caused by gastric metaplasia, detected in paediatric patients with *H. pylori* gastritis, and its occurrence increases with age (Kato et al., 2004).

Epidemiological studies have established a strong causal link between *H. pylori* and gastric cancers, including gastric MALT lymphoma and adenocarcinomas, and there is evidence to support a role for *H. pylori* in transforming normal gastric mucosa to adenocarcinoma. Approximately 80% of gastric adenocarcinomas are related to *H. pylori* infection and subsequent gastritis (Sipponen, 2002). Exposure to *H. pylori* produces a two- to threefold increase in risk of getting gastric cancer. However the majority of those infected with *H. pylori* do not progress to dysplasia and cancer and therefore other factors such as bacterial strain, environment and individual susceptibility also interact in a complex multifactorial process to cause gastric cancer.

H. pylori is also a cause of gastritis in children. As with adult infection, the prevalence of *H. pylori* is seen to be decreasing in developed countries in contrast to developing countries, such as parts of southern and eastern Europe and Asia (Roosendaal et al., 1997; Homan et al., 2012).

There are a number of risk factors associated with *H. pylori* acquisition. Transmission to a child is thought to be from family members, associated with overcrowding, family income, number of children sharing a room, parent's education and increasing age in childhood (Mourad-Baars et al., 2010; Ertem, 2013). Mother to child transmission has been shown to be a significant factor in *H. pylori* colonisation with similarity between types of *H. pylori* in both the mother and child (Hollander et al., 2015).

Many children do not go on to develop the disease but will become carriers, whereas a small proportion display symptoms of *H. pylori* infection. In children symptoms are non-specific but can include epigastric pain, nausea and/or vomiting and anorexia (Homan et al., 2012; Ertem, 2013). *H. pylori* infection in children is associated with antral gastritis and gastric and duodenal ulcers (Sherman, 1994; Mourad-Baars et al., 2010). *H. pylori* gastritis is believed to be progressive but what is not clear is what aspects of the infection in childhood lead to the different *H. pylori*-associated digestive disorders in adult life.

Gastric cancer

Gastric cancer is the fourth most common cancer worldwide (Van Cutsem et al., 2016). Gastric cancer can occur anywhere in the stomach but is divided anatomically as true gastric adenocarcinomas (non-cardia gastric cancers) and gastro-oesophageal junction adenocarcinomas (cardia gastric cancers) (Colquhoun et al., 2015). Gastric cancer has a multifactorial aetiology (cause) with genetic (hereditary) and environmental factors associated with its development. Environmental factors include high salt consumption, low consumption of fruits and vegetables, nitrates, *H. pylori*, obesity, gastro-oesophageal reflux and smoking. Gastric cancer has shown a decline in Western countries in recent years; however, incidence remains high in East Asia, China and Japan (Lawson et al., 2011).

Many people with gastric cancer are asymptomatic and diagnosis is made when the disease is more advanced. Cancer staging considers invasion of the stomach wall structures, lymph node involvement and metastases. Symptoms include anorexia, dyspepsia, weight loss, nausea, vomiting, fatigue and epigastric pain (Lawson et al., 2011). Tumours nearer to the gastro-oesophageal junction and cardia may present with dysphagia.

It is the body and pyloric antrum of the stomach that are at most risk of gastric cancer, because it is here that the epithelium is exposed to acid secretions. Gastric cancers occur from a number of changes in the stomach which can be divided into diffuse and intestinal types. Intestinal-type carcinoma is made up of well-differentiated cell structure and glands, whereas the diffuse type is where cellular change is poorly differentiated and glands are absent (Lawson et al., 2011; Van Cutsem et al., 2016). Intestinal type occurs when brush border and goblet cells replace the normal mucus-secreting gastric mucosa. This is called metaplasia and is susceptible to malignant change. It is believed that gastric cancer progresses from initial chronic gastritis, gastric atrophy followed by intestinal metaplasia, dysplasia and finally cancer. Mucosa-associated lymphoid tissue (MALT) may undergo malignant change causing lymphoma of the stomach.

H. pylori plays an important role in the pathogenesis of chronic gastritis and peptic ulcer diseases and epidemiological evidence has indicated that *H. pylori* is associated with an increased risk of gastric cancer (Heavey and Rowland, 2004; Bornschein et al., 2010; Wang et al., 2014). *H. pylori* infection plays an initiating role in the pathogenesis of gastric cancer by inducing an inflammatory response in the gastric epithelial and immune cells by stimulating inflammatory cytokines. Alterations or mutations in genes are also responsible for regulating cell division such as the inactivation of tumour suppressor genes by *H. pylori*. These alterations or mutations can change factors such as the balance between epithelial cell proliferation and apoptosis. It can bring about increased cell proliferation without a corresponding increase in apoptosis (Heavey and Rowland, 2004; Jones et al., 2006) which can increase the risk of cancer development. In addition *H. pylori* produces a number of substances such as ammonia which impair the immune system and expose the gastric epithelial cells to carcinogens such as nitric oxide. Epstein Barr virus has also been shown to be associated with gastric cancer.

SUMMARY OF KEY POINTS

The stomach
Greatly expanded J-shaped section of the gastrointestinal tract. Functions as a reservoir for food.

Regions of the stomach
1. Cardiac portion – located near the cardiac orifice. The oesophagus joins with the stomach here. It is called the cardiac portion because it lies next to the diaphragm just below the heart.
2. Fundus – dome-shaped region of the stomach, most superior region of the stomach.
3. Body – is the major portion of the stomach that secretes pepsinogen and hydrochloric acid.
4. Pyloric portion – is the most distal portion of the stomach and is responsible for mucus, gastrin and pepsinogen secretion. It terminates in the pylorus which separates the stomach from the duodenum. The middle layer of the muscularis externa (smooth muscle) is thickened here to form a sphincter. This sphincter is normally closed except when acid chyme is being propelled into the duodenum.

The wall of the stomach shows a number of variations from the rest of the gastrointestinal tract.

Epithelium is highly folded forming deep pits called gastric pits. The simple columnar epithelium contains a variety of other cell types:

1. Zymogenic cells (chief cells) – produce pepsinogen a precursor of pepsin.

2. Parietal cells – produce hydrochloric acid and intrinsic factor.
3. Mucous cells – near the lumen they produce standard mucous. Those in the neck of the pit produce a thick alkaline mucous.
4. Enteroendocrine cells – produce a variety of endocrine products, that is gastrin (stimulates HCl secretion), serotonin, somatostatin (inhibits gastrin and HCl release).
5. Muscularis externa – consists of three layers of smooth muscle: the circular, longitudinal and oblique layers.

Factors protecting the stomach lining from gastric juice are as follows:

1. Copious production or a thick, alkaline mucous
2. Epithelial cells are joined at their apical surfaces by tight junctions
3. Epithelium is shed and replaced every 3 days

Functions of the stomach include the following:

1. Temporary storage of food
2. Regulation of release of food into the duodenum
3. Acid secretion and antibacterial action
4. Mechanical digestion with three muscle layers: oblique, circular and longitudinal
5. Chemical digestion with pepsin, lipase
6. Some absorption – water, ions and drugs such as aspirin and alcohol

CHECK ON LEARNING

Stomach
During embryonic development which of the following regions does the stomach develop from: foregut, midgut, hindgut?
Answer – It develops from the foregut.

What effect does the hormone gastrin have on the stomach?
Answer – Gastrin stimulates release of enzymes and acid from the parietal and chief cells glands and stimulates the mixing waves of the stomach muscles.

What effect does the hormone secretin have on the stomach?
Answer – Secretin inhibits gastrin release so inhibits acid and enzyme secretion and inhibits mixing waves of the stomach.

Other than secretin name two other hormones released by enteroendocrine cells that line the duodenum.
Answer – Cholecystokinin (CCK) and gastric inhibitory peptide are released.

What effect does the hormone cholecystokinin have on the stomach?
Answer – It inhibits gastric emptying.

Pepsinogen is the precursor for which digestive enzyme?
Answer – It is the precursor of pepsin.

What are the three phases of gastric secretion?
Answer – The three phases are cephalic, gastric and intestinal.

What type of epithelial cells line the stomach and intestines?
Answer – Columnar epithelial cells line the stomach and intestines.

What region of the stomach contains the highest concentration of gastric glands?
Answer – The body of the stomach contains the highest concentration.

(Continued)

Name the three muscles of the stomach responsible for mechanical digestion and peristalsis.
Answer – The intrinsic, circular, longitudinal and oblique muscles are responsible for mechanical digestion and peristalsis.

What structure allows the stomach to expand as it fills with food?
Answer – Internal folds called rugae allow the stomach to expand.

What is the most important enzyme in gastric digestion?
Answer – Pepsin is the most important.

What is the function of goblet cells?
Answer – Goblet cells produce mucus which protects the epithelial lining from powerful enzymes and acids.

How does entry of chyme into the duodenum slow gastric activity?
Answer – When chyme enters the duodenum through the pyloric sphincter it stimulates the duodenal stretch and chemoreceptors bringing about the enterogastric reflex which inhibits the activity of the myenteric plexus, therefore decreasing gastric motility.

What is the function of the pyloric sphincter?
Answer – The pyloric sphincter is made up of circular smooth muscle and regulates the passage of chyme from the stomach into the duodenum.

CASE STUDY

Peptic ulcer disease

Ben, a 48-year-old company executive, visited his general practitioner (GP) complaining of abdominal pain during the middle of the afternoon. He also describes waking up several times in the night with pain and discomfort. On questioning by the GP Ben explained that he wasn't eating properly because of the pain and he was also producing a dark smelly stool. There are no other problems to report. The GP took a sample of blood to assess full blood count.

The GP referred Ben to the gastroenterologist for investigations into abdominal pain and an appointment was made for an endoscopy. An endoscopy was performed 3 days later. The endoscopy allowed the doctor to observe the gastric mucosa.

The endoscopy also allowed the doctor to remove a tissue sample for examination under the microscope. The endoscopy revealed that Ben had a peptic ulcer. Analysis of the tissue sample showed that Ben also had an infection that was caused by *Helicobacter pylori* bacteria. The results of the full blood count taken by the GP showed that Ben had a slightly low haemoglobin. Ben was prescribed antibiotics for the infection and medication to reduce acid secretion in the stomach. A second endoscopy was ordered for 6 months' time to check the gastric mucosa.

Explanation of normal and abnormal physiology

The following table sets out the normal and altered anatomy and physiology which explains the person's problems.

Normal anatomy/physiology	Altered anatomy/physiology and related problems
Describe the histology of the gastric mucosa. The gastric mucosa is made up of columnar epithelium which specialises in secretion. The stomach epithelium covers the surface of the stomach and has many small openings that extend down into the lamina propria. These are called gastric pits and lead onto gastric glands and are lined with a number of secretory cells. There are four major types of secretory epithelial cells that cover the surface of the stomach: mucous cells, parietal cells (HCl and intrinsic factor), chief cells (pepsinogen) and G cells (hormones).	*What is a peptic ulcer?* Peptic ulcer disease can be defined as the loss of protective cells from the gastric (gastric ulcer) or duodenal lining (duodenal ulcer) down to the submucosa.
Describe the functions of the following components of gastric juice. Hydrochloric acid (HCl) – HCl provides the acid environment that is required for pepsinogen to pepsin and the action of pepsin. Pepsinogen – Pepsinogen is the inactive precursor of the digestive enzyme pepsin. Pepsin – Pepsin is an enzyme that functions in protein digestion. Intrinsic factor – Intrinsic factor aids in the absorption of vitamin B_{12} in the intestine.	*What are the causes of peptic ulcer disease?* Peptic ulcer disease can be attributed to both genetic and environmental factors. They are a problem in both adults and children and can occur at any age. There is evidence to show a strong association between *H. pylori*, gastritis and peptic ulcer development: 90% of all duodenal ulcers and 80% of all gastric ulcers are caused by *H. pylori* infection. Most of the remaining peptic ulcers are caused by long-term usage of certain anti-inflammatory medications, non-steroidal inflammatory drugs (NSAIDs), gastric adenocarcinoma and lymphoma and idiopathic ulcers developing after gastric surgery at sites of anastomosis following radiotherapy.

(*Continued*)

What is the role of the cardiac region of the stomach?
Cardiac region – located near the cardiac orifice. The oesophagus joins with the stomach here. It is called the cardiac portion because it lies next to the diaphragm just below the heart. It has an abundance of mucous-secreting glands that help protect the gastric lining and lubricate the bolus as it enters the stomach through the lower oesophageal sphincter.

What region of the stomach contains the bulk of the gastric glands that produce the enzymes and acids required for chemical digestion?
Main Body

Why is it that the components of gastric juice do not damage the wall of the stomach in the absence of a H. pylori infection?
The cells of the mucous membrane that line the stomach produce a thick, protective mucous that coats the mucous membrane. Also, the mucous secretion is alkaline and therefore neutralises the stomach contents where contact with the mucous membrane occurs.

Why don't most other types of bacteria produce ulcers?
Most bacteria are destroyed by the HCl in gastric juice as they enter the stomach. This represents a chemical barrier to entry, one type of nonspecific defence against infection. *H. pylori* bacteria have the ability to neutralise stomach secretions in their immediate vicinity and thereby bypass the chemical barrier.

What three mechanisms are involved in the regulation of gastric secretions?

Central nervous system

Efferent motor nerves of the sympathetic and parasympathetic pathways of the autonomic nervous system (ANS) synapse with the enteric nervous system plexuses. Parasympathetic innervation has a stimulatory response, increasing motility and secretions and relaxing sphincters. This is mediated through the vagus nerve. Sympathetic innervation has an inhibitory effect decreasing blood flow to the gastrointestinal tract, decreasing secretions and motility and contracting sphincters.

Enteric nervous system

Sensory receptors (chemoreceptors, baroreceptors), short reflex via afferent neurones which synapse with interneurons which process the information and organise a response through motor or efferent neurons, glandular tissue, muscle tissue and endocrine cells. The myenteric plexus and submucosal plexus provide the programmed short reflex responses described above. They are interconnected and stimulate the secretion from gastric glands. These sensory receptors can also stimulate long reflexes to the CNS via the myenteric and submucosal plexuses.

Endocrine system

Entero-endocrine cells dispersed among the mucosal cells of the stomach are stimulated by gastric content releasing hormones into the circulation. These stimulate the secretory cells in the gastric mucosal lining to secrete digestive acids and enzymes.

What is Helicobactor pylori (H. pylori)?
H. pylori is a corkscrew-shaped bacterium found in the stomach lining. It is one of the most common bacterial infections and is responsible for a number of digestive diseases in both children and adults.

How does H. pylori cause a peptic ulcer?
H. pylori infection causes acute and chronic inflammation of the gastric mucosa which is called gastritis. *H. pylori* is recognised as a major aetiology for the development of peptic ulcer disease. The ulcers are caused by gastric metaplasia.

What physiological changes lead to the development of peptic ulcer disease?
An imbalance between mechanisms designed to protect the digestive lining: mucous production, bicarbonate production (neutralise acids) and high rate of epithelial cell replacement and mechanisms in place to assist chemical digestion: acid, pepsin and bile salt production.
If the balance between these mechanisms is disrupted by cellular dysfunction (e.g. overstimulation of the secretory mechanism – dyspepsia), disease (*H. pylori*) or the introduction of toxic substances into the gastrointestinal tract (alcohol, medications) then ulcers can form. Once the defensive barrier is removed the specialist cells of the gastric mucosa are exposed to the corrosive action of acids and enzymes.

Why isn't H. pylori destroyed by the HCl in gastric juice?
H. pylori bacteria have the ability to neutralise stomach secretions in their immediate vicinity and thereby bypass the chemical barrier.

How do antacids, H2 receptor antagonists and proton pump inhibitors (PPIs) work to help ulcers heal?
Antacids act by neutralising or reducing gastric acidity by increasing the pH of the stomach.
H2 receptor antagonists act by preventing histamine from stimulating the gastric parietal cells to secrete hydrochloric acid (e.g. cimetidine and ranitidine).
Proton pump inhibitors suppress the formation of hydrochloric acid from the parietal cell in the gastric epithelium (e.g. omeprazole).

Background: initial investigations

The following table provides the rationale behind the investigations that Ben underwent to diagnose his condition.

Investigation	Result	Rationale
Oesophago-gastro-duodenoscopy (OGD)	Gastric ulcer found	Visualise ulcer area Endoscope can also be used to stop bleeding from the ulcer
Biopsy ulcer – removal of a tissue sample for histopathological examination under a microscope	Presence of *H. pylori* confirmed under a microscope	Test for *H. pylori* and determine whether the ulcer is cancerous
Barium contrast x-rays of the stomach (barium swallow)	Gastric ulcer found, no further ulcers found in the duodenum	Determine the severity and size of an ulcer, which sometimes cannot be completely seen during an endoscopy, particularly if the ulcer is hidden in a fold or further down the duodenum
Full blood count and haemoglobin estimation	Slightly low haemoglobin levels	Peptic ulcer might be bleeding
Serological test for IgG antibodies against *H. pylori*	Positive for IgG	To identify prior infection with *H. pylori*
H. Pylori/urea breath test	Positive	To ascertain urease activity by *H. pylori*. Radioactive urea is ingested by the patient. If *H. pylori* is present it will catalyse the hydrolysis of urea and radioactive carbon dioxide with that detected in breath samples.
Stool antigen test		Alternative to urea breath test for non-invasive detection of *H. pylori*

CLINICAL CHALLENGES

1. Antacids do not effectively heal ulcers but they do relieve symptoms of ulcers by neutralising stomach acid and thereby raising the pH level in the stomach. Find out what antacids are used in your clinical area.

2. Find out how an *H. pylori* infection is managed.

3. Identify signs and symptoms of peptic ulcer disease.

4. Discuss the following complications associated with peptic ulcers: haemorrhage, perforation and gastric outlet obstruction.

Chapter 5

THE SMALL INTESTINE

Specific learning outcomes

- Describe the embryonic development and gross anatomy of the small intestine.
- Describe the histology and physiological function of the small intestine.
- Describe the mechanisms governing motility within the small intestine.
- Describe the mechanisms governing the digestion and absorption of carbohydrates, proteins, fats, minerals, water and electrolytes.
- Discuss the physiological effects of ageing on the structure and function of the small intestine.
- Discuss common developmental abnormalities of the small intestine.
- Discuss common disorders of the small intestine.
- Explain the pathogenesis of common small intestine disorders.
- Compare and contrast the normal physiology of the small intestine with the altered physiology seen with dysfunction of the small intestine.

PRENATAL DEVELOPMENT OF THE SMALL INTESTINE

The major role of the small intestine is completion of digestion and absorption of nutrients. It is here that enzymes liberate basic molecules from more complex ones.

The first section of the intestine after the stomach is the duodenum which initially lies in the midline within the peritoneal cavity. During development it rotates and takes a retroperitoneal (behind the peritoneum) position (see Figure 5.1). The C-shaped loop that is the duodenum is formed from endoderm cells that are part of the foregut and midgut. By week 6, the end of the yolk sac has constricted and separated from the midgut. The midgut then closes and extends into a ventral U-shaped midgut loop.

By week 6 the gut loop protrudes out of the abdomen extending into the umbilical stalk (see Figure 5.1). Further development over the next 2 weeks sees the anterior limb of the midgut loop coiling (rotating by 90°) to form the bulk of the small intestine. The posterior limb of the midgut loop grows to form the remainder of the small intestine and the large intestine. Together the two loops form the duodenum, jejunum and ileum.

During the 10th week the intestines withdraw back into the abdominal cavity, or coelomic, which has now grown large enough to contain it. If the intestinal loops remain external to the abdominal cavity, in the umbilical coelom, this leads to conditions known as omphalocele and gastroschisis (see section on 'Developmental abnormalities of the small intestine'). Following this the intestines continue to grow, rotate a further 180° and differentiate into the specialist cells and structures that make up the small intestine.

The villi, which are responsible for increasing the surface area of the small intestine, develop between weeks 11 and 16. Goblet and immature enteroendocrine cells emerge during weeks 9 and 10. Enzymes such as sucrase, maltase, isomaltase and trehalase are secreted by week 10. Lactase is secreted by week 10 but its activity is very low. Peptidases are secreted by week 10. The small intestine nervous system develops from week 9 with peristalsis able to commence in week 13. The Peyer's patches are specialist epithelial cells, developed from lymphoid cells, which form from endoderm tissue. They provide the intestinal immune system. These appear and develop between weeks 15 and 20. The longitudinal and circular muscles of the small intestine, important for propulsion and segmentation, develop between weeks 6 and 8.

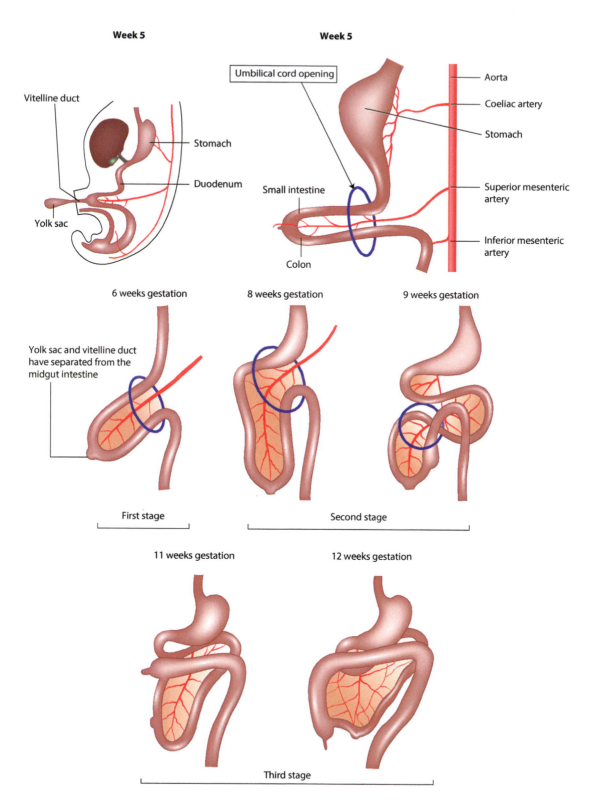

Figure 5.1 Growth and development of the small intestine.

POSTNATAL DEVELOPMENT AND THE ADULT SMALL INTESTINE

Gross anatomy and function

The length of the small intestine in neonates is approximately 200–250 cm. Proportionally, the length of an infant's intestine is greater than that of an adult. The total length of the small and large intestine combined in an infant is six times that of the length of the infant's body. The intestine will experience different rates of growth towards adulthood and these phases of growth are associated with both physiological and dietary changes. Accelerated growth is experienced between 1 and 3 years of age and during adolescence (10–15 years of age). The length of the small intestine in children and adults will be variable.

The small intestine is the longest part of the digestive tract stretching from the pyloric sphincter to the ileocaecal valve where it joins the large intestine (Figure 5.2). The jejunum and ileum are suspended within the abdominal cavity by an extension of the peritoneum called the mesentery which carries blood and nerves to and from this area. The small intestine consists of three sections: duodenum, jejunum and ileum. The duodenum is the shortest section with a length of only 25 cm. It is C-shaped, curving around the head of the pancreas. The duodenum does not produce any digestive enzymes but it does receive enzymes and buffers from the pancreas and bile which is a solution made in the liver and stored in the gallbladder which facilitates the digestion of lipids. These secretions enter into the duodenum via the hepatopancreatic ampulla. In adults the jejunum is approximately 2 meters long and it is here that the majority of digestion and absorption of nutrients takes place. The ileum is the longest section of the small intestine at a length of approximately 3.5 meters. It joins the large intestine at the ileocaecal valve. This valve controls the movement of undigested material into the large intestine.

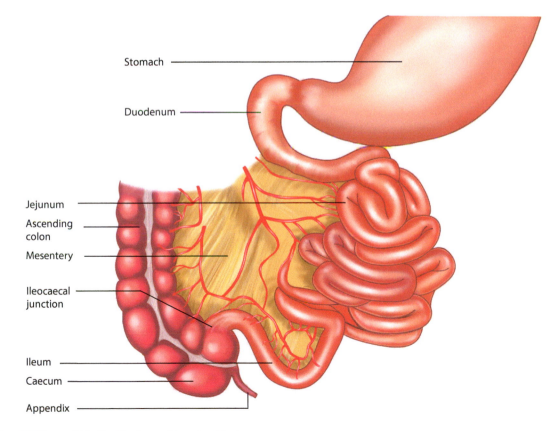

Stomach

Duodenum

Jejunum

Ascending colon

Mesentery

Ileocaecal junction

Ileum

Caecum

Appendix

Figure 5.2 The small intestine: Duodenum, jejunum and ileum.

FUNCTIONAL HISTOLOGY OF THE SMALL INTESTINE

The structure of the small intestine is similar to other regions of the digestive tract except that it has three specialist structures which are adaptions that help define its function. These are plicae, villi and microvilli (Figure 5.3). It is the combination of these structures that greatly increases the surface area for absorption of nutrients. Plicae are circular mucosal folds visible on the inner surface of the small intestine. There are approximately 800 plicae in the small intestine. The circular folds increase the surface area but also help with the mixing of the chyme. Close examination of the surface of the small intestine also reveals millions of projections called villi (finger-like projections) which are approximately 1 mm in height. The simple columnar epithelial cells that line the villi are also made up of absorptive cells that have surfaces which appear like the fibres of a brush, these are called microvilli or brush border fibres which project into the lumen further increasing the surface area for absorption.

There is considerable variation in the number and size of plicae and villi along the length of the small intestine. The number of plicae and villi in the duodenum are small because absorption of nutrients does not take place here. The case is very different in the proximal part of the jejunum because here plicae and villi are very abundant. This is no surprise because the main function of the jejunum is absorption of nutrients. As the small intestine progresses from the jejunum to the ileocaecal valve, less and less nutrients will be available for absorption so the number and size of the plicae and villi will diminish. There are no plicae in the distal section of the ileum.

The single layer of columnar epithelial cells that line the lumen of the small intestine provide a number of essential functions which include assisting in the digestion and absorption of nutrients from the lumen, regulation of water and electrolyte transport and protection against microorganisms within the lumen. The epithelial lining of the small intestine is made up of a diverse range of specialist cells. Stem cells divide to form two types of cell. One of the cells will remain to replenish the stem cell population and the second proliferates and differentiates into one of the four types of epithelial cell (columnar enterocyte cells, enteroendocrine cells, goblet cells and Paneth

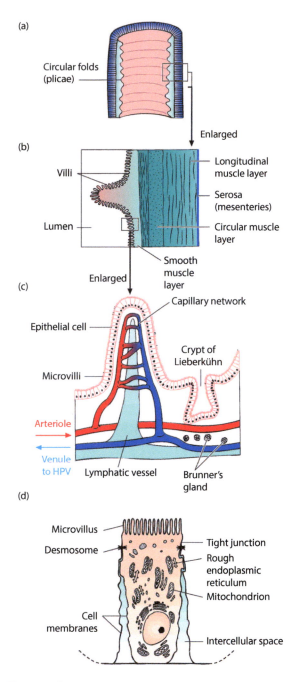

Figure 5.3 Vill. (a) Longitudinal section of duodenum showing circular folds; (b) vertical section through one circular fold; (c) vertical section through one villus; and (d) enlarged intestinal cell.

cells (Figure 5.4). An understanding of the structure and function of these cells is required to understand how the small intestine completes the processes of digestion and absorption of nutrients.

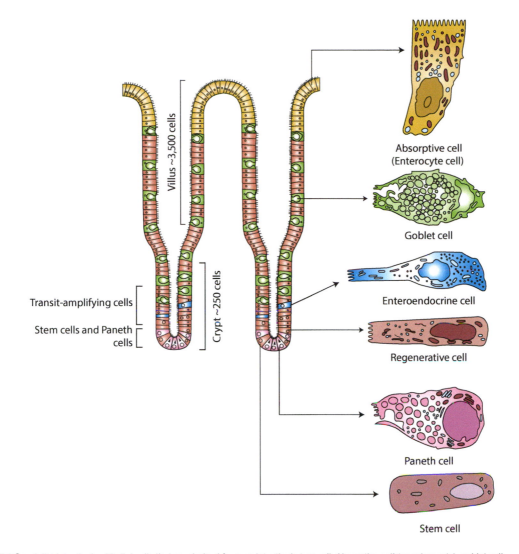

Figure 5.4 Specialist intestinal epithelial cells that are derived from an intestinal stem cell: Absorptive cell (or enterocyte), goblet cell, enteroendocrine cell and Paneth cell.

Goblet cells secrete mucous and are abundant in the crypts of Lieberkühn. Crypts are intestinal glands which can be described as invaginations between the villi. The mucous provides protection against chemical damage from enzymes and mechanical damage caused by friction as chyme moves through the lumen. The enterocytes are involved in both digestion and absorption. Their surfaces are covered with microvilli which play a major role in increasing the surface area. These microvilli form what is often termed a 'brush border' of hair-like fibres. Attached to these are a number of important enzymes which enter into the lumen of the small intestine. These enzymes perform a vital function

of breaking down food material that comes into contact with the brush border. Once these materials are broken down they are then absorbed by the enterocytes. As enterocytes are shed from the villi into the lumen they disintegrate and release their enzymes into the lumen. Within the intestinal glands are enteroendocrine cells which produce intestinal hormones which are released into the lamina propria and diffuse into the capillary blood vessels. These play a role in the coordination of digestive activities, and important ones include gastrin, cholecystokinin (CCK) and secretin. Figure 5.5 provides an overview of regulation of pancreatic and hepatobiliary secretions showing hormonal pathways.

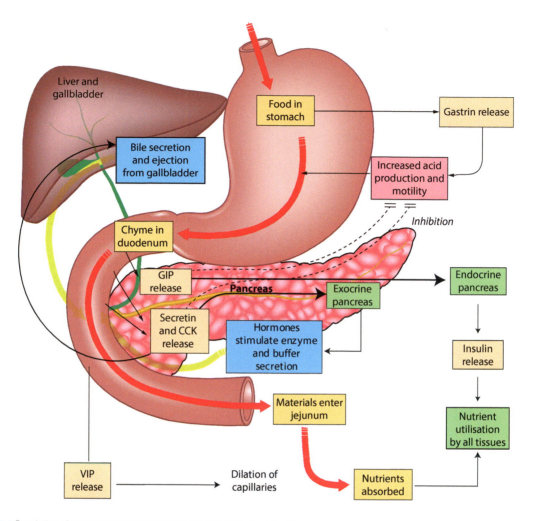

Figure 5.5 Regulation of pancreatic and hepatobiliary secretions: Hormonal pathways.

The crypts of Lieberkühn or intestinal glands extend deep into the lamina propria. The main function of the epithelial cells that line these glands is secretion. At the base of the crypts are the stem cells which are responsible for producing new epithelial cells (Figure 5.4). These stem cells divide to form daughter cells. One daughter cell from each stem cell division is retained as a stem cell. The other stem cells differentiate to form either an enterocyte, enteroendocrine, goblet or Paneth cells which then migrate along the villi towards the tip of the epithelial surface where they are eventually shed into the lumen of the intestine. Once enterocyte epithelial cells are shed they break down and release their intracellular and brush border enzymes into the lumen of the intestine.

The intestinal epithelial lining also acts as a barrier to invasion by microorganisms. It is made up of highly adapted intestinal epithelial cells which are covered with mucus and bactericidal peptides and these cells are also interconnected with tight junctions. This barrier only permits very small numbers of bacteria to penetrate the intestinal epithelium. Paneth cells play a very important role here and their role in digestive defence is explained later. Another type of tissue found in the small intestine that plays a role in intestinal defence is the Peyer's patch. Peyer's patches are collections of lymphoid tissue which can be found in the jejunum but are in much higher concentration towards the end of the ileum. The patches help prevent the invasion of bacteria into the blood supply from the small intestine lumen.

Underneath the intestinal epithelial cells, within each villus, is the lamina propria which contains a network of capillaries and a lymphatic vessel or central lacteal. The nutrients from the lumen of the small intestine move across the epithelium and then diffuse into the capillary network and are transported via the hepatic portal vein to the liver for distribution around systemic circulation. The lacteal (lymph vessel) is responsible for transporting chylomicrons, protein-lipid molecules which are too large to diffuse into the capillaries.

Digestion and absorption of the nutrients is further enhanced by contraction of the muscularis mucosa and the smooth muscles of the muscularis externa whose contractions cause the villi to move backwards and forwards (see section on 'Digestion and absorption of nutrients in the small intestine in adults').

DIGESTIVE DEFENCE

A very important function of the mucosa, which lines the digestive tract, is to provide protection against potential pathogens, harmful toxins and physical injury. The protection is called the digestive barrier. There are two parts to this barrier: intrinsic and extrinsic.

The intrinsic barrier consists of tightly packed epithelial cells which provide a protective wall. Maintenance of this wall is essential because once toxins or pathogens have breached the wall they have free access to the circulatory system allowing them to penetrate all the cells, tissues and organs of the body. There are a number of factors that can lead to a break in the integrity of this wall allowing pathogens and toxins to enter the body, and these include ulcers, inflammatory bowel disease, medications such as aspirin and factors that cause ischaemic damage (sepsis, shock, volvulus, thromboembolism).

Unlike parietal and chief cells in the gastric mucosa, which have plasma membranes resistant to acid erosion, most intestinal epithelial cells are vulnerable to damage from acids. Mucus, part of the extrinsic barrier, provides a level of protection, but as part of the intrinsic barrier the digestive tract relies upon a fast turnover of cells. There are a number of specialised cells that populate the digestive epithelium which are derived from stem cells and these include absorptive enterocytes, mucus-secreting goblet cells,

enteroendocrine cells and Paneth cells. These cells emerge from the stem cells in the base of the intestinal crypts and, apart from Paneth cells, migrate and mature along the epithelium replacing the worn out cells (Figure 5.4). The majority of these cells only live a few days (3–6 days). This rapid turnover ensures that damaged or destroyed epithelial cells are rapidly replaced ensuring maintenance of the gastric barrier.

The extrinsic barrier is contributed to by mucus, bicarbonate, antibiotic peptides and antibodies, hormones, cytokines and prostaglandins.

Mucous cells cover the whole of the digestive tract with mucus. This mucous is synthesised by cells that make up part of the epithelium. Mucous cells are the most abundant secretory cells of the gastric epithelium. They cover the whole of the surface of the stomach and extend down into the gastric glands where 'neck cells' also produce mucous. Mucous cells found throughout the digestive tract produce a bicarbonate-rich mucous that lubricates and protects the epithelium from acids and enzymes and other noxious substances. The carbohydrates on mucin molecules also bind to bacteria which help to prevent epithelial colonisation. Mucous is made up of mucin (protein) and glycoproteins which adheres to the mucosa. Gastric and duodenal epithelial cells also secrete bicarbonate which helps to neutralise acids and maintain a more neutral pH so that enzymes can function.

There are a number of intestinal cells that have innate, non-specific, immune cell activities that are designed to prevent bacteria from leaving the lumen of the intestine, crossing the epithelium and getting into the circulation. These include macrophages, neutrophils and eosinophils that provide a phagocytic function as well as being effector cells. Effector cells are relatively short-lived activated cells that defend the body in an immune response. The phagocytic cells engulf and destroy invading bacteria. Effector cells are stimulated by bacteria to secrete proinflammatory cytokines. Cytokines are produced by activated immune cells and are involved in increasing inflammatory reactions. Dendritic cells are antigen-presenting cells (APCs) and effector cells. APCs process and present antigens and this activates the production of T lymphocytes. Intestinal dendritic cells engulf antigen in either the lamina propria or Peyer's patch and then migrate to the mesenteric lymph node where they interact with naïve T cells and the T cells become sensitised to that particular antigen. Mast cells and natural killer cells are effector cells. Another important group of cells important for intestinal immunity are the Paneth cells. After enterocytes, goblet cells and columnar cells, Paneth cells represent the fourth type of epithelial cell in the small intestine and emerge during the 12th week of gestation. Once developed from the stem cell, Paneth cells migrate to the crypt base and, unlike the other types of epithelial cells the majority of which only live a few days (3–6 days), they have a lifespan of approximately 20 days. Paneth cells are specialised epithelial cells at the base of the crypts and in a healthy individual they are confined to the small intestine. They secrete bacteriocidal peptides, or defensins which have an antimicrobial activity against a number of potential pathogens (gram-positive and gram-negative types of bacteria). Paneth cells also secrete lysozyme and phospholipidase which provides Paneth cells with another line of attack against bacteria, fungi and viruses. These antimicrobial products act on the membranes of microorganisms limiting bacterial growth. Paneth cells contribute to the innate immunity of the small intestine. They also play an important role protecting the stem cells in the crypts (Ayabe et al., 2000). Paneth cells can also be found in the colon of individuals suffering from inflammatory bowel disease. The chronic inflammation associated with the disease causes metaplasia of colonic epithelial cells and Paneth cells develop to help protect the epithelium from bacterial invasion (Cunliffe et al., 2001).

The epithelial plasma cells also contribute to the digestive immune system by producing immunoglobulin A (IgA). This antibody is released into the digestive lumen where it covers much of the epithelium. The luminal IgA only binds to bacteria and other antigens that it has previously been exposed to and is therefore part of the specific immune response.

Prostaglandins are produced within the mucosa and their presence stimulates the production of mucosal mucus and bicarbonate and increases mucosal blood flow. Research has shown that aspirin and other nonsteroidal anti-inflammatory drugs inhibit prostaglandin synthesis and therefore suppress mucous and bicarbonate secretion. This would explain why these drugs have been linked to the development of some ulcers. Epidermal growth factor (EGF) and transforming growth factor-alpha (TGF-alpha) are two peptides believed to play a role in the digestive barrier.

TGF-alpha is secreted by gastric epithelial cells and EGF is secreted from duodenal glands and within saliva. Both these peptides stimulate increased mitosis (cell proliferation) of digestive epithelial cells and also the production of gastric mucous. Other peptides that play an important role in digestive protection are trefoil proteins. These are secreted by goblet cells in the gastric and intestinal mucosa and coat epithelial cells providing resistance to proteolytic effect of enzymes which would otherwise cause destruction of the epithelial cells. It is also believed that trefoil play an important role in tissue repair and protect epithelial cells from toxic substances.

Changes associated with different stages of the lifespan

Peptic ulcer

Peptic ulcer disease can be defined as the loss of protective cells from the gastric (gastric ulcer) or duodenal lining (duodenal ulcer). Peptic ulcer disease is classified in two ways: primary or secondary. Primary or idiopathic peptic ulcer disease occurs where there is no identifiable cause. Secondary peptic ulcer disease is associated with disorders which are known to contribute to ulcer formation. Peptic ulcer disease can be attributed to both genetic and environmental factors and they are a problem in both adults and children and can occur at any age. As discussed in Chapter 4 there is evidence to show a strong association between *Helicobacter pylori*, gastritis and peptic ulcer development.

The pathogenesis of peptic ulcer disease is believed to be an imbalance between mechanisms designed to protect the digestive lining, such as mucous production, bicarbonate production (neutralise acids) and high rate of epithelial cell replacement and other mechanisms in place to assist chemical digestion, including acid, pepsin and bile salt production. If the balance between these mechanisms is disrupted by cellular dysfunction (e.g. overstimulation of the secretory mechanism – dyspepsia), disease (e.g. *H. pylori*) or the introduction of toxic substances into the digestive tract (such as alcohol, medications) then ulcers can form. Once the defensive barrier is removed the specialist cells of the gastric mucosa are exposed to the corrosive action of acids and enzymes.

Stress

Stress can have an impact on the digestive system through a number of different pathways which include hormones, cytokines and neurotransmitters. However the general effect of stress can be summarised by a decrease in the blood flow to the mucosa. This restricts the access of the mucosal cells to oxygen and nutrients causing damage to the specialist cells. A diminished blood supply can reduce mucous production leading to the erosion of the mucosal barrier. This is particularly evident in the stomach and can lead to the formation of ulcers.

SECRETION IN THE SMALL INTESTINE

The secretions that enter the lumen of the small intestine come from two primary sources: mucosa and intestinal glands. An osmotic gradient caused by the hyperosmotic nutrient solution pulls water across the mucosa into the lumen. Mucous is secreted from a number of sources. The goblet cells in the mucosal epithelium secrete mucous. The duodenal glands produce large amounts of mucous when stimulated by: local reflexes, release of hormones from enteroendocrine cells and stimulation by the parasympathetic nervous system. Some of the mucous comes from the Brunner's glands which are found in the first few centimetres of the duodenum embedded in the submucosa. The remainder comes from the crypts of Lieberkühn's (intestinal glands) in the jejunum and ileum. The secretions aid digestion and absorption by lubricating chyme, neutralising acids and providing a solution within which enzymes can function and from which nutrients can be absorbed. The secretions also contain the digestive enzymes peptidases and disaccharidases which come from the disintegration of epithelial cells that are shed from the villi. These enzymes are responsible for the completion of digestion. The small intestine relies heavily upon the secretion of digestive enzymes from the pancreas and bile from the liver to complete the process of digestion so that absorption can take place. See Figure 5.6 for an overview of enzymes involved in digestion.

DIGESTION AND ABSORPTION OF NUTRIENTS IN NEONATES

In order to survive neonates need to have a functioning digestive tract so that they can absorb nutrients. Neonates need to be able to absorb the nutrients within the milk diet available after birth. Neonates

cannot generate all the digestive enzymes required for the diet consumed by adults.

In neonates the intestinal epithelium is relatively permeable, allowing for the absorption of whole carbohydrates and proteins. During the first 4 days after birth the junctions between the epithelial cells of the small intestine narrow and the process of pinocytosis responsible for allowing these large and complex molecules to be absorbed diminishes.

At birth, the concentrations of the brush border enzymes sucrase and maltase are at mature levels. Both infants and adults require brush border disaccharidases (enzymes) to break down dietary disaccharides to monosaccharides. The high activity of brush border enzymes, glucoamylase, sucrose-isomaltase and lactase, enables them to break down lactose and short-chain glucose polymers. Glucoamylase is an enzyme that breaks the bonds near the ends of complex carbohydrates (starches) releasing maltose and free glucose.

Neonates are dependent upon milk feeds and need to have in place the relevant enzymes necessary to absorb nutrients from the milk. Lactose is the most important dietary carbohydrate for neonates. Unlike adults neonates have the capacity to absorb lactose. Lactase (enzyme) activity starts early in gestation between 8 and 9 weeks and then shows a rapid rise in activity during the third trimester in preparation for birth. Weaver et al. (1986) showed that lactase activity is at 98% within 5 days of feeding. Feeding is believed to stimulate the rate of lactase production. After the first week from birth the lactase activity in the neonatal intestine starts to decline and then sucrase activity increases. Sucrase concentrations are relatively stable from birth through to adulthood.

The mechanisms for the transport of monosaccharides across enterocytes are the same in both neonates and adults (Figure 5.7).

Between neonates and adults there are significant differences in the way that proteins are digested and absorbed. Pepsin activity in the stomach of a newborn is low. Although brush border peptidases and pancreatic trypsins and chymotrypsins are present in the neonate, their activity only increases once weaning starts. After birth the neonate relies upon milk feeds to acquire nutrients. Digestion and absorption of milk are enhanced by the release of chymosin, also called rennin. Chymosin coagulates milk protein which has the effect of slowing its progression

(a)

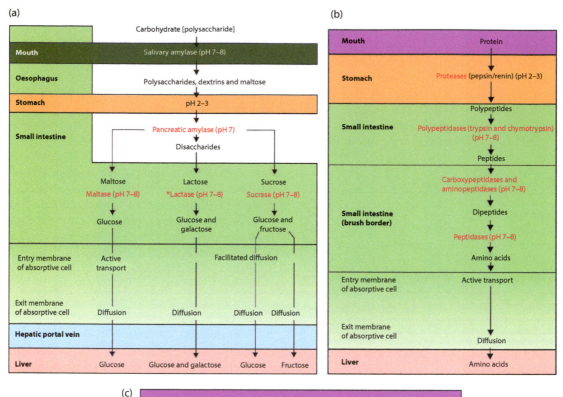

(b)

(c)

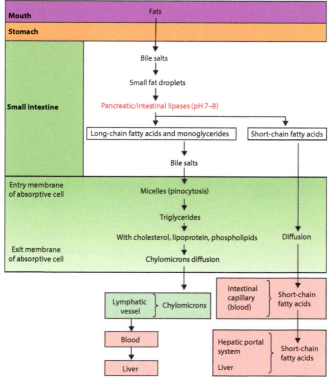

Figure 5.6 Summary of digestion and absorption. (a) Carbohydrate; (b) Protein and (c) Fat.

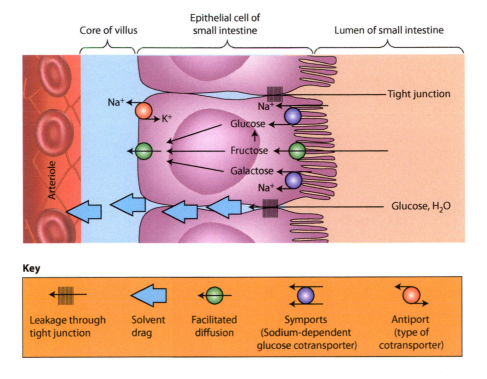

Core of villus — Epithelial cell of small intestine — Lumen of small intestine

Na+
K+
Na+
Glucose
Fructose
Galactose
Na+

Arteriole

Tight junction

Glucose, H₂O

Key

| Leakage through tight junction | Solvent drag | Facilitated diffusion | Symports (Sodium-dependent glucose cotransporter) | Antiport (type of cotransporter) |

Figure 5.7 Absorption of monosaccharides across intestinal epithelial enterocyte cells.

through the stomach providing more time for digestion. Another major difference between neonates and adults is that the neonate intestine is able to transport intact proteins across the mucosa for the first few days after birth. This is very important because it allows the newborn baby to absorb immunoglobulins in colostral milk allowing the baby to acquire passive immunity.

The ability of the small intestine to absorb water, glucose and electrolytes increases through infancy and childhood to adulthood.

DIGESTION AND ABSORPTION OF NUTRIENTS IN THE SMALL INTESTINE IN ADULTS

Absorption of water and electrolytes

For the body to survive, the mucosa of the small intestine must absorb a vast quantity of nutrients and water. A healthy adult will take in approximately 2–2.5 L of fluid a day. Added to this is the large volume of fluid, approximately 6 L, from the secretions of salivary glands, gastric juice, pancreatic juice, bile,

and intestinal juice. By the time this fluid has reached the large intestine 80% will have been absorbed. The most important process that makes absorption from the lumen across the intestinal mucosa possible is the creation of an electrochemical gradient of sodium. Enterocytes maintain a low intracellular concentration of sodium by actively pumping three sodium ions out of the cell in exchange for two. Sodium moves into the cell down a concentration gradient and water moves in association with it. By actively pumping three sodium ions out of the cell in exchange for two this creates a high osmolarity in the interstitial spaces between the enterocytes (Figure 5.8), thus creating the concentration gradient. Water then diffuses in response to the osmotic gradient established by the sodium, in this case into the interstitial space. Water as well as sodium then diffuses into the capillary blood in the villi. The net movement of water across the cell membranes always occurs by the process of osmosis. Osmosis is the movement of water across a selectively permeable membrane from an area of low concentration of dissolved molecules to an area of high concentration of dissolved molecules.

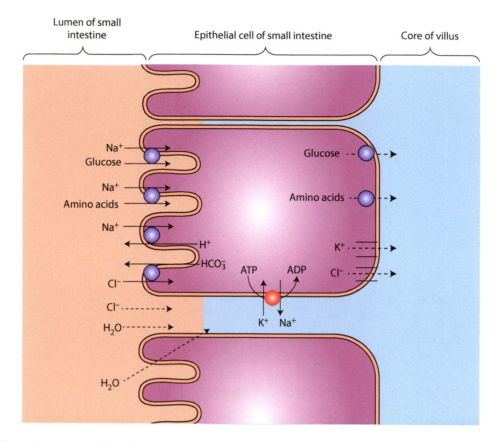

Figure 5.8 Absorption of water and electrolytes across intestinal epithelial enterocyte cells.

Absorption of monosaccharides

Polysaccharide and disaccharide molecules are too large to be absorbed across the intestinal mucosa so they must first be digested to monosaccharides. Starch, a complex carbohydrate (polysaccharide), must first be digested to maltose (disaccharide) by amylase, in pancreatic secretions, before it can be broken down further by brush border enzymes to glucose (monosaccharide). Dietary lactose, sucrose and maltose (derived from starch digestion) come into contact with the brush border enzymes of the epithelial enterocyte cells with the following effect: maltase converts maltose into glucose, lactase converts lactose into glucose and galactose and sucrase convert sucrose into glucose and fructose. These now monosaccharides can be absorbed and taken up by the enterocytes (Figure 5.7). Glucose and galactose move into the enterocyte by a process known as cotransport. Glucose and sodium ions are believed to share the same carrier molecule, which facilitates their transport across the cell membrane

of the enterocyte. As explained earlier through the process of the sodium pump the concentration of sodium ions inside the enterocyte is kept low; therefore, sodium moves into the cell down a concentration gradient and glucose moves in association with it. Sodium is then actively pumped out of the enterocyte into the interstitial spaces between the enterocytes and again glucose moves with it. Both the sodium and glucose molecules then diffuse down a concentration gradient into the capillary blood vessels. Fructose follows a similar pathway into the enterocyte; although this pathway is not influenced by sodium, it requires a different carrier molecule.

It is clear that the absorption of water and monosaccharides is dependent on absorption of solutes of which one of the most important is sodium.

Absorption of amino acids

Proteins are too large to be absorbed so they must be broken down into amino acids. An exception to this rule is found with neonates. For a few days after birth neonates have the ability to absorb intact proteins. This is very important because it allows the new-born baby to absorb immunoglobulins in colostral milk allowing the baby to acquire passive immunity. The process of protein digestion begins in the stomach where pepsinogen, produced by the chief cells, is converted to pepsin. Protein digestion then continues in the small intestine where the duodenum receives pancreatic juice containing the enzymes: trypsin, chymotrypsin and carboxypeptidases. The action of these enzymes breaks down proteins to peptides. The brush borders of the small intestine enterocyte cells have a range of peptidases. These are membrane proteins that further break down the peptides to amino acids. These are then ready for absorption across the enterocyte membrane (Figure 5.9).

The mechanism for the absorption of amino acids is the same as has been described for monosaccharides, that of cotransport. Therefore like monosaccharides amino acid absorption is dependent upon absorption of sodium. Like monosaccharides, once the amino acids have entered the enterocyte they move passively into the capillary blood supply of the villus and are then transported to the hepatic portal vein.

Absorption of fats

The digestion of lipids is more complex than that of proteins or carbohydrates. The majority of lipid that comes from a dietary source is called neutral fat or triglyceride. For lipids to be absorbed two processes need to take place: emulsification and enzyme action. Digestion of lipids begins in the mouth and then continues in the stomach under the action of

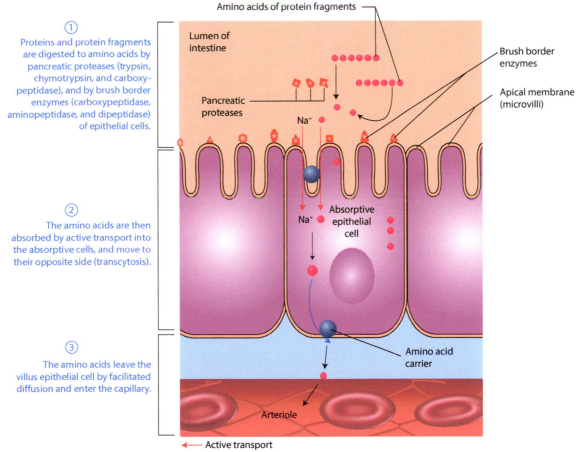

① Proteins and protein fragments are digested to amino acids by pancreatic proteases (trypsin, chymotrypsin, and carboxy-peptidase), and by brush border enzymes (carboxypeptidase, aminopeptidase, and dipeptidase) of epithelial cells.

② The amino acids are then absorbed by active transport into the absorptive cells, and move to their opposite side (transcytosis).

③ The amino acids leave the villus epithelial cell by facilitated diffusion and enter the capillary.

Amino acids of protein fragments

Lumen of intestine

Brush border enzymes

Apical membrane (microvilli)

Pancreatic proteases

Na^+

Na^+

Absorptive epithelial cell

Amino acid carrier

Arteriole

← Active transport

← Passive transport

Figure 5.9 Absorption of amino acids across intestinal epithelial enterocyte cells.

lipases (lipid-digesting enzymes). The bulk of lipid digestion occurs in the small intestine. To assist the process of lipid digestion, bile from the liver, which is stored in the gallbladder, emulsifies lipids. Dietary lipid is insoluble and so must be broken down, and it is this breaking down of the lipid and then holding it in suspension that is called emulsification. This process creates droplets of lipid, therefore increasing the surface area across which lipases can work to liberate the fatty acids. Pancreatic lipase is the main enzyme that causes hydrolysis of triglyceride into monoglyceride and free fatty acids. Lipase is a water-soluble enzyme; therefore, without emulsification lipid digestion would be very difficult. Stable compounds called micelles are formed. These are small round globules consisting of long-chain fatty acids, monoglycerides (a glycerol molecule attached to a single fatty acid) and bile salts. The micelles are absorbed through the enterocytes of the intestinal mucosa (Figure 5.10). The products of lipid digestion, fatty acids and monoglycerides enter the enterocyte by the process of simple diffusion. Once inside the enterocyte, fatty acids and monoglyceride are transported into the endoplasmic reticulum where they are used to manufacture triglyceride. The triglyceride then moves on to the Golgi apparatus where the process continues and the triglyceride is packaged with cholesterol, lipoproteins and other lipids creating compounds called chylomicrons. These chylomicrons, packaged within vesicles, then move to, and fuse with, the plasma membrane. The chylomicrons are then ejected out of the enterocyte cell and enter the lymph system and then eventually blood circulation. Once in the blood circulation chylomicron is separated out into its component parts ready for use by the cells of the body.

Figure 5.11 provides an overview of transport across the intestinal epithelium.

DEVELOPMENTAL ABNORMALITIES OF THE SMALL INTESTINE

Meckel's diverticulum

Within the first two weeks of gestation the primitive yolk sac divides with the larger section forming the primitive gut and the smaller section remaining as a yolk sac close to the placenta. These two sections are connected by a tube, contained within the umbilical cord, called the vitelline duct or omphalomesenteric duct (Figure 5.12) (Malik et al., 2010). The midgut receives nutrition from the yolk sac via the vitelline duct. Under normal development the duct becomes progressively narrower and then disappears by week 6 of gestation. Anomalies occur as a consequence of a failure of the closure and absorption of the vitelline, or omphalomesenteric duct, during the development of the digestive tract (Yamamoto et al., 2003; Tan and Roberts-Thomson, 2006; Malik et al., 2010). A Meckel's diverticulum is a remnant of the vitelline duct or omphalomesenteric duct and is the most common congenital abnormality of the small intestine occurring in approximately 2% of the population (Lu et al., 2001; Malik et al., 2010). It occurs in the terminal ileum 45–90 cm proximal to the ileocaecal valve with the size of the diverticulum varying in size from 1 to 56 cm in length and from 1 to 50 cm in diameter (Malik et al., 2010). It is defined as a blind-ended, sac-like, expanded section of chord that contains all of the layers normally found in the ileum and it also has its own blood supply (Figure 5.13) (Yamamoto et al., 2003). In most cases the diverticulum contains gastric mucosa with parietal and chief cells which secrete hydrochloric acid and produce pepsin. The presence of the acid and protein-digesting enzyme causes mucosal irritation and erosion. This can lead to haemorrhage and perforation (Chan et al., 1999; Malik et al., 2010). There are a number of pathologies associated with Meckel's diverticulum which include volvulus (intestinal obstruction), intussusception, regional enteritis, herniation, diverticulitis, fistula and a number of different types of neoplasm. There are also a number of other associated malformations which include omphalocele (also called exomphalos), anorectal malformations, CNS malformations, oesophageal atresia, cardiovascular malformations and angiodysplasia (Malik et al., 2010).

Omphalocele and gastroschisis

The occurrence of a group of closely associated anomalies called omphalocele, exstrophy of cloaca, imperforate anus and spinal defects (OEIS complex) has been identified (Chen et al., 1997; Kallen et al., 2000; Keppler-Noreuil, 2002; Groner and Zeigler, 2003; Stoll et al., 2008). These anomalies are believed to occur because of a fault with the migration of mesoderm in the caudal part of the embryo that later leads to the infraumbilical mesenchyme and cloacal septum. The incidence of

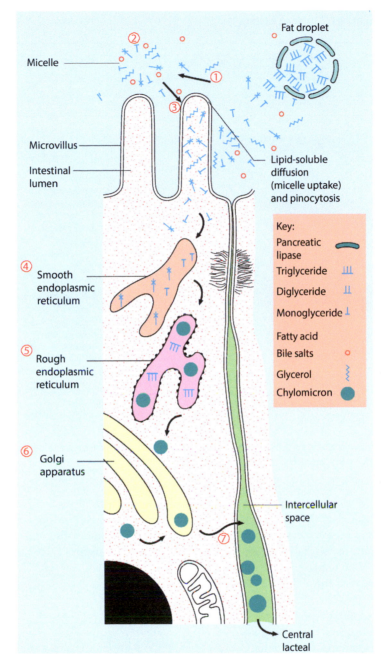

Figure 5.10 Transport of lipids from intestinal lumen through absorptive cells and into the interstitial space. Products of fat (triglyceride) digestion – monoglycerides, fatty acids and glycerol ① – form micelles ② with the bile salts in solution. They enter the absorptive cell by pinocytosis ③ across the microvillus membrane. Within the cell, the products accumulate in the smooth endoplasmic reticulum ④, from which they are passed to the rough endoplasmic reticulum ⑤. There, they are resynthesised into triglycerides and, together with a smaller amount of phospholipids and cholesterol, are stored in the Golgi complex as chylomicrons ⑥ – droplets about 150 nm in diameter. These then leave the cell ⑦.

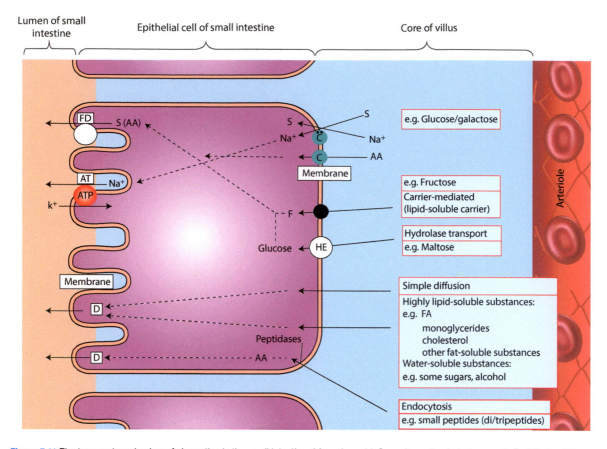

Figure 5.11 The transport mechanism of absorption in the small intestine. AA, amino acid; C, carrier molecule (cotransport); D, diffusion; FA, fatty acid; FD, facilitated diffusion; HE, hydrolysing enzyme; S, sugar, AT, active transport.

OEIS complex is reported by Smith et al. (1992) as 1 in 200,000 to 1 in 400,000 pregnancies.

A lack of mesoderm (one of the three primary germ layers) in the infraumbilical (below the umbilicus) abdominal wall results in omphalocele. With an omphalocele, intestinal loops remain in the umbilical coelom, a space external to the abdominal cavity, and are not repositioned into the abdominal cavity. The intestinal loops are covered with amnion, a thin membranous sac, and peritoneum (Figure 5.14). An omphalocele always has a sac and the umbilical cord arises from the apex of the sac. Omphalocele is associated with a number of other congenital anomalies which suggests a genetic aetiology (Kallen et al., 2000; Stoll et al., 2008). Gastroschisis is different to omphalocele because in gastroschisis there is no sac around the intestinal loops (Figure 5.15). This condition is defined as an intrauterine evisceration (removal of the viscera) of foetal intestine through a paraumbilical anterior abdominal wall defect (Kallen et al.,

2000; Stoll et al., 2008). This defect in the abdominal wall is most commonly found on the right side of the umbilicus. Gastroschisis is rarely associated with major congenital anomalies and is also not believed to have a genetic origin (Table 5.1).

CHANGES ASSOCIATED WITH DIFFERENT STAGES OF THE LIFESPAN

Intussusception

Intussusception can be defined as an invagination or telescoping of a section of one part of the intestine into the next part (Figure 5.16) (Ishida et al., 2002; Lee et al., 2002). It is most common at the junction of the small and large intestine (ileocecal valve). It can occur at any age but is most common in toddlers aged 9–12 months (incidence of 1 in 1200). It is commonly caused by a virus that leads to inflammation and swelling of the mucosa which then prolapses into

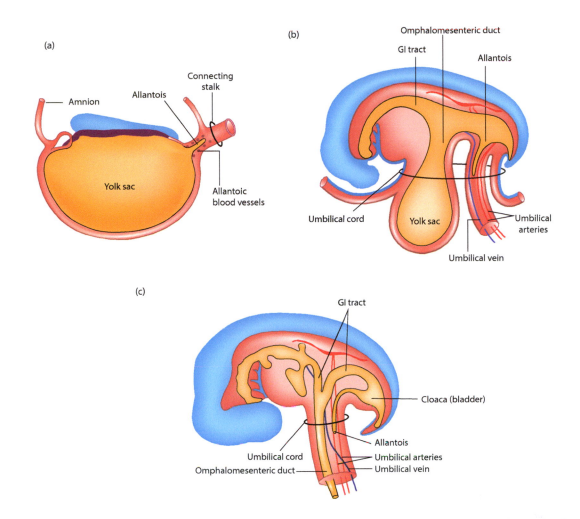

Figure 5.12 Primitive gut: Formation of the Omphalomesenteric duct. (a) **Three-week** embryo; (b) **Four-week** embryo; and (c) **Five-week** embryo.

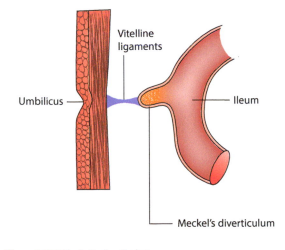

Figure 5.13 A Meckel's diverticulum.

the following section. The invagination causes an obstruction to the passage of dietary residues (Ishida et al., 2002; Lee et al., 2002). Friction caused by the epithelial membranes moving against each other can also cause inflammation, haemorrhage and in some extreme cases perforation of the intestine.

Coeliac disease (CD)

Coeliac disease, also called gluten-sensitive enteropathy, is a chronic systemic autoimmune disorder that occurs in genetically susceptible individuals following the ingestion of gluten-containing products such as wheat, barley and rye. Prolamins and glutens are proteins released during the milling process. Specific prolamins are labelled gliadins (Kumar and Clark, 2000; Fasano and Catassi, 2012; Makharia et al.,

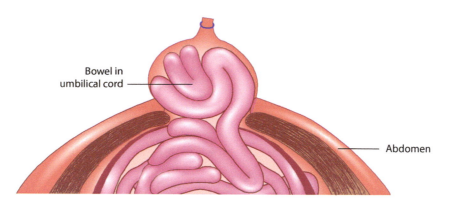

Figure 5.14 Omphalocele: Intestinal loops are covered with amnion, a thin membranous sac, and peritoneum.

2012). Coeliac disease is characterised by a specific serum autoantibody response, injury to the small intestinal mucosa. Clinical presentation of coeliac disease is also wide ranging (Fasano and Catassi, 2012).

Originally it was believed that the hypersensitivity to gluten in coeliac disease was confined only to the intestine and that all other elements of the disease were secondary to malabsorption. However it is now believed that gluten hypersensitivity affects a number of different organs, not just the intestine, and therefore coeliac disease is now classed as a systemic disease (Fasano and Catassi, 2012; Makharia et al., 2012). It is also now generally accepted that there are a wide range of gluten-associated diseases and recent classification includes: 'allergic (wheat allergy), autoimmune (coeliac disease, dermatitis herpetiformis, and gluten ataxia), and possibly immune-mediated (gluten sensitivity)' (Makharia et al., 2012).

Coeliac disease was once thought to be a childhood disease. However research in 1998 suggested that 80% of newly diagnosed individuals are adults and the average age of diagnosis was 44 years (Hin et al.,

1999). What was once thought to be a rare childhood condition affecting 1 in every 10,000 has now been shown by studies carried out in America and Europe to affect people of all ages from anywhere between 1 in 1504 to as many as 1 in 33 individuals (Not et al., 1998; Fasano et al., 2003). The disease is now found in all parts of the world affecting 0.6%–1% of the population worldwide (Fasano et al., 2003). This research also shows wide regional variations within Europe, for example reporting prevalence of 0.3% in Germany and 2.4% in Finland (Mustalahti et al., 2010). Research carried out by Ajit et al. (2006) has shown that coeliac disease is much more common in India than was previously thought with a disease prevalence of 1 in 310 individuals where wheat is a staple food. Prevalence of the disease, generally in developing countries, is also seen to be increasing, and this is believed to be associated with factors such as the adoption of a more Westernised diet and a greater awareness of the disease (Fasano and Catassi, 2012).

For coeliac disease to occur three interrelated elements need to exist: a genetic predisposition, gluten

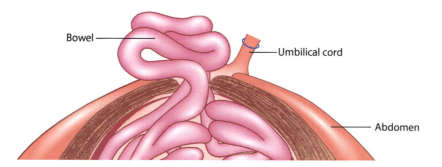

Figure 5.15 Gastroschisis: No sac present around the intestinal loops.

Table 5.1 Outlines the main differences between the two defects: Omphalocele and gastroschisis

	Omphalocele (or exomphalos)	Gastroschisis
Incidence	**1 in 5000**	**1 in 3000**
Aetiology	• Genetic cause is most likely. • Associated with a number of other anomalies. • Occurs early in development (week 10 gestation).	• Genetic cause is unlikely because there are few associated anomalies. • Most likely cause is a nutritional deficit or environmental trigger causing an isolated vascular event late in development.
Site of defect	• Intestinal loops remain in the umbilical coelom and are not repositioned into the abdominal cavity. The intestinal loops are covered with amnion and peritoneum. • Always has a sac and the umbilical cord arises from the apex of the sac.	• Intrauterine evisceration of foetal intestine through a paraumbilical anterior abdominal wall defect is present, nearly always on the right side of the umbilicus. • Never has a sac and the umbilical cord arises from normal place in abdominal wall.
Sac surrounding contents	Sac is present.	Sac is absent.
Health of intestine	• The intestine appears normal. • With a minor omphalocele there might be a small herniation into the umbilical cord (5–8 cm defect). • With a major omphalocele the liver might be exposed and the abdominal and thoracic cavities might be poorly developed.	• Intestine usually becomes shortened, thickened, dilated and is affected by adhesions due to absence of sac and exposure to amniotic fluid.
Associated anomalies	• Genitourinary abnormalities. • Chromosomal abnormalities (trisomy 13, 18 or 21). • Cardiac defect (30%–40%). • Beckwith-Wiedemann syndrome (10%). • Premature (10%).	• 60% of infants are of low birth weight.
Complications	• Volvulus • Intestinal atresia • Stenosis • Malrotation	• Poor gut motility • Volvulus • Intestinal atresia • Stenosis • Malrotation

Source: Kallen K et al. 2000. *American Journal of Medical Genetics* 92:62–68; Smith NM et al. 1992. *Journal of Medical Genetics* 29:730–732; Stoll C et al. 2008. *American Journal of Medical Genetics Part A* 146(10):1280–1285; Wilson RD, Johnson MP. 2004. *Fetal Diagnosis and Therapy* 19:385-398; Ledbetter DJ. 2006. *Surgical Clinics of North America* 86:246-260; Chen CP et al. 1997. *American Journal of Perinatology* 14:275–279; Groner JI, Zeigler MM. 2003. *Newborn Surgery*, 2nd edn. London: Arnold, pp. 629–636; Keppler-Noreuil KM. 2002. *American Journal of Medical Genetics* 107:72–76.

in the diet and an immune-mediated response. There then follows a pattern of events which can be summarised in the following stages (Figure 5.17): the appearance of coeliac antibodies, the development of intestinal enteropathy, the onset of symptoms (localised and systemic) and then the development of complications. The length of time over which these stages occur varies from weeks to decades (Fasano and Catassi, 2012). The precise mechanism of damage is not clear but it is believed that an immunogenetic mechanism is likely. Individuals with certain genetic groups will generate a stronger than usual response to gliadin. This genetic susceptibility is associated with the presence of human leukocyte antigen (HLA) alleles HLA-DQ2 or HLA-DQ8 and HLA-DQ2 found in 90% of individuals with coeliac disease (Agrawal et al., 2000; Green and Jabri, 2003; Trynka et al., 2011). When an individual with these alleles consumes food containing glutens it causes a T-cell–mediated immune response and chronic inflammation (Green and Jabri, 2003). Once in the proximal small intestine the gliadin element of gluten is absorbed into the lamina propria and binds with receptors on the T cell which results in the release of antibodies. These antibodies trigger the release of leukocytes and cytokines which then destroy the microvilli of the intestinal mucosa (Young and Thomas, 2004). The existence of anti-gliadin antibodies in the blood of individuals is used as a screening mechanism for coeliac disease. Other substances screened for include immunoglobulin IgA. Blood tests also include a specific antibody test for tissue transglutaminase (Dieterich et al., 1998; Sulkanen et al.,

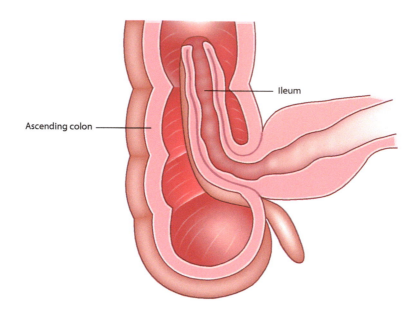

Figure 5.16 Intussusception: Infolding of the terminal ileum into the ascending colon.

1998; Fanciulii et al., 2000; McPhillips, 2000; Fasano and Catassi, 2012; Silvester and Duerksen, 2013). This was recently recognised as the main antibody involved in coeliac disease. The immune response and associated inflammation cause the mucosa to become flat in appearance as the microvilli and villi are damaged. The mucosa becomes thicker as crypt hyperplasia occurs (increased production and growth of the crypt cells). This will also interfere with absorption. Damage or destruction of the microvilli and brush border disrupts the action of brush border enzymes and the absorption of nutrients. This leads to a number of malabsorption problems which become progressively worse unless gluten is removed from the diet.

Coeliac disease can present in different ways at different stages of the lifespan. Presentation in adults can be non-specific and therefore can be confused with other digestive complaints such as ulcerative colitis and Crohn's disease. This makes diagnosis difficult and therefore leads to problems establishing prevalence. Presentation in infants normally occurs between the ages of 6 and 12 months. These infants present with anorexia, abdominal distention, diarrhoea, failure to thrive, offensive stool and muscle wasting (Green and Jabri, 2003). The symptoms that cause the parents to take the infant to their GP are closely associated with the infant being introduced to cereal products in their diet (Fasano et al., 2003).

Older children and adults present with symptoms unrelated to the digestive tract, older children presenting with problems such as failure to thrive, anaemia and neurological problems (Green and Jabri, 2003). Adults present with rheumatoid arthritis, dermatitis, chronic hepatitis, iron deficiency anaemia, neurological dysfunction, osteoporosis, stunted growth and reproductive problems (Xola et al., 1995; Shaker et al., 1997; Hin et al., 1999; McPhillips, 2000; Fasano and Catassi, 2001; Kong, 2003).

Crohn's disease

Crohn's disease is a chronic autoimmune inflammatory bowel disorder that appears to be caused by a defective immune response to intestinal flora in genetically susceptible hosts which involves both the innate, non-specific, and the acquired specific immune response (Sartor, 1994, 1997, 1999, 2001; Bouma and Strober, 2003).

Prevalence of Crohn's disease has been reported at 5–10 people per 100,000 (Carter et al., 2004) and it is believed to be steadily increasing. In 2006 Rampton and Shanahan (2006) reported the prevalence of Crohn's disease at 1 in 1000 people in Europe and the United States and in 2008 they reported the prevalence at 1 in 250 people (Rampton and Shanahan, 2008). The disease affects people at all stages of the lifespan but is most common in the age range 10–40

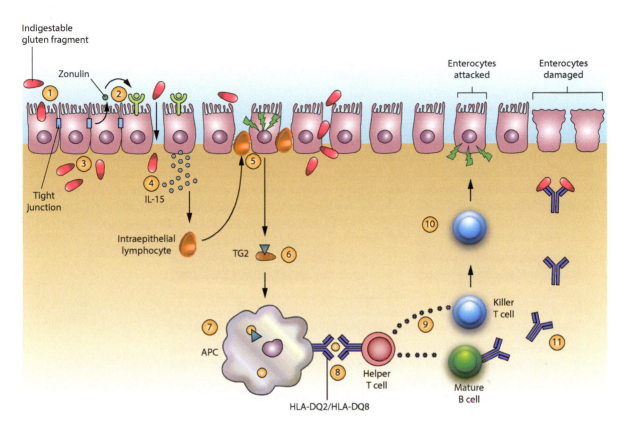

Figure 5.17 Coeliac disease: Immune response. (1) Indigestable fragment of gluten taken up by enterocyte; (2) Gluten stimulates enterocyte to release zonulin causing tight junctions to open up; (3) Gluten passes between enterocytes; (4) Gluten stimulates enterocytes to secrete interleukin-15 (1L-15) which activates intraepithelial lymphocytes (immune cells); (5) Areas of damage; (6) Damaged enterocytes release tissue transglutaminase (TTG), an enzyme which modifies the gluten; (7) Modified gluten taken up by antigen presenting cell (APC); (8) APC joins the modified gluten to HLA molecules and display the resulting complexes to Helper T cells; (9) Helper T cells that recognise the complexes secrete molecules that attract the immune cells that attack enterocytes; (10) Killer T cells attack enterocytes; (11) B cells release antibodies that target gluten causing further damage.

years (Carter et al., 2004; Rampton and Shanahan, 2008). The disease can affect any part of the digestive tract from the mouth to the anus. The area most often affected is the terminal ileum and the ileocaecal region (Jewell, 1998). Pathogenesis of Crohn's disease can be attributed to three interrelated factors: genetic, environmental and immunological.

Genetic factors

Family studies and epidemiological studies into monozygotic and dizygotic twins have shown that genetics has a very clear role to play in the development of inflammatory bowel disease (IBD) (Tysk et al., 1991). Studies by Satsangi et al. (1994) and Probert et al. (1993) showed that for individuals with Crohn's disease there was an increased prevalence of

IBD in relatives. A study carried out by Bennett et al. (1991) found that 12 out of 33 children born to parents where Crohn's disease was present were affected by the disease. A number of studies have confirmed the involvement of the *CARD15/NOD2* gene in the aetiology of Crohn's disease (Annese et al., 2003; Bairead et al., 2003; Cavanaugh et al., 2003; Rogler, 2004). Mutations on the *CARD15* gene on chromosome 16 are believed to be associated with 20%–30% of cases of Crohn's disease. However research carried out by Linde et al. (2003) also showed that homozygous carriers (e.g. genotype TT or tt) of the *CARD15/NOD2* mutation can be healthy, indicating that genetic factors are not the sole determinant of Crohn's disease and that environmental factors must also have an influence.

Environmental factors

One of the most important environmental triggers that seems to affect the pathophysiology of Crohn's disease is food. Sakamoto et al. (2005) and Tsujikawa et al. (2001) found that diets that contained a lot of fat and sugar accelerated the onset of Crohn's disease. A number of studies have also suggested that intestinal flora play a key role in triggering the onset of inflammation. It is believed that the adherence and invasion of pathogenic *Escherichia coli* (*E. coli*) into the intestinal mucosa brings on the development of the disease (Fellermann et al., 2003). Under normal circumstances the body's innate defence mechanisms would prevent bacteria crossing into the intestinal mucosa. However Fellermann et al. (2003) believes that the mutated and defective *CARD15/NOD2* gene identified earlier could lead to a breakdown in the body's innate defence responses leading to the invasion of bacteria into intestinal mucosa, bringing about an inflammatory response.

Immunological abnormalities

Genetics and environmental factors are believed to be initiating factors for Crohn's disease although the exact aetiology is unknown. What is understood is that in some way regulation of mucosal immunity malfunctions leads to a prolonged inflammatory response in the gut (Figures 5.18 and 5.19) (Sartor,

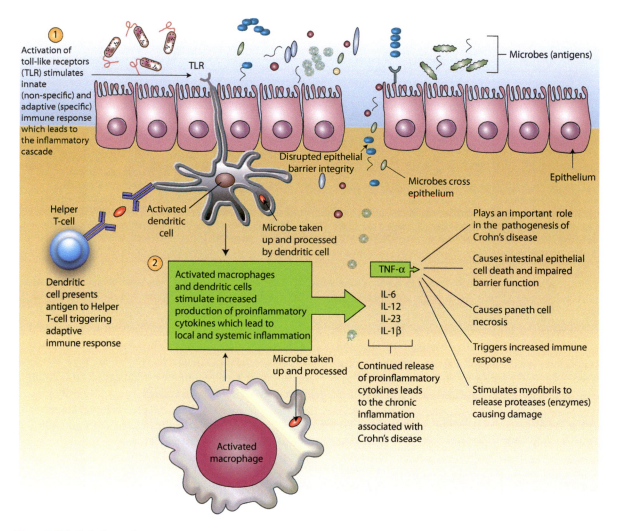

Figure 5.18 Crohn's disease: Immune response.

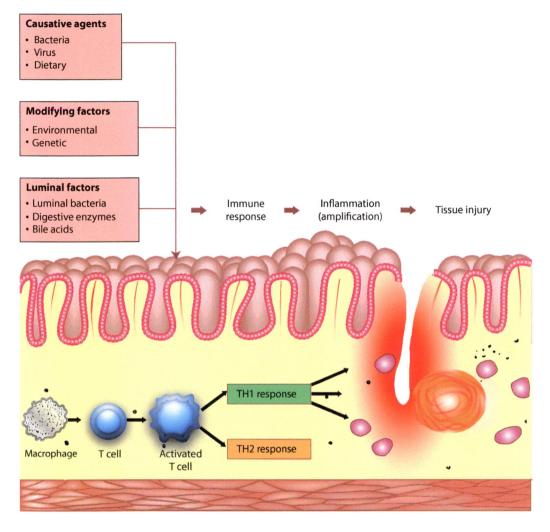

Figure 5.19 Crohn's disease: Tissue injury.

1994, 1999, 2001; MacDonald et al., 2000; Bouma and Strober, 2003). An overly aggressive cell-mediated response to intestinal flora is believed to be the main cause of the chronic inflammation seen in patients with Crohn's disease. However the cells providing the innate immune response are also believed to play an important role in the pathogenesis of the disease. Intestinal flora lie at the boundary between the intestinal lumen and the systemic circulation and will take the opportunity to invade and cause infection if the mucosa is damaged. When such an invasion occurs the normal response is inflammation. According to Sands (2007) the key factor that differentiates individuals with Crohn's from normal individuals is the inability to regulate the inflammatory state and return it to a condition of normal controlled intestinal inflammation. Individuals with Crohn's disease will develop uncontrolled and chronic inflammation as the body fails to shut down the inflammatory response.

SUMMARY OF KEY POINTS

The small intestine

1. Receives acid chyme from the stomach
2. Place where digestion is completed and absorption occurs on the villi which line the surface of the small intestine
3. Is divided up into three regions: duodenum, jejunum, ileum.

The duodenum

1. Starts at the pyloric sphincter and then connects with the jejunum, the C shape surrounds the head region of the pancreas
2. Connects with the sphincter of Oddi (or hepatopancreatic sphincter) which controls the movement of pancreatic juice and bile into the duodenum
3. The duodenal epithelial cells show variation from the rest of the digestive tract:
   i. The submucosa contains Brunner's glands which secrete alkaline mucous which neutralises the acid-rich chyme from the stomach.
   ii. The mucosa of the proximal portion of the duodenum has very few plicae and villi but towards the distal end of the duodenum the numbers of plicae and villi significantly increase.

The jejunum

1. Has large numbers of plicae circularis and villi designed to maximise the surface area to assist with digestion and absorption
2. Has intestinal crypts (crypts of Lieberkühn) which are deep invaginations of the lamina propria that contain many different cell types:
   i. Goblet cells producing mucous
   ii. Enterocytes (epithelial cells) releasing membranous enzymes that complete digestion: aminopeptidases break down peptides to amino acids, disaccharidases (includes maltase, sucrase, lactase) break down disaccharides to monosaccharides, for example maltose to glucose
   iii. Enteroendocrine cells producing hormones such as cholecystokinin and secretin

iv. Paneth cells secreting defensins that disrupt microbial cells membranes
v. Stem cells located at the base of crypt producing the specialist epithelial cells
vi. Worn out enterocyte epithelial cells bring to the surface enzymes, for example enterokinase, an enzyme that activates pancreatic enzymes

Ileum

1. Very few plicae or villi, but otherwise the structure is virtually the same.
2. Most of the nutrients have been absorbed.
3. Concentrations of lymphoid nodules, also referred to as Peyer's patches, are found in the submucosa, especially at the distal end of the ileum.

Absorption in the small intestine

1. Absorption into enterocytes is by cotransport for glucose and amino acids; facilitated diffusion for fructose; simple diffusion for glycerol, fatty acids, cholesterol and fat-soluble vitamins.
2. Electrolytes such as Na, K, Cl and HCO_3 are absorbed which create an osmotic gradient that facilitates the absorption of water.
3. Movement in the small intestine: There are two types:
   i. Segmentation: localised contractions of the circular muscle that mixes the chyme. Contractions are rapid in the duodenum (approximately 12/min) and then become slower in the ileum (approximately 8/min).
   ii. Mass movement is a term given to describe powerful peristaltic contractions that occur in the small and large intestines. They occur three or four times a day, usually coinciding with meal times. After a meal, distension of the stomach and the duodenum brings about duodenal colic reflexes, coordinated by nerve plexuses; these reflexes bring about a significant increase in intestinal activity and movement along the small intestine.

CHECK ON LEARNING

Small intestine

Where are the stem cells found that replace worn out intestinal epithelial cells?
Answer – They are found in intestinal crypts.

What is the function of intrinsic factor?
Answer – It binds with vitamin B_{12} and facilitates the absorption of B_{12} at the terminal ileum.

What effect does the hormone secretin have on the stomach?

Answer – Secretin inhibits gastrin release so it stops acid and enzyme secretion and stops mixing waves of the stomach.

Other than secretin name two other hormones released by enteroendocrine cells that line the duodenum.
Answer – Two other hormones are cholecystokinin (CCK) and gastric inhibitory peptide.

What three structures increase the surface area of the small intestine to maximise the absorption potential of nutrients?

(Continued)

Answer – They are plicae circularis, villi and microvilli.

How does the structure of the intestinal epithelium enhance the function of the intestine?
Answer – The epithelium of the intestine consists of columnar epithelium made up of a single layer of cells which aids secretion and absorption of nutrients.

What would be the effect of the arrival of chyme in the duodenum that was rich in fat?
Answer – Cholecystokinin is released from the enteroendocrine cells into circulation and is transported via the circulatory system to the gallbladder where it stimulates the release of bile into the duodenum to emulsify the fats.

There are specialised sites in the ileum that produce leukocytes designed to help protect the body from harmful pathogens. What are these specialised sites called?

Answer – They are called Peyer's patches which are lymphoid nodules.

What is the function of the ileocaecal valve?
Answer – The ileocaecal valve is made up of circular smooth muscle and regulates the passage of chyme from the ileum to the large intestine.

Why do mucous glands in the submucosa of the duodenum produce alkaline mucous?
Answer – They do so to neutralise the acid chyme. Intestinal enzymes cannot work in an acid environment.

In which section of the small intestine does the majority of absorption occur?
Answer – It occurs in the jejunum.

CASE STUDY

Coeliac Disease
Sarah is 16 years old referred by her GP to gastroenterology out-patients department complaining of weight loss, chronic fatigue, needing to eat every 2–3 hours and loose stools and flatulence and abdominal bloating. Allergy testing demonstrated a severe allergy to gluten. Blood results showed anaemia.

Explanation of normal and altered physiology
The following table sets out the normal and altered anatomy and physiology which explains the person's problems.

Normal anatomy/physiology	Altered anatomy/physiology and related problems
The epithelial lining of the small intestine is made up of columnar epithelial cells.	*What type of disorder is coeliac disease?* Coeliac disease is a chronic systemic autoimmune disorder. It is an inherited genetic disorder that causes dysfunction of the immune system where exposure to certain antigens (in this case glutens) produces antibodies (autoantibodies) that attack and destroy the body's own epithelial cells (in this case the small intestine).
How does this cell structure, as opposed to stratified squamous epithelium, enhance the function of the intestine? Columnar epithelium is made up of a single layer of cells which aids secretion and absorption of nutrients.	
How do Peyer's patches in the small intestine help protect the body? Peyer's patches are specialised sites of lymphoid nodules in the ileum that produce leukocytes designed to help protect the body from harmful pathogens.	
What are sources of vitamin B_{12}? Dietary vitamin B_{12} is released from ingested proteins in the stomach through the action of pepsin and acid.	*What three interrelated factors need to exist for coeliac disease to occur?* 1. A genetic predisposition 2. Gluten in the diet 3. An immune-mediated response
What function does vitamin B_{12} perform? Vitamin B_{12} is required for the maturation of erythrocytes and deficiency leads to anaemia. It is also required for the healthy functioning of nerve fibres.	

(Continued)

What structures of the small intestine increase the surface area for absorption?
Plicae circularis, villi and microvilli.

The epithelial lining of the small intestine is covered in enterocytes.

What is their role in the completion of chemical digestion and absorption?
Enterocytes (epithelial cells) release membranous enzymes that complete digestion: aminopeptidases break down peptides to amino acids, disaccharidases (includes maltase, sucrase, lactase) break down disaccharides to monosaccharides, for example maltose to glucose.

What role do the parietal cells play in facilitating the absorption of vitamin B_{12}?
Intrinsic factor is produced by the parietal cells. It is a glycoprotein that binds to vitamin B_{12} in the terminal ileum of the small intestine. This binding forms a complex which binds with receptors on the ileal wall allowing transfer of vitamin B_{12} across the ileal wall into the blood.

Describe the process by which water and electrolytes move across the epithelial membrane.
Movement occurs because of the generation of an electrochemical gradient of sodium. Enterocytes maintain a low intracellular concentration of sodium by actively pumping three sodium ions out of the cell in exchange for two. This creates a high osmolarity in the interstitial spaces between the enterocytes, thus creating a concentration gradient. Water then diffuses in response to the osmotic gradient established by the sodium into the interstitial space. Water as well as sodium then diffuses into the capillary blood in the villus.

Sarah has been diagnosed with malnutrition secondary to coeliac disease.

What is causing the malnutrition?
Inflammation caused by the immune system damages or completely destroys the villi which impairs the ability of the intestinal cells to absorb nutrients causing malabsorption and malnutrition. This would explain Sarah's weight loss and chronic fatigue.
Intestinal malabsorption can lead to deficiencies and low blood levels of protein, iron, calcium, vitamin B_{12}, folate, vitamin D and vitamin K. These deficiencies, in turn, can lead to other blood test abnormalities such as iron deficiency anaemia and prolonged prothrombin time (measures how quickly blood clots). Malabsorption can also lead to steatorrhea (excess fats in the stool).

Why might Sarah be suffering from iron deficiency anaemia?
Iron is an important component of haemoglobin in red blood cells. When iron is deficient, production of red blood cells is impaired, and anaemia develops. Iron deficiency anaemia can occur either through loss of blood (with its iron-containing red blood cells) or lack of intestinal iron absorption.

Why is Sarah at risk of osteopenia (low bone mineral density)?
Because of deficiencies of vitamin D and calcium.

Why is Sarah experiencing chronic diarrhoea?
Damage to the intestinal villi limits the absorption of nutrients and water. The nutrients and water remain in the lumen of the bowel. Accumulation of excessive dietary nutrients in the intestinal lumen can lead to an osmotic diarrhoea. Nutrients that remain in the lumen of the bowel exert an osmotic effect, retaining water in the lumen and causing an osmotic diarrhoea.

Background – initial investigations
The table below provides the rationale behind the investigations that Sarah underwent to diagnose this condition.

Investigation	Result	Rationale
Oesophago-gastro-duodenoscopy (OGD) and removal of tissue biopsies from duodenum	Confirmed damage to and destruction of intestinal villi and the presence of high numbers of lymphocytes	Inflammation caused by an immunological reaction damages the intestinal villi and increases the number of lymphocytes
Antibody tests	Antibody tests confirm the presence of abnormally high levels of antibodies specific for coeliac disease: endomysial, anti-tissue transglutaminase and anti-gliadin antibodies	In patients with coeliac disease, anti-gliadin antibody is an antibody produced against gliadin in the diet and endomysial and anti-tissue transglutaminase antibodies are antibodies produced against the body's own tissues.
Full blood count serum vitamin B_{12} Red blood cell folate (folic acid)	Low haemoglobin Low serum vitamin B_{12} Low folic acid	Anaemia – caused by iron deficiency anaemia

CLINICAL CHALLENGES

1. Discuss with your supervisor/mentor if family members should be screened for coeliac disease.
2. Discuss why Sarah might have a prolonged prothrombin time (blood test that measures how quickly blood clots).
3. Symptoms among patients with coeliac disease can vary greatly – discuss other symptoms that Sarah could experience if she continued to ingest glutens in her diet.

CASE STUDY

Crohn's Disease

Tom, a 14-year-old boy, was referred to a paediatric gastroenterologist because of recurrent episodes of abdominal pain, abdominal distension, poor appetite, fatigue, nausea, vomiting and bloody diarrhoea. Physical examination identified that height and weight for his age group was low and examination also showed there was evidence of delayed growth.

Explanation of normal and altered physiology

The following table sets out the normal and altered anatomy and physiology which explains the person's problems.

Normal anatomy/physiology	Altered anatomy/physiology and related problems
List the different mechanisms of protection for the digestive system. Acid secretions – stomach Antibacterial secretion – saliva Immunoglobulins – saliva Mucous – protective barrier Rapid turnover of cells – replace worn out cells Tightly packed epithelial cells – protective wall Non-specific (innate) phagocytes – macrophages, neutrophils, eosinophils engulf and destroy invading bacteria Specific immune response – activation of T lymphocytes by antigens that cross the epithelium Paneth cells secrete bacteriocidal peptides, or defensins which have an antimicrobial activity against a number of potential pathogens Epithelial plasma cells produce immunoglobulin A (IgA). Luminal IgA (antibody) only binds to bacteria and other antigens that it has previously been exposed to and is therefore part of the specific immune response.	*What is Crohn's disease?* Mouth to anus – An autoimmune disorder that appears to be caused by a defective immune response to intestinal flora in genetically susceptible hosts which involves both the innate, non-specific, and acquired specific immune response. It can affect all sections of the digestive tube lining from the mouth to the anus.
Glucose and amino acids move into the enterocyte by a process known as cotransport. *Describe the process for the absorption of fats in the small intestine from the intestinal lumen to the blood circulation.* Fatty acids and monoglycerides enter the enterocyte by the process of simple diffusion. They are then transported into the endoplasmic reticulum where they are used to manufacture triglyceride. The triglyceride then moves on to the Golgi apparatus where it is packaged with cholesterol, lipoproteins and other lipids-creating compounds called chylomicrons. These chylomicrons, packaged within vesicles move to, and fuse with, the plasma membrane where they are ejected out of the enterocyte cell and enter the lymph system and then eventually blood circulation.	*Why is Tom experiencing fatigue, and showing signs of malnutrition and delayed development?* The abdominal pain and diarrhoea can cause reduced food intake. Recurrent inflammation, damage and destruction of intestinal epithelial cells can lead to insufficient brush border enzymes and poor absorption of nutrients across the intestinal epithelium. Inflammation in the large intestine can reduce absorption of water and vitamins across the large intestine epithelium. The loss of protein secondary to severe inflammation and the production of inflammatory exudates can cause malnutrition. The loss of iron through mucosal haemorrhage and the loss of electrolytes through diarrhoea can lead to malnutrition. Disruption of B_{12} absorption in the terminal ileum due to epithelial cell inflammation, damage and destruction contributes to anaemia.

(Continued)

How does movement occur in the small intestine?
Segmentation – localised contractions of the circular muscle that mixes the chyme (approximately 12/min in the duodenum slowing to approximately 8/min in the ileum)
Mass movement is a term given to describe powerful peristaltic contractions that occur in the small and large intestines. They occur three or four times a day, usually coinciding with meal times. After a meal, distension of the stomach and the duodenum brings about duodenal and colic reflexes, coordinated by nerve plexuses. These reflexes bring about a significant increase in intestinal activity and movement along the small intestine.

Describe three functions of the large intestine.

1. Bacteria digest protein and produce vitamin B and K.
2. Cells of the epithelium absorb water, ions and vitamins.
3. Faeces is formed ready for defaecation.

What types of receptors are found in the mucosal lining?
Baroreceptors
Chemoreceptors
Thermal receptors
Nociceptors

Describe the structure and function of visceral and parietal peritoneum.
Structure – the abdominal (or peritoneal) cavity is lined by parietal peritoneum. The organs of the digestive system are surrounded by visceral peritoneum. Both consist of thin serous membranes made up of mesothelium which are covered by a thin fluid layer called transudate (peritoneal fluid).
Function – reduces friction between cavities and the surfaces of organs; anchors organs to body wall.

What is causing Tom's abdominal distension?
Narrowing of the intestinal lumen due to inflammation or the development of strictures can lead to obstruction of the flow of the contents through the intestine. When the intestine is obstructed chyme and gases from the stomach and the small intestine cannot pass into the colon leading to symptoms of severe abdominal cramps, nausea, vomiting and abdominal distention.

Why is Tom suffering with frequent episodes of diarrhoea?
Diarrhoea is a common clinical symptom associated with Crohn's disease. In Crohn's disease regulation of mucosal immunity malfunctions lead to a prolonged inflammatory response in the gut. Inflammatory secretions increase the volume of fluid into the intestinal lumen causing an inflammatory diarrhoea.
Destruction or damage to the epithelial cells responsible for absorbing water and nutrients can also lead to an additional fluid volume in the intestine.

What could be the causes of abdominal pain in patients suffering from Crohn's disease?
Damage or destruction of the intestinal epithelial cells can lead to the development of ulcers. These ulcers can perforate the intestinal wall and create a fistula (tunnel) between the intestine and adjacent organs and lead to the development of abdominal abscesses. These can cause symptoms of abdominal pain and pyrexia.
The abdominal pain can also be caused by the abdominal distention (see above).

What acute life-threatening complications are associated with Crohn's disease?
Perforation of the intestine
Obstruction of the intestine

Background – initial investigations

The table below provides the rationale behind the investigations that Tom underwent to diagnose this condition.

Investigation	Result	Rationale
Blood tests	Low Hb Low B_{12} and zinc Elevated platelet count Elevated white cell count Elevated erythrocyte sedimentation rates (ESR) – (norm. ESR: males <50 years is 0–15 mm/hr, females <50 years is 0–20 mm/hr) Hypoproteinaemia Low blood electrolytes	Anaemia – caused by either iron deficiency or haemorrhage Low B_{12} – caused by inflammation of the terminal ilium Low zinc – caused by losses from inflammatory exudate and diarrhoea – can cause delayed growth in children Elevated platelets – caused by inflammation Elevated WCC – caused by infection Elevated ESR – caused by inflammation Low protein and electrolytes – caused by diarrhoea

(Continued)

Barium x-ray studies	Barium x-rays confirmed ulcerations and narrowing in the small intestine	Establishes the distribution, nature, and severity of the disease
Oesophago-gastro-duodenoscopy	Detected ulcers and extensive areas of inflammation in the duodenum and jejunum	Endoscopy used to visualise changes to stomach and small intestine mucosa
Colonoscopy (more accurate than barium x-rays)	Detected small ulcers and small areas of inflammation in the colon and terminal ileum	Allows direct visualisation of the rectum, large intestine and terminal ileum to assess the degree of inflammation Allows for small tissue samples (biopsies) to be taken and sent for examination under the microscope to confirm the diagnosis of Crohn's disease
Tissue biopsy (via colonoscopy)	Biopsies of the duodenum showed blunting of the villi and chronic inflammation consistent with Crohn's disease	Allows for small tissue samples to be taken and sent for examination under the microscope to confirm the diagnosis of Crohn's disease
Computerised axial tomography (CAT or CT)	CT of abdomen showed dilated loops of small and large intestine; no abscesses or fistula detected	Allows for imaging of the entire abdomen and pelvis; useful in detecting abscesses

CLINICAL CHALLENGES

1. What are the differences between Crohn's disease and ulcerative colitis?
2. In what circumstances would surgery be used for patients with Crohn's disease?
3. What is the aim of pharmacological management of Crohn's disease?
4. What are the nutritional options available to manage Tom's malnutrition and delay in growth?

Chapter 6

THE ACCESSORY ORGANS: PANCREAS, LIVER AND GALLBLADDER

Specific learning outcomes
- Describe the embryonic development and gross anatomy of the pancreas, liver and gallbladder.
- Describe the histology and physiological function of the pancreas, liver and gallbladder.
- Explain the mechanism and regulation of hepatobiliary and pancreatic secretions.
- Discuss the physiological effects of ageing on the structure and function of the pancreas, liver and gallbladder.
- Discuss common developmental abnormalities of the pancreas, liver and gallbladder.
- Discuss common disorders of the pancreas, liver and gallbladder.
- Explain the pathogenesis of common hepatobiliary and pancreatic disorders.
- Compare and contrast the normal physiology of the hepatobiliary and pancreatic systems with the altered physiology seen with dysfunction of these systems.

THE PANCREAS

Prenatal development of the pancreas

The pancreas develops from two pancreatic buds (dorsal and ventral) which in turn have developed from the septum transversum which forms from a concentration of mesenchyme tissue (from mesodermal cells) that develops within the caudal part of ventral mesentery of the foregut. During the fourth week of gestation the dorsal bud emerges first (Figure 6.1) and grows more rapidly than the ventral bud and extends behind the duodenum into the dorsal mesentery. As the duodenum grows it rotates and transports the ventral pancreatic bud to the dorsal mesentery where it fuses with the dorsal bud during the seventh week. The dorsal bud generates the body and tail of the pancreas. The ventral bud generates the head and uncinate (part of the head of the pancreas) processes of the pancreas. The duct systems fuse together so that the gland drains through the Wirsung's duct (or main pancreatic duct) into the papilla of Vater. The duct that connects the accessory papilla to the main duct remains as the Santorini duct (or accessory pancreatic duct). During the foetal period the islet cells differentiate from the pancreatic bud endoderm. These cells go on to develop into the specialist endocrine islet cells that produce the hormones insulin and glucagon that regulate blood glucose levels, and the exocrine acini and duct cells that play a role in completing digestion. Insulin can be secreted from week 10 gestation.

Postnatal development and adult pancreas
Gross anatomy and function

The exocrine (enzyme) function of the pancreas starts at birth whereas the endocrine function (hormones: insulin and glucagon) can be identified between 10 and 15 weeks' gestation and onwards as they play a role in foetal development.

Postnatally the pancreas plays a vital role in secreting enzymes from acini cells which are required to digest starches and proteins and alkaline juices from duct cells. These alkaline juices are required to neutralise the acidic environment in the duodenum so that enzymes in the small intestine can work.

It is not until late infancy that the exocrine function of the pancreas becomes fully developed. Pancreatic amylase is produced by the acini cells from birth but it is not released into the duodenum until 4–6 months. The low activity of amylase in newborns is compensated for by the high activity of brush border enzymes, glucoamylase, sucrose-isomaltase and lactase, which are able to break down lactose and short-chain glucose polymers.

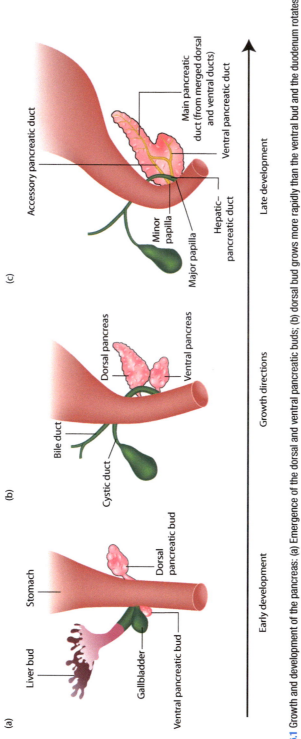

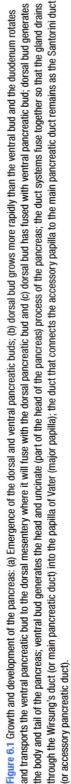

Figure 6.1 Growth and development of the pancreas: (a) Emergence of the dorsal and ventral pancreatic buds; (b) dorsal bud grows more rapidly than the ventral bud and the duodenum rotates and transports the ventral pancreatic bud to the dorsal mesentery where it will fuse with the dorsal pancreatic bud and (c) dorsal bud has fused with ventral pancreatic bud; dorsal bud generates the body and tail of the pancreas; ventral bud generates the head and uncinate (part of the head of the pancreas) process of the pancreas; the duct systems fuse together so that the gland drains through the Wirsung's duct (or main pancreatic duct) into the papilla of Vater (major papilla); the duct that connects the accessory papilla to the main pancreatic duct remains as the Santorini duct (or accessory pancreatic duct).

Infant pancreatic lipase production starts at 30 weeks' gestation and, in relation to adults, remains low until the first year of life. Pancreatic lipase and bile salt-dependent lipase are active in the small intestine and convert the triglyceride to monoglyceride which can then be absorbed. Pancreatic lipase does not hydrolyse (digest) breast milk effectively and so milk digestion is reliant upon the activity of salivary and gastric lipase. Pancreatic and bile salt-dependent lipase are unable to penetrate the phospholipid component of the milk fat globule membrane and hydrolyse triglycerides. Therefore the partial hydrolysis of fat in the stomach is a prerequisite for the completion of digestion and absorption of fatty acids and monoglycerol in the small intestine. Bile salts also contribute to the breaking down of the milk fat globule membrane.

The release of pancreatic proteases (protein digesting enzymes) begins from 26 weeks' gestation. The activity of these enzymes is low at birth and steadily increases until 8 months. The activity of proteases can be linked to the stages of development. In early infancy the milk diet does not contain complex proteins so there is a limited requirement for proteases. This means that protein digestive activity in the stomach of a newborn is low. However compensation for this is provided by pancreatic trypsins and chymotrypsins and intestinal enteropeptidases which have a higher activity in the newborn. Intestinal protein digestion through pepsin activity is fully developed in infants at 3–8 months of age (DiPalma et al., 1991).

In adults when food in the stomach has reached the correct acid pH and 'soup'-type consistency it is ready to be ejected into the duodenum. When it reaches the duodenum two changes must take place for digestion and absorption to be completed. First the acid chyme must be neutralised so that enzymes can work, and second the proteins, fats and carbohydrates must be broken down so that they are small enough to be absorbed across the mucosa. The pancreas plays a vital role in both of these processes. The pancreas functions as both an exocrine and an endocrine gland. Within the pancreas are cells called islets of Langerhans. The islets only make up approximately 1% of the cells of the pancreas. These cells contain beta cells that secrete insulin and alpha cells that secrete glucagon, hormones that regulate glucose and lipid metabolism. However it is the pancreas's exocrine function and its contribution to digestion and absorption that are explored here.

Functional histology of the pancreas

The pancreas is a pink, elongated organ with a head, which is surrounded by the C-shaped duodenum, a body and a tail (Figure 6.2). It lies posterior to the stomach and projects out laterally from the duodenum towards the spleen. The pancreas is enclosed within a thin transparent membrane of connective tissue (visceral peritoneum). The majority of the pancreatic tissue is made up of exocrine cells which produce enzymes and buffers. The exocrine function is performed by cells called acini (a single cell is called an acinus) and epithelial cells (Figure 6.2). Acini are packed with membrane-bound secretory granules, or zymogen granules, that contain the enzymes. The epithelial cells line the ducts within the pancreas. They produce a watery secretion, rich in bicarbonate, with a pH of 7.5–8.8 which serves to dilute and buffer the acids within the chyme that enter into the duodenum. The enzymes from the acini cells are released into intralobular ducts which then join with the pancreatic duct. The pancreatic duct is responsible for transporting these secretions to the duodenum through the duodenal papilla. The main pancreatic duct fuses with the common bile duct before it joins the duodenum.

Pancreatic secretions (exocrine secretions)

There are two types of secretions from the pancreas: enzymes and bicarbonate. The bicarbonate neutralises acids in the duodenum and the enzymes help complete the process of digestion by breaking down nutrients into basic molecules so they can be absorbed across the small intestine mucosa. The three major enzymes produced by the pancreas that are vital for completion of digestion are proteases, lipase and amylase.

A number of proteases are produced by acini cells in the pancreas. Two important ones are trypsin and chymotrypsin. As with pepsin in the stomach, these enzymes are manufactured in the inactive forms of trypsinogen and chymotrypsinogen to prevent autodigestion of pancreatic tissue. Trypsinogen is converted to the active trypsin by the enzyme enterokinase which is secreted by intestinal enterocyte epithelial cells. Once formed trypsin also has the effect of activating trypsinogen and chymotrypsinogen.

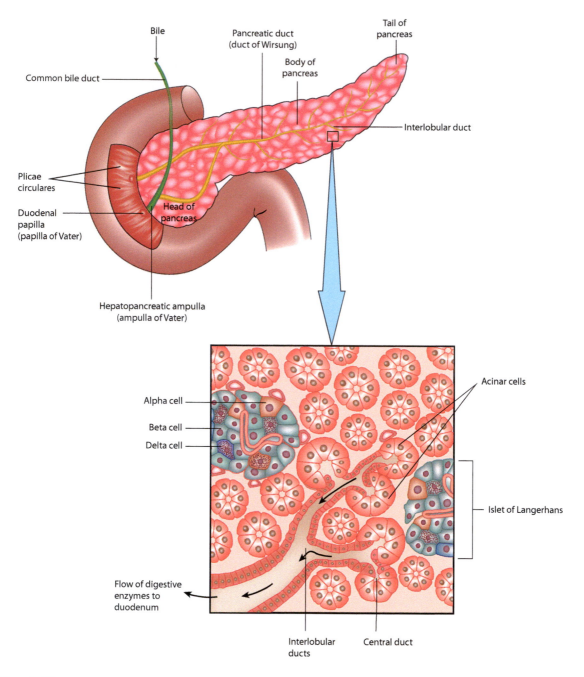

Figure 6.2 The pancreas.

Both trypsin and chymotrypsin destroy the peptide bonds linking amino acids together. This serves to break down polypeptides to peptides, therefore making peptide chains shorter, but these proteases cannot break down the peptides to the single molecule amino acids. This role is largely performed by peptidases. This is an enzyme released from the brush border membrane of the intestinal enterocyte epithelial cells.

Food material entering the small intestine contains complex lipids in the form of tryglycerides. These lipids are too large to be absorbed directly into the intestinal mucosa. The enzyme pancreatic lipase is responsible for converting tryglycerides into monoglyceride and free fatty acids. The digestion of lipids requires the presence of bile salts, generated by the liver. These salts emulsify the fats increasing the surface area across which the enzymes can work. These molecules are then small enough to be absorbed. Digestion of lipids is therefore dependent upon secretion from both the liver and the pancreas. Weight reduction medications have utilised this process to help manage obesity. For example drugs such as Orlistal (Xenical) interfere with the production of pancreatic lipase inhibiting the breakdown of lipids, thereby reducing the uptake of lipids into circulation.

Pancreatic secretions also contain pancreatic amylase responsible for converting dietary starch to maltose (disaccharide) and then the enzyme maltase, released from the brush border membrane of the intestinal enterocyte, converts maltose to glucose (monosaccharide) where it then becomes small enough to be absorbed and transported across the epithelial membrane.

Regulation of pancreatic secretions

Regulation of pancreatic secretions is by neural and hormonal pathways. The pancreas is innervated by the vagus nerve when anticipation of food generates a low level of stimulation of the pancreas. This means that the pancreas starts to synthesise enzymes before food enters the stomach. The major stimulus for secretion from the pancreas comes from hormones released by entero-endocrine cells lining the duodenum: cholecystokinin, gastrin and secretin (see Figure 5.5).

As chyme enters the duodenum the presence of partially digested proteins and fats stimulates enteroendocrine cells to release cholecystokinin into the lamina propria which then diffuses into the circulation and arrives at the pancreas, and binding with receptors on the acinar cells stimulating them to release pancreatic enzymes. The presence of the acid chyme entering into the duodenum stimulates enteroendocrine cells to release secretin. This hormone targets the epithelial duct cells lining the pancreatic ducts stimulating them to release a watery secretion, rich in bicarbonate, with a pH of 7.5–8.8 which serves to dilute and neutralise the acids within the chyme that enter into the duodenum.

The presence of peptides and amino acids in the stomach together with parasympathetic neural activity stimulates the release of gastrin by the entero-endocrine G cells in the gastric mucosa. As well as stimulating gastric secretion and motility, gastrin also serves to stimulate the acinar cells to release pancreatic enzymes.

Developmental abnormalities of the pancreas

Pancreas divisum

There are a number of abnormalities of the pancreatic duct system which include pancreas divisum and the rarer annular pancreas. During the second month of gestation the pancreas is formed from the fusion of dorsal and ventral buds (or anlage) (Figure 6.3). The ventral bud emerges with the biliary system and goes on to form the inferior and posterior section of the pancreatic head. The dorsal bud forms the remaining part of the head and the body and tail of the pancreas. During normal development the duct systems fuse together so that the gland drains through the Wirsung's duct into the papilla of Vater. The duct that connects the accessory papilla to the main duct remains as the Santorini duct. If embryological development stops at the middle stage the ventral part remains separate from the dorsal part and becomes an isolated ventral pancreas. This condition is called pancreas divisum (see Figures 6.3 and 6.4) (Nishino et al., 2006; Spicak et al., 2007). When this occurs there is only one pathway for pancreatic drainage and this is through the Santorini duct to the accessory papilla. With only this pathway available for pancreatic drainage, pressure can build up causing obstructive pancreatic pain and pancreatitis (Spicak et al., 2007). Recurrent acute pancreatitis and chronic pancreatitis are the main manifestations of this condition. Pancreatic divisum is also associated with pancreatic cancer (Nishino et al., 2006).

Annular pancreas

Annular pancreas is a rare congenital malformation that occurs due to incomplete rotation of the pancreatic ventral bud during embryogenesis. The ventral and dorsal parts fuse through a circumferential branch. This abnormal ring of pancreatic tissue encircles the second part of the duodenum (Figure 6.5). The anomaly is believed to be the result of incomplete migration of the ventral pancreatic bud during embryogenesis. Other congenital anomalies associated with annular pancreas are intestinal

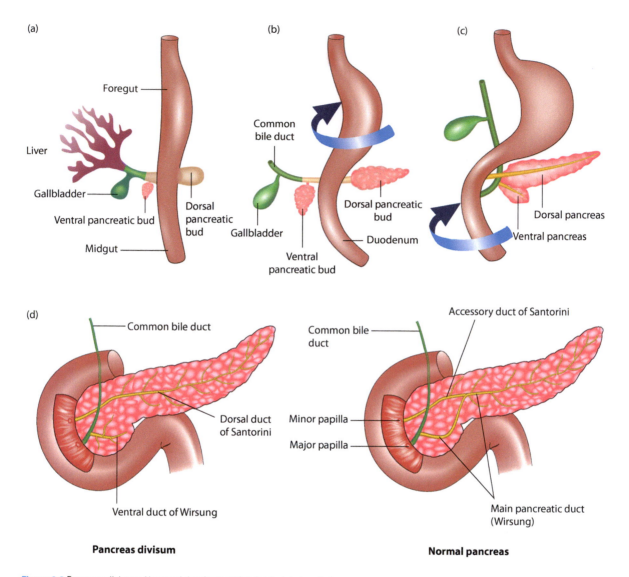

Figure 6.3 Pancreas divisum: Abnormal development leaving isolated ventral pancreas.

rotation, trisomy 21 (Down syndrome), cardiac defects, tracheoesophageal fistulae, duodenal atresia and pancreas divisum.

Changes associated with different stages of the lifespan

Cystic fibrosis

Cystic fibrosis (CF) is a multisystem genetic disorder. It is caused by mutation of the cystic fibrosis transmembrane conductance regulator (CFTR) gene on chromosome 7 which was discovered in 1989 (Riordan et al., 1989; Rommens et al., 1989) leading to an understanding of the underlying pathophysiology found in CF epithelial tissues which includes the intestine, pancreas, sweat glands and the airway (Marino et al., 1991; Strong et al., 1994). According to the World Health Organization (WHO, 2015) incidence in the United Kingdom is 1 in 2600; in the United States it is 1 in 3500. Ireland has the highest incidence of cystic fibrosis at 1 in 1800. Cystic fibrosis is characterised by the excessive buildup of viscous secretions which mainly affects the respiratory and digestive systems contributing to growth

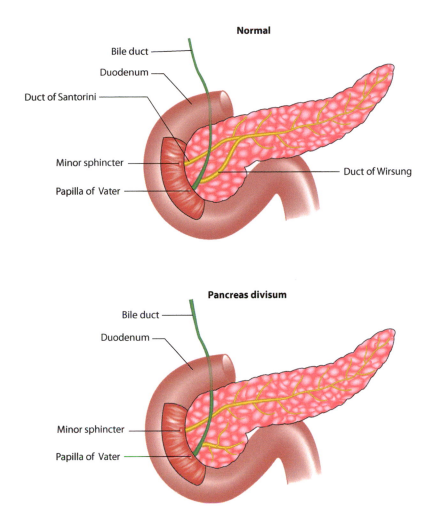

Figure 6.4 Pancreas divisium: One pathway, rather than two, for pancreatic drainage.

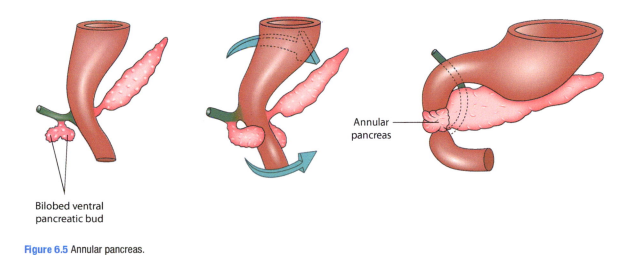

Figure 6.5 Annular pancreas.

deficits, chronic respiratory infection, progressive lung tissue damage and premature death. VanDevanter et al. (2016) review of research found that 'structural abnormalities and dysfunction in the digestive and respiratory systems were observed prenatally, in infants, and throughout childhood among children with CF, including bowel, pancreatic, and liver abnormalities, nutritional deficiencies, growth deficits, airway anomalies, inflammation, pulmonary dysfunction, infection, and pulmonary exacerbations' (p. 149). Newborns with CF can have serious pancreatic insufficiency and digestive complications related to their disease (Scaparrotta et al., 2012). In the pancreas, chloride conductance in the apical membrane of pancreatic duct cells is affected (Marino et al., 1991; Strong et al., 1994; O'Sullivan and Freedman, 2009). CFTR regulates the movement of electrolytes (chloride and bicarbonate ions) and water across the epithelial membrane. The loss of CFTR function, caused by mutations of the gene, leads to the development of pancreatic dysfunction and the development of lesions (Marino et al., 1991; Strong et al., 1994; O'Sullivan and Freedman, 2009). The CFTR functions as a chloride ion channel. Under healthy circumstances acid in the duodenum stimulates the release of secretin from the enteroendocrine cells that line the duodenum. Secretin, via blood circulation, stimulates pancreatic duct cells to release bicarbonate (HCO_3^-)-rich isotonic fluid into the duct lumen. Loss of CFTR function means that the duct cells cannot secrete chloride or bicarbonate and water into the lumen of the pancreatic duct. This leads to the secretions in the pancreatic duct becoming viscous, reducing flow through the duct and leading to protein precipitation in the duct (Kopelman et al., 1988; Naruse et al., 2002; O'Sullivan and Freedman, 2009). This leads to obstruction, pancreatic dysfunction and pancreatic insufficiency by blocking acinar secretion. Acinar cells gradually become replaced with cysts, fibrous tissue and fat. This eventually disrupts the function of the islets reducing the production of insulin and other islet hormones.

Acute pancreatitis

Acute pancreatitis is a condition characterised by inflammation of pancreatic tissue. The prevalence of acute pancreatitis in England is 10 per 100,000 (Goldacre and Roberts, 2004). In Norway, Germany and Netherlands it is 16–20 per 100,000 (Eland et al., 2000; Lankisch et al., 2002; Gislason et al., 2004) and in the United States it is 32–44 per 100,000 (Frey et al., 2006; Fagenholz et al., 2007). Recent studies have attributed this variation in incidence to alcohol consumption but this is now under debate. The increasing incidence of obesity, and obesity-associated gallstones, is believed to be related to the growing incidence of pancreatitis (Shaffer, 2006). Approximately 80% of cases of acute pancreatitis are attributed to gallstones and alcohol abuse (Whitcomb, 2006; Forsmark and Baillie, 2007). Pathogenesis includes biliopancreatic reflux, obstruction of the pancreatic exocrine secretion by gallstones, biliary sludge or neoplasm. Causes other than gallstones and alcohol include structural abnormality such as pancreas divisum, metabolic disorders, infection and genetic defects (Arendt, 1989a,b; Kemppainen and Puolakkainen, 2007).

Chronic pancreatitis

There are many aetiologies of chronic pancreatitis. In Western countries the most common cause in adults is chronic alcohol abuse (Jarnagin, 2013). The incidence of chronic pancreatitis in Europe and Western countries is approximately 6–7 per 100,000 population (Mitchell et al., 2003; Spanier et al., 2008; Jupp et al., 2010). Similar incidences have been reported in other regions of the world (Wang et al., 2009; Yadav, 2011) although a high incidence has been reported in Asian countries, especially in Japan and India (Garg, 2012). Worldwide the overall prevalence of chronic pancreatitis has recently been reported to be increasing, and it is believed that this is likely to be due to increasing alcohol consumption together with the introduction of more effective diagnostic techniques (Jarnagin, 2013).

Chronic pancreatitis is caused by inflammation of pancreatic tissue which leads to the progressive and irreversible destruction of exocrine and endocrine glandular parenchyma. A major cause of chronic pancreatitis is attributed to alcohol abuse (Gukovskaya et al., 2006). Alcohol has been shown to induce apoptosis (programmed cell death) in many different types of tissues in the body such as hepatocytes, neurons and intestinal epithelial cells. However studies of cell death pathways in the pancreas carried out by Gukovskaya et al. (2006) and Fortunato et al. (2006) have shown that chronic alcohol intake inhibits rather than induces apoptosis.

Although apoptosis is inhibited, the disruption of the cell death pathway and the mechanisms involved exacerbate parenchymal cell necrosis, thereby predisposing the person to the development of chronic pancreatitis. The parenchyma is replaced with fibrotic tissue.

THE LIVER

The liver carries out an important secretory and excretory function in relation to digestion mainly in respect to the synthesis and secretion of bile. The liver performs many other functions but only those relating to digestion are considered here. In order to understand this function it is important to consider the histological structure.

Prenatal development of the liver and biliary tree

The liver develops from a region called the transverse septum (collection of mesodermal cells). This region is where the ectoderm of the amnion meets the endoderm of the yolk sac externally and where the foregut meets the midgut internally. The transverse septum, as it grows, differentiates to form the hepatic diverticulum and the primordium from which the liver and gallbladder emerge (Figure 6.6). The liver appears at the end of week 3 or early in week 4 of gestation. The liver develops rapidly between weeks 5 and 10 taking up the majority of the abdominal cavity.

The hepatic diverticulum produces the parenchyma (functional cells) of the liver, specialised liver

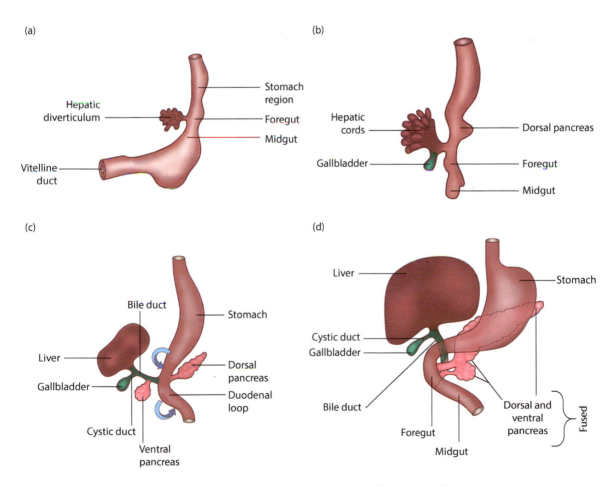

Figure 6.6 Growth and development of the liver and biliary tree. (a) Four weeks; (b and c) Five weeks; (d) Six weeks gestation.

cells called hepatocytes, and the epithelial lining of the biliary tract. The hepatocytes are arranged into a series of plates in the mesenchyme tissue (from mesodermal cells) of the transverse septum. The differentiating glandular tissue, as well as forming plates, is also bathed with vitelline and umbilical veins to form hepatic sinusoids. These form canal-type structures that are lined by the hepatocytes. The splanchnic mesenchyme (structure created during embryogenesis) in the transverse septum also forms the stroma, the connective tissue that makes up the liver capsule (or Gilson's capsule), the falciform ligament (attaches the liver to the abdominal and diaphragm wall), and the hematopoietic (blood-forming) tissue of the liver. Mature Kupffer cells are macrophages found in the lumen of hepatic sinusoids. Primitive macrophages arise in the yolk sac and then differentiate into foetal macrophages. These then enter the blood circulation and migrate to the developing liver. The connective tissue and smooth muscle of the biliary tract also develop from this mesenchyme. The formation of bile begins in week 12. Breast milk is already emulsified so bile will not be needed until the infant starts to take solid food.

Hepatocytes extend into the septum transversum and the connection between the hepatic diverticulum and the foregut narrows. This narrowing leads to the formation of the bile ducts. An outgrowth of the bile duct forms the cystic duct which then extends into the gallbladder. Via the common bile duct the hepatic and cystic duct can deliver bile to the duodenum.

Postnatal development and adult liver
Gross anatomy and functional histology

The liver is found in the abdominal cavity. It is in contact with the diaphragm superiorly. The largest section lies in the right hypochondriac and epigastric regions and the remainder extends across to the left hypochondriac. It is covered by a transparent membrane called the visceral peritoneum (serosa) which is continuous with the abdominal peritoneum. The liver is divided into four lobes: anteriorly there are the right and left lobes which are separated by the falciform ligament. Posteriorly the caudate and quadrate lobes can be identified (Figure 6.7). Connective tissue throughout the liver divides the lobes into approximately 100,000 liver lobules. This connective tissue also acts as a form of scaffolding providing support for the many blood vessels, lymph vessels and bile ducts. The liver lobules are the structural units of the liver. Each lobule consists of a hexagonal arrangement of plates of hepatocytes which radiate out from a central vein which is at the centre of the lobule (Figure 6.8). The hepatocytes make contact with blood in the sinusoids which are canal-like ducts lined with fenestrated endothelial cells. The gap between the endothelium and the hepatocytes is called the *space of Disse*. The fenestrated endothelial cells (gaps in the endothelium) allow plasma to drain between the cells forming lymph (Figure 6.9). The majority of the lymph that enters the lymphatic circulation comes from the liver. Kupffer cells are also found within the sinusoids. These are phagocytic cells which engulf pathogens. For example some bacteria can cross the epithelium if it is damaged and Kupffer cells attack and destroy these. Kupffer cells also remove cell debris and any damaged red blood cells.

Blood supply of the liver

Blood leaving the small intestine is rich in absorbed nutrients. It travels via the superior mesenteric vein to the hepatic portal vein where it then enters the liver. And 75% of the blood entering the liver is venous blood which enters via the hepatic portal vein. The remaining 25% of blood is arterial blood and this enters the liver via the hepatic artery. Blood enters the liver at the porta hepatis (doorway to the liver) via the hepatic artery and the hepatic portal vein. The blood enters the liver lobules via portal triads (Figure 6.10). There are six portal triads, one for each corner of the hexagonal-shaped lobule. A portal triad consists of a branch of the hepatic artery, the hepatic portal vein and the bile duct. When blood enters the lobule via the portal triad, venous and arterial blood becomes mixed as it drains into sinusoids. Sinusoids are ducts in the liver tissue which function like 'canals' transporting the blood to the hepatocytes. As blood flows through the sinusoids it comes into contact with hepatocytes which then absorb nutrients and secrete synthesised molecules. If there is an excess of nutrients these are removed and stored and if there is a deficiency of nutrients these are released or synthesised by the hepatocytes. From sinusoids blood then flows into the central vein, hepatic vein and then into the vena cava.

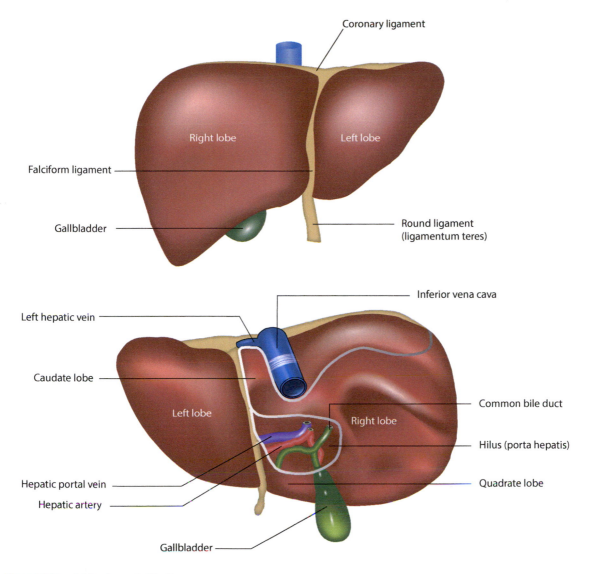

Figure 6.7 Prenatal development of the liver.

Formation and functions of bile

One of the functions of hepatocytes is to produce bile. Bile consists of water, electrolytes, bile acids, cholesterol, phospholipids and bilirubin. Bile plays a key role in the digestion of fats within the small intestine. Bile is secreted by hepatocytes into canaliculi which transport bile out of the lobule where it drains into bile ductules, interlobular bile ducts and then collects in the right and left hepatic ducts outside the liver. These then join up to form the common hepatic duct (Figure 6.11). As bile flows through the bile ducts the ductal epithelial cells (cholangiocytes) that line its surface modify the bile by secreting a watery, bicarbonate-rich secretion. This secretion plays an important role in neutralising the acid environment in the duodenum so that pancreatic and small intestine enzymes can function. The bile then either flows via the common bile duct emptying into the duodenum or it enters the cystic duct and is stored in the gallbladder. The gallbladder stores and concentrates bile between meals and overnight. Bile will remain within the gallbladder until its release is triggered by the contraction of the walls of the

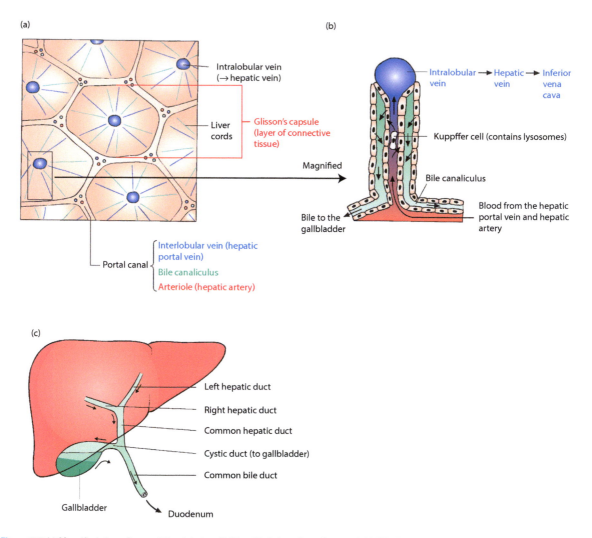

Figure 6.8 (a) Magnified view of several liver lobules. (b) Magnified view of one liver cord. (c) Bile ducts.

gallbladder. During the time that bile remains in the gallbladder, water and some electrolytes are absorbed causing the bile to become more concentrated.

In neonates bile acid production is low. Bile acids are conjugated with the amino acids taurine or glycine to form bile salts. Breast milk provides a rich supply of taurine so in infancy conjugation with taurine occurs more readily.

Bile performs two key functions. It contains bile salts which are vital for the digestion and absorption of fats and fat-soluble vitamins. Bile also removes waste products such as bilirubin from the body as a component of faeces.

Bile salts make up one of the most important constituents of bile. They are water-soluble derivatives

of cholesterol. Two important bile acids are produced in the liver: cholic acid and chenodeoxycholic acid. These are conjugated (made soluble) to an amino acid to produce the conjugated form that is released into the canaliculi (Figure 6.12). Bile acids perform two important functions. First they help to break down, or emulsify (not digest), fat globules to smaller fat droplets. This helps to increase the surface area across which the enzyme lipase can work to digest fats. When bile salts have completed their function they are released back into the lumen of the small intestine and are transported with chyme to the terminal ileum. The majority of bile acids are reabsorbed across the terminal ileum epithelium into blood and are then transported via the hepatic

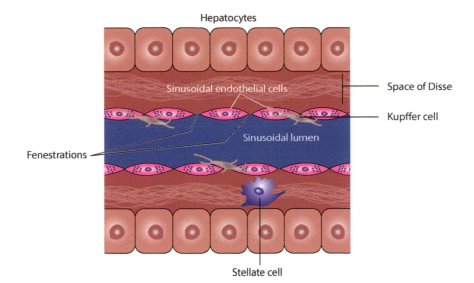

Figure 6.9 Fenestrated endothelial cells.

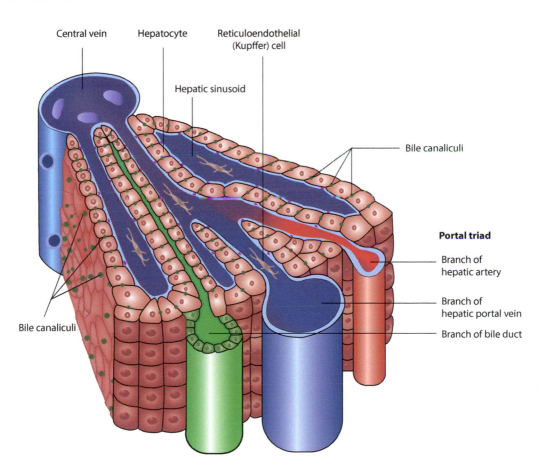

Figure 6.10 Portal triads.

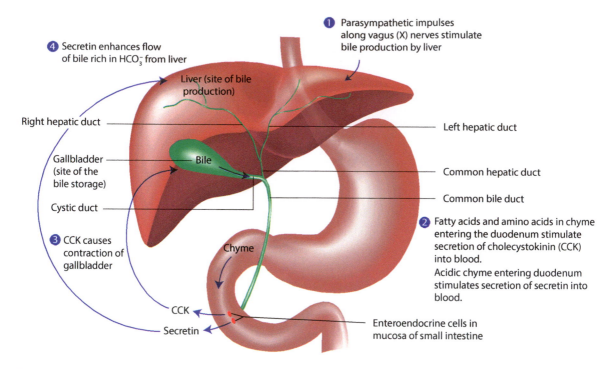

Figure 6.11 Pathway of bile secretion.

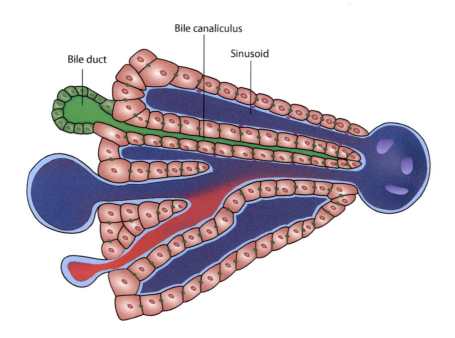

Figure 6.12 Canaliculus: Transport of bile from hepatocytes.

portal vein to the sinusoids in the liver lobules. Here the bile salts are then taken up by the hepatocytes and are effectively recycled so that they can be secreted again as an important constituent of bile. The continuous recycling of bile acids is known as the enterohepatic circulation (Figure 6.13). In early infancy the secretion of bile salts into the small intestine is much reduced. This has the effect of reducing the digestion of fats, and in particular long-chain fatty acids. This should not present a problem for breastfed infants as breast milk contains fats that are already emulsified.

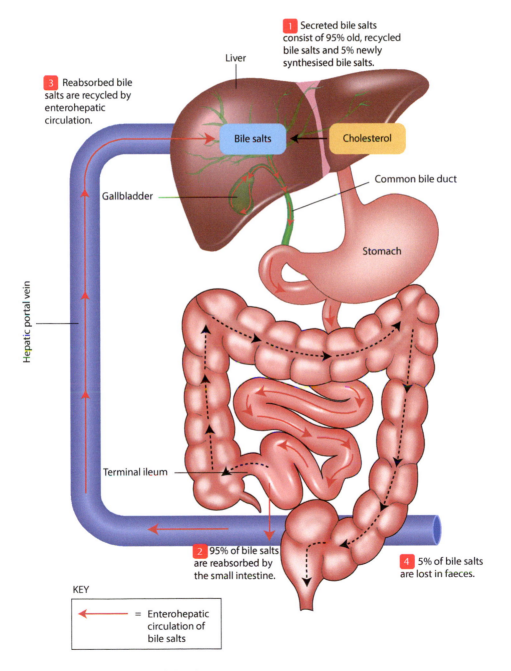

1 Secreted bile salts consist of 95% old, recycled bile salts and 5% newly synthesised bile salts.

Liver

3 Reabsorbed bile salts are recycled by enterohepatic circulation.

Bile salts

Cholesterol

Common bile duct

Gallbladder

Stomach

Hepatic portal vein

Terminal ileum

2 95% of bile salts are reabsorbed by the small intestine.

4 5% of bile salts are lost in faeces.

KEY

← = Enterohepatic circulation of bile salts

Figure 6.13 Enterohepatic circulation: Recycling of bile salts.

The secretion of bile provides an important mechanism for removing waste products from the body. One important substance eliminated in this way is bilirubin. Bilirubin is a by-product of the breakdown of haemoglobin (Figure 6.14). Phagocytic cells in the liver (Kupffer cells) and throughout the body break down and recycle the molecular components of haemoglobin. One of these components is heme. This is converted by the phagocytes into bilirubin. This is then released into the plasma and is carried around by albumin. Free bilirubin is then removed from albumin and is absorbed by the hepatocytes. Within the hepatocytes, bilirubin becomes conjugated bilirubin.

This process converts insoluble bilirubin into a soluble form so it can leave the hepatocytes and be secreted into the canaliculi and become a component of bile. It is then transported along the hepatobiliary tract to the duodenum. Bacteria in the intestine break down the bilirubin, and it is the by-products of this which give faeces its distinctive colour.

The inability of the liver to remove bilirubin from the body can lead to a yellow discolouration of the skin. The clinical term for this is jaundice. In neonates this can be caused by the faster turnover of red blood cells as compared to adults. Where the rate of bilirubin production is higher than the liver

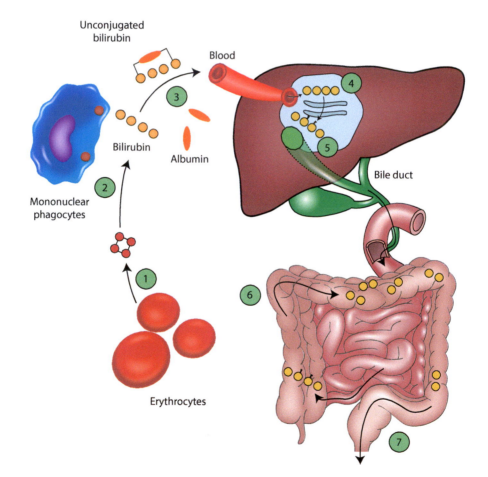

Figure 6.14 Formation of bilirubin from the breakdown of haemoglobin: (1) As erythrocytes disintegrate (process of haemolysis) the haemoglobin is degraded or separated into globin, iron and heme; (2) heme is degraded to biliverdin by the enzyme heme oxygenase in the mononuclear phagocytes (macrophages); (3) biliverdin is subsequently reduced to bilirubin by the enzyme biliverdin reductase; (4) circulating bilirubin (insoluble) is bound to albumin and subsequently taken up by the hepatocytes; (5) to make it soluble, bilirubin undergoes conjugation, a reaction catalysed by the enzyme bilirubin UDP-glucuronyl transferase (UDPG); (6) conjugated bilirubin (soluble) is excreted into bile and reaches the bowel and (7) bilirubin glucuronides (conjugated form) are deconjugated by colonic bacteria and eliminated in the faeces.

can manage, this can result in jaundice. In neonates an immature liver can also mean that the hepatocytes are unable to conjugate (make soluble) bilirubin. Bilirubin needs to be soluble in order for it to be excreted from the hepatocytes (live cells) into the canaliculi. If the bilirubin cannot be conjugated it binds to albumin, is circulated in blood and gets deposited in the skin, sclera and mucous membranes (see section on 'Hyperbilirubinaemia').

Age-related changes affecting the liver

There are a number of age-related changes that affect the liver. These include thickening and reduced sinusoidal fenestration of the liver endothelial cells, collagen deposition, causing a reduction in hepatocyte function and increased numbers of fat stellate cells. The liver mass and blood flow in the older person are also reduced and this causes a reduction in the rate of drug clearance. Ageing also affects the Kupffer cells making them less responsive (Jansen, 2002; Hilmer et al., 2005).

Age-related changes have functional implications for the liver. Reduced sinusoidal perfusion impairs hepatic clearance of waste macromolecules that takes place in liver sinusoidal endothelial cells. Loss of fenestrations leads to impaired transfer of lipoproteins from blood to hepatocytes, which results in hyperlipidemia (Hilmer et al., 2005). The liver is the central organ for lipoprotein metabolism. Lipoproteins transfer from the hepatic sinusoidal capillary lumen across the hepatic sinusoidal endothelium into the space of Disse. From here they are taken up by the hepatocytes. Impaired transfer of lipoproteins is a major risk factor for the development of atherosclerosis. There are a wide range of substances found in blood that are metabolised by the liver so age-related changes in the hepatic sinusoid and microcirculation can have significant systemic implications for ageing and diseases associated with old age.

Developmental abnormalities of the liver

Hyperbilirubinaemia

Hyperbilirubinaemia is the excessive accumulation of bilirubin in the body. Although the neonate liver is immature it can perform the same functions as an adult liver albeit less effectively. This means the neonate liver is at risk of hyperbilirubinaemia. Bilirubin is generated from the breakdown of

haemoglobin (Figure 6.14). The process begins with macrophages breaking down heme (blood pigment) to biliverdin. This is then broken down to bilirubin. Unconjugated or indirect bilirubin is insoluble and cannot therefore be excreted so it binds to plasma albumin and is transported to the liver hepatocytes where it is metabolised into conjugated or direct bilirubin which is soluble. Conjugated bilirubin is soluble so when it is in this form it can be excreted into bile and transported to the duodenum. Once in the small intestine the conjugated bilirubin is then metabolised by the bacterial flora to produce urobilin and stercobilin. It is stercobilin that gives stool its distinctive colour.

Prenatally the placenta performs the function of removing bilirubin. Ineffective clearance of bilirubin in the neonate liver leads to jaundice or icterus (Behrman et al., 2000; Newman et al., 2006). There are a number of possible causes of hyperbilirubinaemia in neonates. The mechanism of deconjugation in the liver turning insoluble bilirubin to a soluble form can be impaired. The inability of the newborn's liver to effectively process bilirubin is termed physiological jaundice. Delayed passage of bilirubin-rich meconium could lead to increased deconjugation, absorption and circulation of bilirubin (Dennery et al., 2001). The neonate requirement for high levels of red blood cells together with the fragility and short lifespan of these red blood cells can lead to excessive bilirubin levels leading to hyperbilirubinaemia. Conditions that lead to the increased rate of breakdown of red blood cells, such as polycythaemia, can also lead to hyperbilirubinaemia. It can also be caused by slow production of plasma proteins in the immature liver. This means there is reduced capacity for unconjugated bilirubin to be transported to the liver. Unconjugated bilirubin therefore becomes elevated leading to hyperbilirubinaemia.

Changes associated with different stages of the lifespan

Hepatitis infection

Hepatitis refers to inflammation of the liver that can be caused by a number of factors which can be classified under the headings: infectious and non-infectious. Infectious factors include viral, bacterial, fungal and parasitic organisms, and non-infectious factors include alcohol, drugs, autoimmune and metabolic diseases. Hepatitis can lead to fibrosis (scarring of liver tissue), cirrhosis and cancer of the liver.

According to the WHO (2015) the most common cause of hepatitis in the world is viral hepatitis. There are five main hepatitis viruses which are referred to as types A, B, C, D and E. Hepatitis B and C together are the most common cause of liver cirrhosis and cancer (WHO, 2015).

Hepatitis A and E are usually caused by ingestion of contaminated food or water. Hepatitis B, C and D usually occur as a result of parenteral contact with infected body fluids. Routes of transmission for these viruses are normally following receipt of contaminated blood or blood products or through the use of contaminated equipment during an invasive medical procedure. Hepatitis B transmission is through sexual contact; from mother to baby at birth, from family member to child.

Hepatitis C (HCV) is the most common form of viral hepatitis in the United Kingdom (WHO, 2015). It is a small envelope virus that contains RNA. Once the virus has gained entry to hepatocytes (liver cells) it causes hepatitis (inflammation) and cirrhosis (fibrosis). HCV infection and alcohol abuse are the two most common causes of chronic liver disease in Western Europe and North America. An estimated 170 million people worldwide and 3.9 million in the United States have been infected with the hepatitis C virus (HCV) (Alter et al., 1999; WHO, 2015). In Western countries, up to 50% of cases of end-stage liver disease have alcohol as a main aetiological factor (Orholm et al., 1985). Approximately 15%–20% of chronic alcoholics develop cirrhosis over a 20–30 year period.

Infection with HCV is associated with factors such as IV drug use, blood transfusions and needlestick injuries. HVC is spread through direct parenteral inoculation, transplantation of an infected organ, perinatal exposure or sexual contact. Hepatocytes infected by the HCV virus are destroyed by the immune system but in some cases not all the virus is destroyed. The HCV virus can also mutate very quickly and suppress the cell-mediated immune response (Darling and Wright, 2004). These factors mean the virus can persist leading to chronic hepatitis and then eventually liver cirrhosis. Over a period of 20–30 years, 20% of patients infected with HCV progress to cirrhosis (Seeff, 2002).

Alcoholic fatty liver, acute alcoholic hepatitis and alcoholic cirrhosis

The three most commonly recognised forms of alcoholic liver disease (ALD) are alcoholic fatty liver (steatosis), acute alcoholic hepatitis and alcoholic cirrhosis (Arteel et al., 2003; Mazen and Morgan, 2003; Bruha et al., 2012). Approximately 80% of individuals who regularly consume excessive amounts of alcohol develop steatosis, 10%–35% develop alcoholic hepatitis, and approximately 10% will develop cirrhosis. An alcohol-related fatty liver is characterised by an accumulation of fatty deposits in the hepatocytes (steatosis). Alcoholic hepatitis is characterised by inflammation and necrosis of liver cells. Alcohol causes an accumulation of water within the cells (hepatocyte ballooning). It is believed that 15–20 years of excessive drinking is required for alcoholic hepatitis to develop.

Simple steatosis is characterised as being a reversible state following a period of abstinence from alcohol. However with continued abuse, it too, can induce fibrogenesis (Reeves et al., 1996). Up to 20% of the patients with simple steatosis are likely to develop fibrosis or cirrhosis within a period of 10 years (Teli et al., 1995a). Steatohepatitis is characterised as a condition that is usually only found in some alcoholics where a fibrogenic process has taken place which can induce changes leading to cirrhosis. Steatohepatitis is also reversible (Poynard, 2000), however it is likely that some evidence of fibrosis is likely to remain (Mu et al., 2010). Steatohepatitis, in particular, often coincides with liver cirrhosis in active alcoholics and is a frequent cause of decompensation of cirrhosis (Stewart and Day, 2004).

The most severe form of alcoholic liver injury is alcoholic cirrhosis (fibrosis of the liver). In this condition liver cells are replaced with fibrous tissue which restricts blood and biliary flow through the liver leading to the development of portal hypertension, jaundice, damage to hepatocytes and eventual liver failure. Pathogenesis of alcoholic liver disease is characterised by the development of collagen deposits in the space of Disse and around the central veins which causes an acceleration of the cirrhosis. The collagen deposits eventually form bridges between central veins and portal tracts isolating groups of hepatocytes which leads to the development of the characteristic uniform nodules found on its surface. As the cirrhosis progresses regenerative processes lead to the development of larger and more irregular-shaped nodules further isolating groups of hepatocytes, narrowing the hepatic veins, restricting blood flow and leading to other problems such as portal hypertension (Arteel et al., 2003; Mazen and Morgan, 2003).

In people with cirrhosis of the liver where functionality is impaired and there is associated decompensated cirrhosis prognosis is poor. Decompensated liver disease often presents with symptoms and complications which include jaundice, portal hypertension, variceal haemorrhage, ascites and hepatic encephalopathy. People who stop taking alcohol but have decompensated cirrhosis (i.e. associated complications) have a 5-year survival at a rate of 60% against the 30% survival rate in those who continue in the abuse (Diehl, 2002). The mortality rate for severe alcoholic hepatitis is up to 50%.

Nonalcoholic fatty liver disease (NAFLD)

Nonalcoholic fatty liver disease (NAFLD) is a term that describes a wide range of liver disease that includes steatosis (a fatty liver), non-alcoholic steatohepatitis (NASH) to cirrhosis (fibrosis of the liver). Fat accumulation in the hepatocytes is common to all stages of NAFLD and is a significant contributing factor in the development of hepatitis (inflammation) and related fibrosis. Impaired responsiveness to insulin is believed to be a significant factor causing the accumulation of fat in NAFLD (Teli et al., 1995b; Angulo, 2002; Sakurai et al., 2007). NAFLD and NASH occur in individuals who do not consume excessive amounts of alcohol. NAFD is also associated with a number of metabolic abnormalities which include obesity, type 2 diabetes and dyslipidemia, all of which are important risk factors for cardiovascular disease (Sakurai et al., 2007).

Nonalcoholic steatohepatitis (NASH) is characterised by inflammation (hepatitis) of the liver with fat accumulation (steatosis) in the absence of significant alcohol consumption (Sanyal, 2002; Neuschwander-Tetri and Caldwell, 2003). Although considered a mild condition it can progress to cirrhosis. NASH is believed to be a common cause of unexplained cirrhosis in Western countries. The incidence of NASH has been shown to increase with increasing prevalence of obesity (Sanyal, 2002; Neuschwander-Tetri and Caldwell, 2003). Steatohepatitis, once considered to be rare in children, is now accepted as a significant childhood liver disease (Roberts, 2002). Its increasing significance is believed to be attributed to rising levels of childhood obesity which has shown to be associated with NAFLD.

THE GALLBLADDER

Prenatal development of the gallbladder

The gallbladder, in adults, is the site of bile storage and concentration. The bile is released into the duodenum to emulsify fats.

The development of the liver, gallbladder and biliary tree begins at the fourth week of gestation as a ventral bud, or hepatic diverticulum, from the most caudal part of the foregut (Lamah et al., 2001). As the diverticulum grows its connection with the foregut narrows to form the external hepatic bile duct. The hepatic diverticulum extends into the septum transversum and divides into two parts as it grows between the layers of the ventral mesentery: the larger cranial part (pars hepatica) is the primordium of the liver and the second part is the smaller ventral invagination (pars cystica) (Lamah et al., 2001) which forms a vacuole that expands to form the gallbladder. Its stalk becomes the cystic duct.

Postnatal development and adult gallbladder
Gross anatomy and function

Between meals bile travels down the cystic duct and is stored in the gallbladder. The gallbladder is a green pear-shaped muscular sac. It consists of a fundus, body and neck. The fundus protrudes from the underside of the liver. The gallbladder stores and concentrates bile by removal of non-essential solutes and water, leaving bile acids and bile pigments. The muscle walls of the gallbladder remain partially contracted most of the time. These contractions become much more vigorous when chyme enters the duodenum. The presence of fats in the duodenum stimulates enteroendocrine cells that line the duodenum to release the hormone cholecystokinin (see Figure 5.5 for an overview of digestive tract hormones). Cholecystokinin travels via blood circulation to the gallbladder bringing about contraction of the muscles in the walls of the gallbladder and the common bile duct allowing secretion of bile into the cystic duct, along the common bile duct and joining the pancreatic duct at the duodenal ampulla before emptying into the duodenum. A muscular sphincter called the pancreaticohepatic sphincter (sphincter of

Oddi) encircles the lumen of the common bile duct and is only open in the presence of cholecystokinin. Once in the small intestine the bile emulsifies fats and aids absorption of fat-soluble vitamins.

Developmental abnormalities of the gallbladder

Gallbladder agenesis

Gallbladder agenesis (GBA) is a rare congenital abnormality in which the gallbladder fails to develop during embryogenesis (Bennion et al., 1988; Cabajo et al., 1997; Lamah et al., 2001; Yoldas et al., 2014). Failure of the pars cystica to develop results in agenesis of both the gallbladder and the cystic duct. The existence of the condition within families suggests that there are familial hereditary forms of GBA (Wilson and Deitrick, 1986). Reported incidence ranges from 10 to 75 per 100,000 population (Richards et al., 1993) and only 413 cases were reported in 1999 (Singh et al., 1999). Of individuals with gallbladder agenesis, 23% will go on to develop symptoms that suggest bile tract disease (Wilson and Deitrick, 1986; Richards et al., 1993). Individuals experience right upper quadrant abdominal pain (90% of cases), nausea and vomiting (66% of cases), intolerance to fatty food (37% of cases), dyspepsia (30% of cases) and jaundice (35% of cases) (Vijay et al., 1996; Baltazar et al., 2000). Gallbladder agenesis has also been associated with a number of digestive, skeletal, cardiovascular and genito-urinary malformations (Coughlin et al., 1992; Goel et al., 1994; Singh et al., 1999; Dell'Abate et al., 2000; Sriram et al., 2001). Associated digestive malformations include imperforate anus, duodenal atresia, malrotation and pancreas divisum, the pathogenesis of which are explained in this chapter under the relevant sections.

Changes associated with different stages of the lifespan

Gallstones (cholelithiasis)

Cholelithiasis is a common condition. It affects 5%–22% of people in Western countries (Everhart et al., 1999; Aerts and Penninckx, 2003). Volzke et al. (2005) reported 10%–20% of Europeans and Americans have gallstones. Gallbladder disease is the leading cause of digestive-related hospital admissions in Western populations (Sandler et al., 2002) and cholelithiasis is one of the most prevalent diseases.

However, although relatively common, only 10%–30% of people with gallstones go on to develop clinical symptoms such as biliary colic or other digestive symptoms associated with the disease (Keus et al., 2006). Shaffer (2005) also found an increase in the prevalence of gallstones with age. Shaffer reported that of women 70–79 years of age 57% have evidence of gallstones or have a history of cholecystectomy (Shaffer, 2005). Gallstones form when the concentration of cholesterol or bilirubin exceeds the solubility in the bile salt and phospholipid-rich bile. The formation of bile by the hepatocytes is the mechanism by which the liver removes excess cholesterol from the body. Bile consists of lipids, bile salts, phospholipids and cholesterol. The plasma membranes of hepatocytes have transporter proteins called ABC transporters which allow the movement of these lipids, in solution, through the membrane into the canalicular lumen (Oude Elferink et al., 2006).

The composition of hepatic bile is further modified by the bicarbonate and chloride-rich secretions of bile duct epithelial cells (cholangiocytes) that line the bile duct. This mechanism results in the movement of water into the bile helping to dilute it. The flow of bile is driven by the osmotic pressure of solutes secreted by the hepatocytes and the bile duct epithelial cells. This secretory process involves the pumping of solutes against a concentration gradient, requiring the expenditure of adenosine triphosphate (ATP). This process increases the concentration of electrolytes in bile leading to the osmotic attraction of water into the bile (Oude Elferink, 2003). Dysfunction of these pumps leads to impaired bile flow (cholestasis) further increasing the risks of cholelithiasis. There are a number of inherited cholestatic diseases, caused by mutations in genes, which are characterised by dysfunction of the secretory pump process (Oude Elferink, 2003). Dysfunction of the pumping mechanism in the bile duct epithelial cells is a characteristic of the disease cystic fibrosis.

There are two types of gallstones: cholesterol stones and pigment stones. A predominant 80% of gallstones consist of cholesterol crystals and are formed within the gallbladder (Figure 6.15). There are three mechanisms that contribute to cholesterol gallbladder stones, of which cholesterol supersaturation of bile, and gallbladder hypomotility (Paumgartner and Sauerbruch, 1991) are two. Proteins such as mucin and aminopeptidase may also allow cholesterol

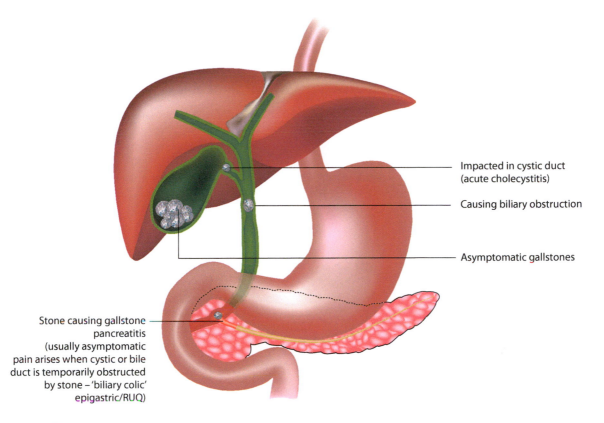

Impacted in cystic duct
(acute cholecystitis)

Causing biliary obstruction

Asymptomatic gallstones

Stone causing gallstone
pancreatitis
(usually asymptomatic
pain arises when cystic or bile
duct is temporarily obstructed
by stone – 'biliary colic'
epigastric/RUQ)

Figure 6.15 The gallbladder.

crystals to precipitate, a process known as nucleation (Afdhal et al., 1995).

Cholesterol is insoluble in water and its solubility is dependent upon the detergent properties of bile salts and phospholipids. An excess of biliary cholesterol in relation to bile salts and phospholipids can result from hypersecretion of cholesterol, or from hyposecretion of bile salts or phospholipids. The most common cause of supersaturation is cholesterol hypersecretion (Einarrson et al., 1985; Nisell et al., 1985). Hypersecretion could be caused by increased hepatic uptake of cholesterol, commonly associated with obesity, or increased hepatic synthesis of cholesterol. In non-obese individuals the development of cholesterol-rich gallstones is associated with reduced bile salt circulation within the liver.

The other 20% of gallstones consist of pigment stones. Pigment stones are caused by anything that elevates unconjugated (insoluble) bilirubin levels reducing the solubility of bile in the gallbladder causing precipitation of calcium bilirubinate (Allen et al., 1981). Excessive levels of unconjugated bilirubin can be caused by haemolytic anaemias or ineffective erythropoiesis (red blood cell production) which leads to excessive secretion of bilirubin from the liver (Lee and Ko, 1999).

Obstetric cholestasis

Stasis of bile can be triggered by pregnancy and this is termed obstetric cholestasis or intrahepatic cholestasis of pregnancy (Maringhini et al., 1987; Milkiewicz et al., 2002; Milkiewicz et al., 2003; Oude Elferink, 2003; Jorge et al., 2015). Obstetric cholestasis is a reversible type of cholestasis that can develop in the third trimester and usually resolves after birth (Oude Elferink, 2003). It is believed that individuals have an inherited genetic susceptibility to obstetric cholestasis where inherited gene mutations result in genetic hypersensitivity to oestrogen. Obstetric cholestasis affects 0.1%–1.5% of pregnancies in Europe and 9.2%–15.6% in South American countries (Milkiewicz et al., 2003). Symptoms include pruritus (intense sensation of itching) and jaundice (yellowing of the skin) and the condition is also associated with increased foetal mortality in late pregnancy and early delivery (Milkiewicz et al., 2003; Oude Elferink, 2003). Obstetric cholestasis is believed to be characterised by a reduction in bile formation caused by elevated levels of oestrogen during the last trimester. Oestrogen is believed to inhibit the canalicular transport mechanisms reducing the secretion of bile across the hepatocyte membrane causing bile stasis (Milkiewicz et al., 2002; Milkiewicz et al., 2003; Oude Elferink, 2003).

Other factors that can lead to cholestasis include rapid weight loss and total parenteral nutrition (TPN). Reduced intake of nutrients, particularly fats, associated with rapid weight loss diets suppresses the stimulation for the production and secretion of bile (Shiffman et al., 1991). TPN is a method of feeding used when there is dysfunction or disease of the digestive tract. TPN delivers nutrients in their basic molecular form, e.g. monosaccharides, amino acids, directly into the circulatory system via a central intravenous line. This method of delivery bypasses the digestive system and therefore disrupts the normal regulatory processes that stimulate the production and secretion of bile.

SUMMARY OF KEY POINTS

Pancreas

The pancreas sits posterior to the stomach.

It is made up of three lobes – the head, the middle and the tail.

The head connects to the duodenum, the entry into the small intestine.

The pancreas is both an endocrine gland and an exocrine gland.

Its endocrine function involves the secretion of the hormones insulin and glucagon from islet cells to regulate blood glucose levels. The exocrine function involves secretion of enzymes from acini cells that aid in the digestion of fats and proteins in the small intestine.

The exocrine glands secrete directly into the pancreatic duct.

Endocrine glands secrete hormones directly into the bloodstream.

The common bile duct from the liver is shared with the duct from the exocrine pancreas, which connects to the duodenum.

Acinar cells manufacture and secrete digestive 'juices' into the main pancreatic duct.

There are two types of secretions from the pancreas into the pancreatic duct – enzymes and bicarbonate. The bicarbonate neutralises acids in the duodenum and the enzymes help complete the process of digestion by breaking down nutrients into basic molecules so they can be absorbed across the small intestine mucosa. The three major enzymes produced by the pancreas that are vital for completion of digestion are proteases, lipase and amylase.

Bicarbonate – neutralises the acidity of the chyme arriving from the stomach increasing the pH from 1 to 8.

Pancreatic proteases – such as trypsin and chymotrypsin break down polypeptides to peptides. Peptidases, enzymes released from the brush border membrane of the intestinal enterocyte epithelial cells, break down peptides to amino acids, single molecules which can then be absorbed.

Pancreatic lipase converts tryglycerides into monoglyceride and free fatty acids.

Pancreatic amylase converts dietary starch to maltose (disaccharide).

There are several different types of cells that comprise the endocrine islets, these are as follows:

1. Alpha cells – Produce glucagon, which raises the level of blood glucose. Glucagon stimulates the conversion of glycogen into glucose in the liver (glycogenolysis). It also converts fat and protein into intermediate metabolites, which eventually are converted to glucose (gluconeogenesis).
2. Beta cells – Produce insulin which lowers the level of blood glucose. Insulin regulates the metabolisation of carbohydrates in the blood, as well as affecting the metabolisation of fats, and how the liver manages glucagon.
3. Delta cells – Produce somatostatin which inhibits the release of specific hormones. Somatostatin reduces the rate of absorption of food from the contents of the small intestine. Somatostatin is secreted by the hypothalamus and the small intestine as well.

Liver

The largest section of the liver lies in the right hypochondriac and epigastric regions of the abdominal cavity and the remainder extends across to the left hypochondriac.

The liver is in contact with the diaphragm superiorly.

The liver is divided into four lobes – anteriorly there are the right and left lobes which are separated by the falciform ligament and posteriorly the caudate and quadrate lobes.

Connective tissue throughout the liver divides the lobes into approximately 100,000 liver lobules. This connective tissue also acts as a form of scaffolding providing support for the many blood vessels, lymph vessels and bile ducts.

Liver lobules are the structural units of the liver.

Each lobule consists of a hexagonal arrangement of plates of hepatocytes which radiate out from a central vein which is at the centre of the lobule.

Hepatocytes are cells that make up between 70% and 80% of liver mass and carry out important metabolic and secretory functions and therefore have a high concentration of cellular organelles such as endoplasmic reticulum (smooth and rough) and Golgi apparatus for secretory functions.

Hepatocytes also have high numbers of mitochondria to provide energy to support the many metabolic functions on the liver.

Hepatocytes lie adjacent to endothelial cells which form the walls of the sinusoids.

Sinusoids are canal-like ducts lined with fenestrated endothelial cells.

The gap between the endothelium and the hepatocytes is called the 'space of Disse'.

The fenestrated endothelial cells (holes in the endothelium) allow plasma to drain between the cells forming lymph.

Blood supply of the liver

Blood enters the liver via the hepatic portal vein and hepatic artery at the porta hepatis (doorway to the liver). It then enters into the liver lobules (hexagonal shape) through six portal triads.

Blood entering the liver lobules travels along sinusoids (canal like structures) transporting the blood to the liver cells.

As blood flows through the sinusoids it comes into contact with hepatocytes which then absorb nutrients and secrete synthesised molecules.

From sinusoids blood then flows into the central vein, hepatic vein and then into the vena cava.

The many functions of the liver can be grouped under the following headings:

1. Storage – e.g. glucose, fat-soluble vitamins, minerals
2. Detoxification – e.g. drugs, alcohol, toxins, hormones
3. Phagocytes – pathogens, damaged cells
4. Synthesis – e.g. plasma proteins, amino acids (albumin, clotting factors).

The **main** role of the liver in terms of digestion is the production and secretion of bile.

Bile consists of water, electrolytes, bile acids, cholesterol, phospholipids and bilirubin. The primary functions of bile are to

1. Deodorise faeces – Bilirubin is converted to urobilinogen by bacteria in the colon.
2. Activate enzymes – The bile duct secretes bicarbonate-rich fluid to help neutralise acids in the duodenum.
3. Emulsify fats – Bile salts break down fats in preparation for action of lipase. The bile salts are then recycled.
4. Remove waste products from the body – Bilirubin (by-product from the breakdown of haemoglobin) is excreted in bile.

Gallbladder

It is located in the right hypochondriac region.

It is pear shaped and can be divided into three sections – fundus, corpus (or body) and the neck.

The fundus is a round blind-ended sac-like structure that normally extends beyond the liver's margin. It contains most of the smooth muscle of the organ.

The corpus (or body) is the main storage area for bile. It contains most of the elastic tissue and tapers into the neck.

The neck curves and is responsible for delivering bile to the cystic duct.

The function of the gallbladder is to store and release bile, a fluid made by the liver.

Bile contains bile salts formed in the liver from cholesterol, bile pigments (bilirubin and biliverdin) derived from haemoglobin, cholesterol and phospholipids.

Bile emulsifies (breaks down) fats.

The presence of fats in the duodenum stimulates enteroendocrine cells to release the hormone cholecystokinin into the circulatory system and on arrival at the gallbladder causes contraction of the gallbladder smooth muscle and bile is released.

Bile travels down the cystic duct, joining the common bile duct and then the pancreatic duct at the ampulla of Vater before delivering the bile into the duodenum through the major duodenal papilla of Vater where it mixes with chyme and begins the process of breaking down fats.

Most bile salts are reabsorbed in the small intestine and recycled to the liver.

CHECK ON LEARNING

Pancreas

What is trypsinogen and what does it do?
Answer – It is secreted from the pancreas; it helps digest proteins.

What enzymes are produced by the pancreas?
Answer – Proteases, lipases, amylases and nucleases are enzymes produced by the pancreas.

Where are the stem cells found that replace worn out intestinal epithelial cells?
Answer – Intestinal crypts.

What role does the pancreas play in creating the right environment in the duodenum so that enzymes can function?
Answer – Duct cells in the pancreas secrete bicarbonate which travels down the pancreatic duct entering the duodenum and neutralising the acid chyme, creating the right pH for enzyme activity.

Entero-endocrine cells in the duodenum produce the hormones, secretin and cholecystokinin. What effects do these hormones have on the pancreas?
Answer – Secretin causes the pancreas to release bicarbonate into the duodenum, and cholecystokinin causes the pancreas to release enzymes into the duodenum.

Liver

What is the liver's role in digestion?
Answer – The liver produces bile that emulsifies (breaks down) fats. Emulsification increases the surface area for the action of lipases which digest fats.

Describe the process for the conversion of red blood cells to bilirubin.
Answer – Haemoglobin breaks down into four polypeptide chains called globins. Each globin separates from its heme group, and each heme group further decomposes into iron and biliverdin, and biliverdin is converted into bilirubin.

Why does bilirubin need to be converted from unconjugated to conjugated bilirubin?
Answer – Unconjugated bilirubin is insoluble so it cannot be excreted. In the liver cells (hepatocytes) it is metabolised into conjugated bilirubin which is soluble. The process is called deconjugation. Conjugated bilirubin is soluble so it can be excreted into bile and transported to the duodenum.

Gallbladder

What is the function of the gallbladder?
Answer – It stores and concentrates bile.

Entero-endocrine cells in the duodenum produce the hormone cholecystokinin. What effect does this hormone have on the gallbladder?
Answer – Cholecystokinin causes the gallbladder to contract releasing bile into the biliary ducts and then into the duodenum.

Explain the pathway that bile takes from the gallbladder to the duodenum.
Answer – The pathway is as follows: cystic duct, common bile duct, hepatopancreatic ampulla and sphincter, duodenal papilla and duodenum.

CASE STUDY

Neonatal Jaundice

Sarah gave birth to her first child Michael. Sarah had a normal and uneventful pregnancy. Sarah is married to Tom; both are healthy with no significant past medical history. Sarah went into labour at 10 a.m. which was 1 day after her due date. Delivery was uncomplicated and both mother and baby Michael were comfortable. Two days later Sarah and Michael were released from the maternity unit. That evening Sarah noticed that Michael's eyes were yellow. Sarah phoned the maternity unit and spoke to the paediatrician. Sarah and Michael were recalled back to the unit and on examination the paediatrician informed Sarah and Tom that Michael has physiological neonatal jaundice.

The paediatrician explained to Sarah and Tom that neonatal jaundice is quite a common condition in neonates and that physiological jaundice is the most common type. The paediatrician explained that with this type the jaundice is the result of normal destruction of old or worn foetal red blood cells but an inability of the newborn's liver to process bilirubin effectively, a chemical produced when red blood cells are destroyed. This means the bilirubin accumulates in the blood leading to the yellow colouring of the eyes and the skin.

Michael's serum bilirubin levels are found to be quite high: 20 mg/dL, and the paediatrician informed Sarah and Tom that Michael needs phototherapy. It was decided that the phototherapy could be managed at home with daily testing of serum bilirubin levels. Phototherapy was successful, and 4 days later when the bilirubin levels dropped to less than 15 mg/dL the treatment was discontinued.

Explanation of normal and altered physiology

The following table sets out the normal and altered anatomy and physiology which explains the person's problems.

(*Continued*)

Normal anatomy/physiology	Altered anatomy/physiology and related problems
How is bilirubin removed prenatally? Prenatally the placenta performs the function of removing bilirubin.	*Explain two other causes of neonatal jaundice other than physiological jaundice.*
Where are old or worn out foetal red blood cells destroyed? The liver is responsible for the removal of old or worn out red blood cells from the circulation. Macrophages break down haemoglobin.	1. Increased haemolysis, e.g. polycythemia, Rh incompatibility. 2. Deficient conjugation of bilirubin (unconjugated hyperbilirubinaemia), e.g. breastfeeding – breast milk contains substances that interfere with conjugation. 3. Decreased excretion of bilirubin (conjugated hyperbilirubinaemia), e.g. biliary atresia, neonatal hepatitis.
What is the normal sequence of steps in the breakdown of haemoglobin? Haemoglobin breaks down into four polypeptide chains called globins. Each globin separates from its heme group and each heme group further decomposes into iron and biliverdin. Much of the biliverdin is converted into bilirubin. Unconjugated bilirubin travels in plasma, bound to albumin and enters the liver cells. Unconjugated bilirubin is insoluble so it cannot be excreted. In the liver cells (hepatocytes) it is metabolised into conjugated bilirubin which is soluble. The process is called deconjugation. Conjugated bilirubin is soluble so it can be excreted into bile and transported to the duodenum.	*What type of jaundice does Michael have?* Physiological jaundice. *What is the cause of excess bilirubin in normal physiological neonatal jaundice?* The excess bilirubin is not due to an abnormal level of red blood cell destruction. It is due to the inability of the young liver cells to conjugate bilirubin, or make it soluble in bile, so that it can be excreted and removed from the body by the digestive tract.
The liver excretes both biliverdin and bilirubin in bile. The bile is stored in the gallbladder and released into the small intestine. *What happens to bilirubin when it enters the intestine?* Once in the intestine the conjugated bilirubin is then metabolised by the bacterial flora to produce urobilin and stercobilin. It is stercobilin that gives stool its distinctive colour. The bilirubin is then eliminated with faeces.	*What causes the yellow colouration of Michael's skin and the sclera of his eyes?* The yellow coloration of the skin and sclera of the eyes are due to the accumulation of bilirubin in adipose tissue and its adherence to collagen fibres. This inability is corrected, usually within 1 week, as the liver cells synthesise the conjugation enzymes.
Bile salts perform two important functions. One function is to break down, or emulsify fat globules to smaller fat droplets. *What happens to bile salts when they have completed this function?* When bile salts have completed their function they are released back into the lumen of the small intestine and are transported with chyme to the terminal ileum. The majority of the bile salts are reabsorbed across the terminal ileum epithelium into blood and are then transported via the hepatic portal vein to the sinusoids in the liver lobules. Here the bile salts are then taken up by the hepatocytes and are effectively recycled so that they can be secreted again as an important constituent of bile.	*What affect can jaundice have on Michael's nervous system if the jaundice worsens?* High levels of bilirubin in the blood can cause destruction of nervous tissue and brain damage. *Describe a treatment for neonatal jaundice.* Phototherapy alters the chemical form of bilirubin, making it easier for the liver to excrete.

(Continued)

Background – initial investigations

The table below provides the rationale behind the investigations that Michael underwent to diagnose this condition.

Investigation	Result	Rationale
Full blood count Measurement of levels of specific types of bilirubin (conjugated/unconjugated)	Michael's bilirubin levels are 20 mg/dL 25 mg/dL is critical Serum unconjugated 12–25 mg/dL in healthy full-term is an indication for phototherapy	Jaundice usually becomes apparent when total bilirubin levels exceed 5 mg/dL; however, the clinical significance of bilirubin levels depends on postnatal age in hours. A bilirubin level of 12 mg/dL may be pathologic in an infant younger than 48 hours but is benign in an infant older than 72 hours. Discontinuation of home phototherapy is safe once the total serum bilirubin level has decreased to less than 15 mg/dL in healthy full-term infants older than 4 days.
Blood group and rhesus factor	Negative for antibodies	Detect antibodies against RBC seen in ABO/Rh incompatibility that may cause cellular damage and haemolytic anaemia.
Reticulocyte count	Normal levels of reticulocyte	Useful if the infant is anaemic to measure red blood cell production. Raised levels in cases of haemolysis.

CLINICAL CHALLENGES

1. What are the side effects of phototherapy?
2. What care should be provided during treatment with phototherapy?
3. What factors would you need to consider when explaining this condition to parents?

Chapter 7

THE LARGE INTESTINE

Specific learning outcomes
- Describe the embryonic development and gross anatomy of the large intestine and rectum.
- Describe the histology and physiological function of the large intestine and rectum.
- Describe the mechanisms governing motility within the large intestine and defaecation.
- Describe the processes governing absorption of water, electrolytes, vitamins and minerals.
- Describe the process governing the formation of faeces and defaecation.
- Discuss the physiological effects of ageing on the structure and function of the large intestine and rectum.
- Discuss common developmental abnormalities of the large intestine and rectum.
- Discuss common disorders of the large intestine and rectum.
- Explain the pathogenesis of common colonic and rectal disorders.
- Compare and contrast the normal physiology of the large intestine with the altered physiology seen with dysfunction of the large intestine.

The large intestine is the last stage of the journey for food residue (chyme). The functions of the large intestine can be summarised into three processes: absorption of water and electrolytes, formation and storage of faeces and fermentation of indigestible molecules such as cellulose by microbes in the colon.

PRENATAL DEVELOPMENT OF THE LARGE INTESTINE

The large intestine develops at a faster rate than the small intestine during the prenatal period but after birth this rate is reversed.

The ascending colon and the first two thirds of the transverse colon develop from the midgut. (Figure 7.1 shows where the large intestine develops from and Figure 7.2 shows overview growth and development during embryogenesis.) The remainder of the transverse colon, the descending colon, sigmoid colon, rectum and upper section of the anal canal develop from the hindgut. The endoderm of the hindgut forms the epithelial membrane and glands from the end of the midgut to the upper section of the anal canal. The lower section of the anal canal including the mucosa and glands develops from a structure called the proctoderm or anal pit. The lower part of the hindgut expands forming the cloaca. During week 4 of gestation the cloaca becomes divided by the development of a band of mesenchymal cells called the urorectal septum (tissue that grows into the cloaca). The upper section of the divided cloaca becomes the anal canal and the lower section becomes the rectum. Once the urorectal septum is formed the cloacal membrane divides into an anterior urogenital membrane and a posterior anal membrane. Towards the end of the seventh week the anal membrane breaks down and forms the anal opening. The cloacal membrane ruptures at the end of week 8 making the hindgut continuous with the outside of the embryo through the anus (Figure 7.3).

The longitudinal and circular muscles that make up the muscularis layers of the digestive tract develop from week 8. The early nervous system that innervates the gut wall begins to develop in week 5 but does not become fully mature until 6 months. The enteroendocrine cells responsible for secreting hormones into the lamina propria and circulation form from week 10. Goblet cells emerge around week 12. Brush border enzymes start to be secreted into the large intestine from around week 10. The rate of secretion increases up to week 20 and then secretion begins to reduce. Villi are initially found in the large intestine but these disappear after 12 weeks.

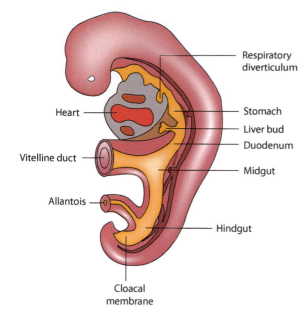

Figure 7.1 Growth and development of the large intestine: Showing midgut and hindgut locations.

POSTNATAL DEVELOPMENT AND THE ADULT LARGE INTESTINE

In a neonate the large intestine is approximately 40 cm in length. There will be a degree of variability regarding the length in children and adults but it is approximately 150 cm.

Gross anatomy

The large intestine starts at the point where chyme enters through the ileocaecal valve into the caecum (Figure 7.4). The opening of the ileocaecal value is controlled by the gastroileal reflex and the hormone gastrin. Food entering the stomach stimulates pressure receptors which trigger a neural response resulting in relaxation of the ileocaecal valve. The presence of nutrients in the stomach stimulates the release of the hormone gastrin which travels via the blood circulation leading to relaxation of the valve.

There are seven sections that make up the large intestine and they are caecum, ascending colon, transverse colon, descending colon, sigmoid colon, rectum and anus.

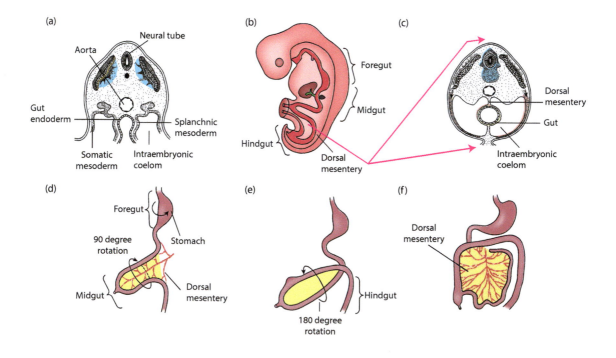

Figure 7.2 Growth and development of the large intestine: An overview. (a) 3 weeks gestation; (b and c) 5 weeks gestation; (d) 6-8 weeks with 90 degree rotation; (e) 10 weeks with 180 degree rotation and (f) 12 weeks gestation.

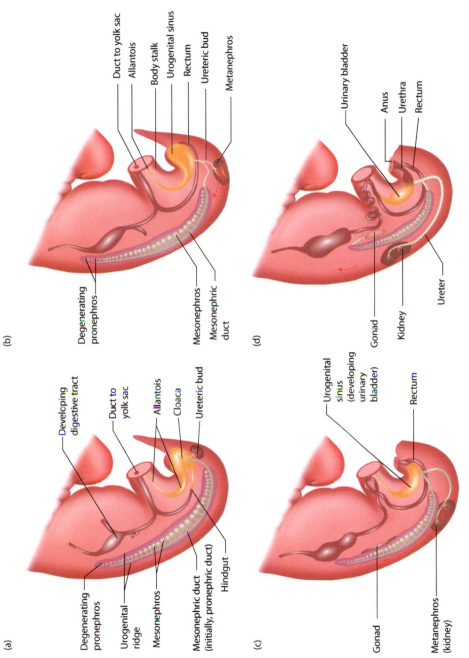

(a)

Degenerating pronephros

Developing digestive tract

Urogenital ridge

Duct to yolk sac

Mesonephros

Allantois

Cloaca

Mesonephric duct (initially, pronephric duct)

Ureteric bud

Hindgut

(b)

Degenerating pronephros

Duct to yolk sac
Allantois
Body stalk
Urogenital sinus
Rectum
Ureteric bud
Metanephros

Mesonephros
Mesonephric duct

(c)

Gonad

Urogenital sinus (developing urinary bladder)

Rectum

Metanephros (kidney)

(d)

Urinary bladder

Anus
Urethra
Rectum

Gonad

Kidney

Ureter

Figure 7.3 Formation of the anus. (a) Week 5; (b) Week 6; (c) Week 7; (d) Week 8.

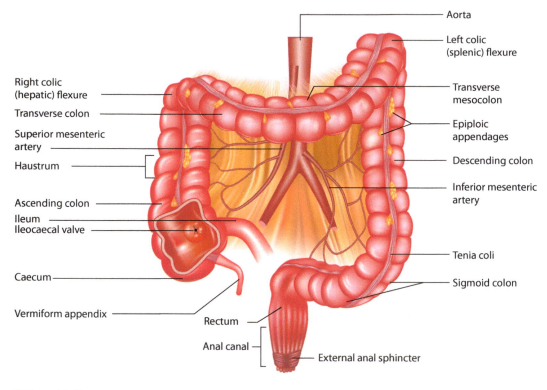

Aorta

Left colic (splenic) flexure

Right colic (hepatic) flexure

Transverse colon

Transverse mesocolon

Superior mesenteric artery

Epiploic appendages

Haustrum

Descending colon

Inferior mesenteric artery

Ascending colon

Ileum

Ileocaecal valve

Tenia coli

Caecum

Sigmoid colon

Vermiform appendix

Rectum

Anal canal

External anal sphincter

Figure 7.4 Large intestine.

The caecum lies beneath the ileocaecal valve and is continuous with the ascending colon. It has a 'pouch'-like structure and it is here that the process of compaction of chyme begins. The 'worm-like' structure that extends from the caecum is called the vermiform appendix. The appendix has a concentration of lymphoid tissue and is described as an organ of the lymphatic system. The appendix also provides a reservoir ideal for the multiplication of the microbes found within the large intestine. Food residue in the caecum moves up the ascending colon along the right lateral and posterior wall to the right colic (hepatic) flexure and then turns and becomes the transverse colon extending across the abdomen laterally from right to left. The transverse colon joins the descending colon at the left colic (splenic) flexure moving inferiorly along the left side of the abdomen where it joins the sigmoid colon. This is a short 'S'-shaped section of the colon that terminates in the rectum.

The main function of the rectum is the temporary storage of faecal matter. To help the rectum perform this function effectively it has an expandable structure. The rectum also has three lateral curves

or rectal valves which slow down the progression of faeces in the rectum (Figure 7.5). The rectal mucosa is made up of simple columnar epithelial cells (Figure 7.6). There are no villi or enzymes but an abundance of goblet cells serve to ease the passage of faeces and protect the lining from toxic substances produced by bacterial action. The arrival of faecal matter in the rectum triggers distention of the rectal walls bringing about the 'call to stool' or the urge to defaecate. The last section is the anorectal canal, the point at which waste material in the form of faeces leaves the body. The anorectal canal starts where the rectum penetrates the levator ani muscle (Figure 7.7). This region contains longitudinal folds called anal columns which then join transverse folds which mark the end of the simple columnar epithelial cells and the beginning of stratified squamous epithelial cells. The anorectal canal has two sphincters which control the movement of faeces out of the body, the internal and external sphincters, made up of circular bands of muscle. The internal sphincter is smooth muscle and is controlled by the parasympathetic system and is therefore not under voluntary control. The external

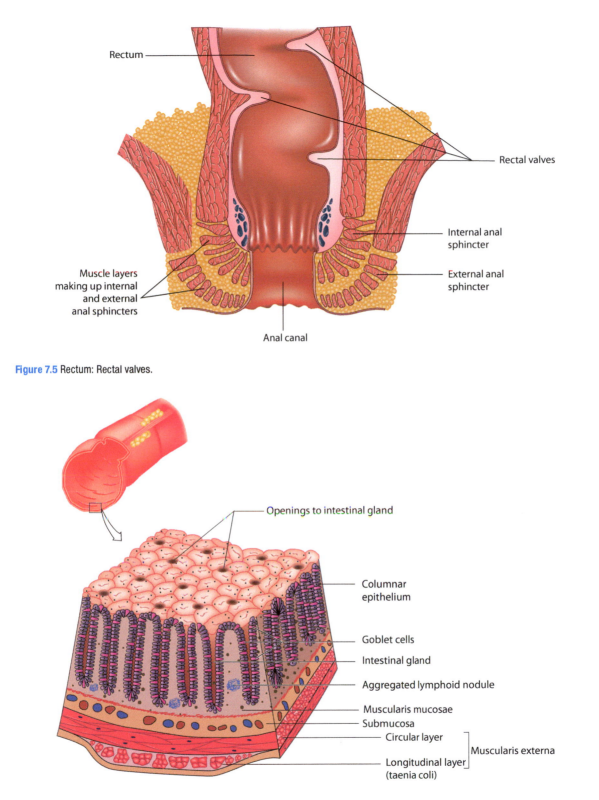

Figure 7.5 Rectum: Rectal valves.

Figure 7.6 Microscopic anatomy of the large intestine.

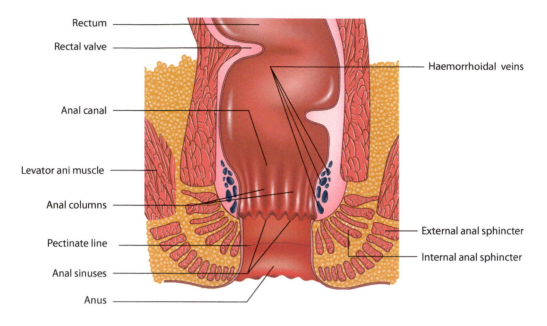

Figure 7.7 Anorectal canal.

anal sphincter is skeletal muscle and is therefore under voluntary control. The anal columns contain anal sinuses with an abundance of mucous-producing cells. When compressed by the passage of faeces down the anal canal these sinuses release mucus which further aids the passage of faeces out of the body. These squamous epithelial cells become keratinised at the margins where faecal matter leaves the body.

Functional histology

The histology of the large intestine shares many features of the small intestine. However there are differences and those differences reflect the specialist functions of the large intestine. In the small intestine the longitudinal muscle completely encircles the lumen, whereas in the colon it does not and instead is gathered into three bands called taenia coli, a unique feature of the large intestine. Increased tone of the taenia coli along the colon produces another unique feature called haustra. Haustra look like pouches and are separated by folds in the intestinal mucosa.

The large intestine has thinner walls than the small intestine and the mucosa is devoid of villi. This means there is much less surface area available for absorption. The surface of the mucosa is flat with many small holes leading to intestinal glands which extend deep into the lamina propria. These glands contain stem cells which replicate to produce the specialist cells that line the epithelium. The most abundant cells that line the epithelium are mucous-producing goblet cells. The secretion of mucous is triggered by short reflexes. Pressure and chemical receptors are stimulated by the presence of food residues in the large intestine bringing about short reflexes, coordinated by the nerve plexuses within the submucosa, resulting in secretion of mucous from the goblet cells. The mucous helps make the intestinal lining 'slippery' and also serves to lubricate faeces as it becomes more formed and compacted. The mucous also helps protect the epithelial lining from toxins produced by bacteria and the abrasive nature of formed stool. No enzymes are produced in the large intestine. Any digestion that does take place is carried out through bacterial action.

MOVEMENT WITHIN THE LARGE INTESTINE

According to Obermayr et al. (2013) neural development in the intestine is not fully mature until 5 years of age. The frequency of stool is variable across the lifespan due to developmental and physiological changes. This variability is also influenced by diet factors. Stool frequency during the first week after birth ranges from 1 to 9 stools per day. This is reduced to 1–7 stools between the second and twentieth weeks.

Meconium is produced in the immature intestines from about the 16th week of gestation. It is soft, greenish-black and consists of bile pigments, epithelial cells, mucus, swallowed amniotic fluid and fatty acids. The passing of meconium after birth is an indication that the lower intestines are patent. Postnatally, meconium is passed for approximately 2 days after birth. As the baby feeds the colour of the stool changes from greenish-black to greenish-brown which indicates the whole of the digestive tract is patent. When lactation is fully established the stool is soft and yellow.

There are two major processes that regulate the movement of food residue through the large intestine: mass movement and segmentation.

The passage of food residues along the colon shows considerable variation. The movement from the caecum up the ascending colon and in the transverse colon is similar to the process of segmentation seen in the small intestine. The presence of food residues in the haustra produces segmenting like contractions which move the contents backwards and forwards between the haustra. This process is called 'haustral shuttling' (Figure 7.8). This has the effect of slowing down the movement of food residues through the ascending and transverse colon, thereby providing more time for water and electrolytes to be absorbed by increasing the length of time the residues are exposed to the mucosa. These contractions are less significant in the descending and sigmoid colon and serve to mould the faeces into its generally recognised formed shape.

A second process of motility seen in the colon is mass movement. Mass movement is a term given to describe powerful peristaltic contractions that occur in the colon. These contractions occur three or four times a day, usually coinciding with mealtimes. After a meal, distension of the stomach and the duodenum trigger gastrocolic and duodenal colic reflexes, co-ordinated by nerve plexuses. These reflexes bring about a significant increase in colonic activity. Mass movement pushes faeces into the rectum, which is usually empty. Distension of the rectum stimulates the defaecation reflex. Defaecation is largely a spinal reflex mediated via the pelvic nerves and results in reflex (involuntary) relaxation of the internal anal sphincter followed by voluntary relaxation of the external anal sphincter.

Defaecation

During infancy and early childhood defaecation is an involuntary act. Defaecation changes from involuntary to voluntary as a learned behaviour. The movement of dietary residue into the rectum stimulates the sensory receptors in the rectal walls. Sensory stimulation leads to an autonomic nervous system response bringing about relaxation of the internal anal sphincter causing defaecation to occur. Rectal stimulation leads to contraction of the external anal sphincter allowing the person to choose when to defaecate. Figure 7.9 presents the physiology of defaecation.

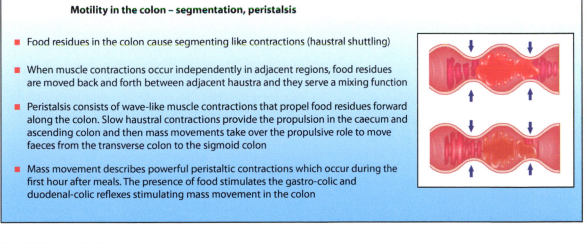

Motility in the colon – segmentation, peristalsis

- Food residues in the colon cause segmenting like contractions (haustral shuttling)

- When muscle contractions occur independently in adjacent regions, food residues are moved back and forth between adjacent haustra and they serve a mixing function

- Peristalsis consists of wave-like muscle contractions that propel food residues forward along the colon. Slow haustral contractions provide the propulsion in the caecum and ascending colon and then mass movements take over the propulsive role to move faeces from the transverse colon to the sigmoid colon

- Mass movement describes powerful peristaltic contractions which occur during the first hour after meals. The presence of food stimulates the gastro-colic and duodenal-colic reflexes stimulating mass movement in the colon

Figure 7.8 Haustral shuttling.

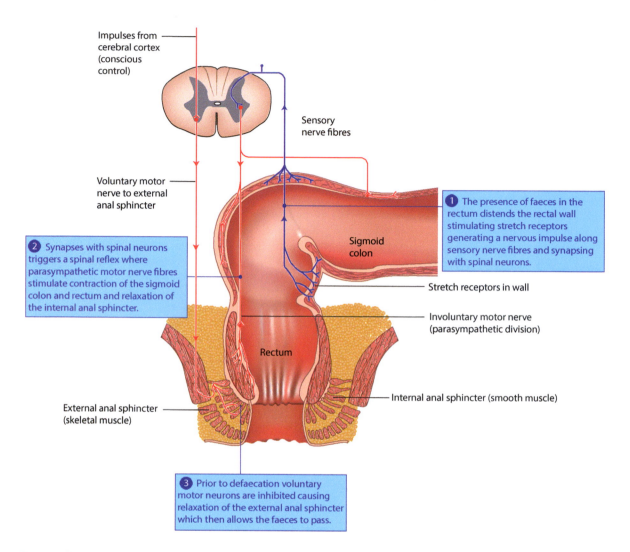

Impulses from cerebral cortex (conscious control)

Sensory nerve fibres

Voluntary motor nerve to external anal sphincter

1 The presence of faeces in the rectum distends the rectal wall stimulating stretch receptors generating a nervous impulse along sensory nerve fibres and synapsing with spinal neurons.

2 Synapses with spinal neurons triggers a spinal reflex where parasympathetic motor nerve fibres stimulate contraction of the sigmoid colon and rectum and relaxation of the internal anal sphincter.

Sigmoid colon

Stretch receptors in wall

Involuntary motor nerve (parasympathetic division)

Rectum

Internal anal sphincter (smooth muscle)

External anal sphincter (skeletal muscle)

3 Prior to defaecation voluntary motor neurons are inhibited causing relaxation of the external anal sphincter which then allows the faeces to pass.

Figure 7.9 Physiology of defaecation.

ABSORPTION FROM THE LARGE INTESTINE

A key function of the colon is to absorb water and electrolytes (sodium and chloride ions). Sodium absorption and anion exchange are believed to be poorly developed at birth but improve rapidly during the first year of life. This would explain why infants produce a very watery stool and why infants are more at risk from fluid and electrolyte imbalances.

The mechanism for water and electrolyte absorption is essentially similar to that seen in the small intestine. To summarise this process: sodium ions are transported from the intestinal lumen across the epithelium by the action of the sodium pump. The epithelial cells of the colon maintain a low intracellular gradient of sodium by pumping three sodium ions out of the cell for every two that come in. Sodium therefore moves into the cell down a concentration gradient and water goes with it. Sodium is then actively pumped out of the cell into the interstitial spaces and the water again goes with it. The sodium and water then diffuse into the capillary blood vessels that supply the colon tissues. Chloride ions are absorbed by exchange with bicarbonate. Secretion of bicarbonate into the intestinal lumen also serves to neutralise acids manufactured through the process of microbial fermentation.

There are a number of other substances that the colon absorbs. Microbial activity in the colon generates a number of important water-soluble vitamins. These include vitamin K which the liver needs to manufacture clotting factors, biotin which is needed for glucose metabolism and vitamin B_5 which is needed for the synthesis of steroid hormones and some neurotransmitters.

Microbial fermentation

Up until birth the foetal gut is sterile. After birth the neonate is exposed to bacteria and the gut quickly becomes colonised. The bacteria play an important role in the hydrolysis and fermentation of undigested carbohydrates which can then be used as an energy source. The large intestine does not produce any enzymes however the resident bacteria do, and it is these bacterial enzymes, such as cellulase, that can digest the complex carbohydrates not digested in the small intestine. Bacteria enter the colon via the anus and through the small intestine. Common colonic bacteria found in early infancy include enterobacter, bifidobacteria, bacteriodes and clostridium. Following weaning the resident colonic bacteria change to the type of flora found in adults.

Cellulose is a common component of our diet but we do not produce the enzyme cellulase which is needed to break it down. Bacteria in the gut produce this enzyme resulting in the production of the following substances: fatty acids, lactic acids, methane, hydrogen and carbon dioxide. Fermentation is therefore a major source of flatus in humans. Nitrogen, oxygen, carbon dioxide, hydrogen and methane are the primary gases that make up flatus. These gases do not give off an odour. The gases responsible for the distinctive odour flatus provides only make up a small part of flatus and they are hydrogen sulphide, scatols and indols. The make-up and volume of flatus are very much dependent upon what a person eats.

DEVELOPMENTAL ABNORMALITIES OF THE LARGE INTESTINE AND ANAL REGION

Intestinal malrotation and associated volvulus

Intestinal malrotation is a birth defect involving a malformation of the intestinal tract (Pickhardt and Bhalla 2002; Gamblin et al., 2003). During embryonic development the digestive tract starts as a straight tube and after 10 weeks' gestation the tube makes two rotations. Intestinal malrotation occurs when the tube does not make these turns (Figure 7.10a). This birth defect presents in a broad range of clinical manifestations based on different anatomical configurations ranging from abnormal intestinal position, to complete nonrotation, to reverse rotation (Kapfer and Rappold, 2004). Neonates will present with bilious vomiting, bloody stools and failure to thrive. Infants present with recurrent abdominal pain, intestinal obstruction, malabsorption, vomiting, common bile duct obstruction, abdominal distension and failure to thrive. Intestinal malrotation can lead to volvulus (twisted intestine) (Figure 7.10b) causing intestinal obstruction and in severe cases intestinal ischaemia and necrosis as the blood supply is interrupted. In adults in the extreme manifestation of intestinal malrotation, that is, with an associated volvulus, patients may present with a high-grade bowel obstruction and intestinal ischaemia (Palepu et al., 2007).

There are three types of volvulus: midgut, caecal and sigmoid volvulus. A midgut volvulus is diagnosed when there is a twisting of the small bowel around its mesenteric artery axis resulting in intestinal obstruction and an interruption of blood circulation leading to bowel ischaemia and necrosis (Papadimitriou et al., 2011). Volvulus of the small intestine is relatively uncommon and is associated with some form of a malrotation (Roggo and Ottinger, 1992). A midgut volvulus can be primary, that is without any underlying cause, or secondary to birth defects or acquired conditions. Small bowel volvulus is potentially life threatening, because of the risks of intestinal ischaemia, and therefore requires immediate surgical intervention. Primary midgut volvulus is more frequent in children and young adults and is rarely present in adults in whom secondary volvulus is more prevalent (Papadimitriou et al., 2011; Chi Ho Y, 2012). The annual incidence of midgut volvulus is smaller in Western countries (1.7–5.7 per 100,000 population) and larger in Africa and Asia (24–60 per 100,000 population) (Iwuagwu and Deans, 1999).

Volvulus in adults tends to occur most commonly in the sigmoid colon (70%–80%) and caecum (10%–20%) (Roggo and Ottinger, 1992). A colonic volvulus is diagnosed when part of the colon twists on its mesentery, resulting in obstruction. The main types

(a)

(b)

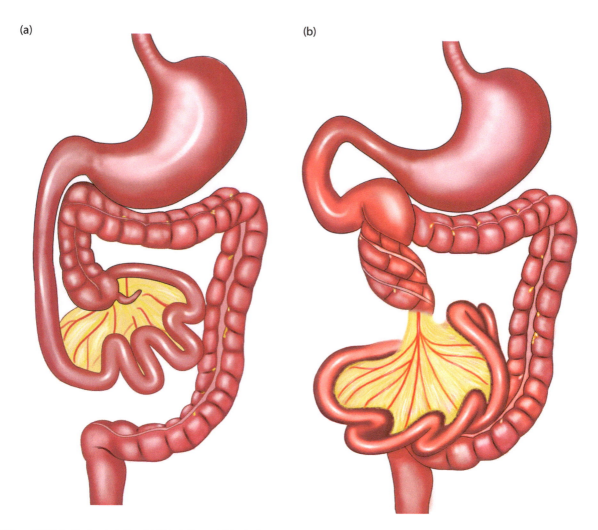

Figure 7.10 Intestinal malrotation. (a) Malrotation and (b) volvulus.

of colonic volvulus are sigmoid volvulus and caecal volvulus (Elsharif et al., 2012; Lianos et al., 2012). In the United States colonic volvulus is responsible for approximately 5% of all cases of intestinal obstruction and 10%–15% of all cases of large-bowel obstruction. In these populations, the most common site of large-bowel torsion is the sigmoid colon (80%), followed by the caecum (15%), the transverse colon (3%) and the splenic flexure (2%) (Halabi et al., 2014).

Anorectal malformations

Anorectal malformations are defects that occur in the 5th–7th weeks of gestation and are characterised by abnormal development of the anus and rectum and affect 1 in 5000 neonates (Pena and Levitt, 2006;

Levitt and Pena, 2007). Anorectal malformations can lead to the development of a number of abnormalities: the rectum may not connect to the anus, the anal passage may be narrow or in the wrong location, a membrane may cover the anal opening or the rectum may connect to the urinary tract or reproductive system via a fistula with no anal opening present (Pena and Levitt, 2006; Levitt and Pena, 2007). During the sixth week the structures that will eventually become the rectum and anus develop from an expanded section of the caudal hindgut called the cloaca. The cloaca then becomes divided by the growth of a band of mesenchymal cells called the urorectal septum (tissue that grows into the cloaca). The upper section of the divided cloaca becomes the anal canal and the lower section becomes the rectum. Once the urorectal septum is formed the cloacal membrane divides into an anterior urogenital membrane and a posterior anal membrane. Towards the end of the seventh week the anal membrane breaks down and forms the anal opening. The majority of anorectal malformations are a consequence of the abnormal partitioning of the cloaca by the urorectal septum. Figure 7.11 shows the different types of anorectal malformations (Pena and Levitt, 2006; Levitt and Pena, 2007). Imperforate anus

(see Figure 7.11d) is one of the more common developmental congenital malformations and it is characterised by the absence of a normal anal opening.

Exstrophy of cloaca

Exstrophy of cloaca is a rare congenital malformation that affects the lower abdominal wall structures. The cloaca is the part of the embryo that develops into these structures. A neonate with cloacal exstrophy is born with a section of the large intestine

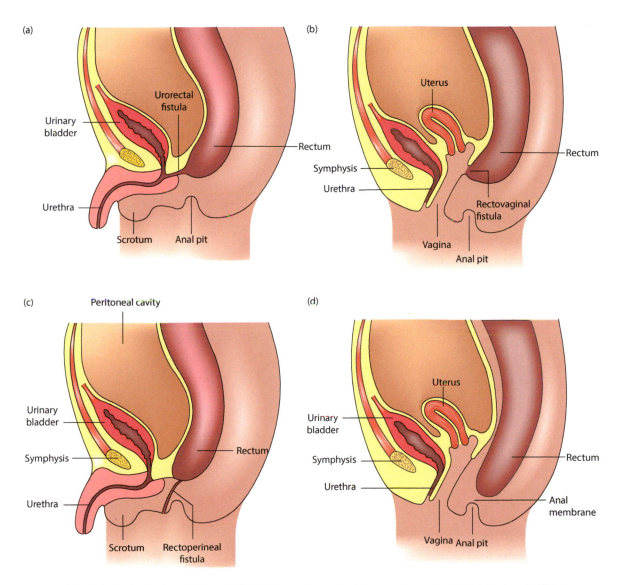

Figure 7.11 Gastrointestinal embryology. (a) Urorectal fistula (abnormal connection between rectum and urethra); (b) rectovaginal fistula (abnormal connection between rectum and vagina); (c) rectal atresia (abnormal narrowing/stenosis); and (d) imperforate anus (absence of a normal anal opening).

sitting outside the body (Warner and Ziegler, 2000). It occurs once in every 200,000–400,000 births (Manzoni and Hurwitz, 1998). There are a number of different theories that explain the embryological occurrence of exstrophy of cloaca. What these theories seem to suggest is that there is a defect in gastrulation in the caudal part of the embryo which affects the tail-folding of the embryo and this explains an oversized cloaca membrane (Manzoni and Hurwitz, 1998; Kallen et al., 2000). Gastrulation involves a series of cell migrations to positions where they will form the three primary cell layers: ectoderm, endoderm and mesoderm. The development of an oversized cloacal membrane creates a wedge effect which serves as a mechanical barrier to mesodermal migration. This results in the impaired development of the abdominal wall. Exstrophy of the cloaca occurs when the wedge effect occurs before the formation of the urorectal septum at week 6 (Smith et al., 1992; Kallen et al., 2000; Lund and Hendren, 2001).

Hirschsprung's disease

Hirschsprung's disease is a congenital motility disorder characterised by the absence of ganglion (nerve) cells (aganglionosis) of the myenteric and submucosal plexus (enteric nervous system) in the variable lengths of the digestive tract (Amiel and Lyonnet, 2001; Brooks et al., 2005). During embryonic development (5th–12th weeks' gestation) ganglion cells formed from the ectoderm germ layer start their growth in the mouth and finish in the anus forming ganglia between the muscle layers along the length of the digestive tract. In the large intestine this process starts at the top of the colon and ends at the rectum. In Hirschsprung's disease, this process does not finish and the ganglia do not form along the entire length of the colon (Figure 7.12). This can affect small or large sections of the colon. Studies carried out in the United States and Denmark estimated the incidence to be one case per 1500–7000 births (Russell et al., 1994; Meza-Valencia et al., 2005). Approximately

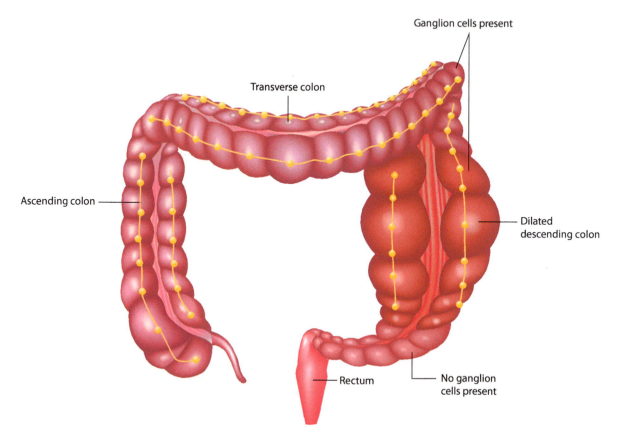

Figure 7.12 Hirschsprung's disease.

20% of infants will have one or more associated abnormalities involving the neurological, cardiovascular, urological and digestive system (Ryan et al., 1992). The absence of nerve cells in the digestive tract results in a failure to pass meconium, chronic severe constipation and colonic distention in the neonatal period (Iwashita et al., 2003). The lack of innervations of these cells stunts peristalsis, restricting propulsion of dietary residues along the colon. Dietary residues accumulate causing distension of the bowel.

CHANGES ASSOCIATED WITH DIFFERENT STAGES OF THE LIFESPAN

Diarrhoea

Damage or destruction of digestive epithelial cells leads to diarrhoea. Diarrhoea is a common clinical symptom defined by an increase in the volume of stool which commonly occurs when intestinal movement is too rapid for the absorption of water. The increase in volume can be attributed to a number of factors:

1. Inflammation or infection of the intestinal mucosa
2. Osmotic diarrhoea
3. Motility disorder

Inflammation or infection of the intestinal mucosa

The digestive system has a very robust defence against pathogens. However, sometimes these defences break down which can lead to damage and destruction of epithelial cells resulting in a secretory and inflammatory diarrhoea. Pathogens in the digestive system can cause diarrhoea in a number of ways. Some pathogens, like *Clostridium difficile* (*C. difficile* bacterium), a gram-positive spore-forming bacillus, are non-invasive (do not enter cells) but secrete toxins that stimulate fluid secretions from epithelial cells (McFarland, 2005). Others, like rotavirus (virus) and salmonella (rod-shaped gram-negative bacteria), are invasive and when they enter intestinal epithelial cells they trigger an immune response which leads to increased secretion into the lumen of the small intestine generating an inflammatory diarrhoea.

C. difficile is the most common bacterial cause of infectious diarrhoea in hospitalised patients (Bartlett, 2006; D'Souza, 2007). In the last 10 years, the number of patients diagnosed with *C. difficile*-related infections, such as *C. difficile*-associated diarrhoea (CDAD), has increased sixfold in England and Wales (D'Souza, 2007). *C. difficile* is one of a number of bacterial infections that have the ability to produce enzymes that can digest or damage the intestinal mucosa (Hopkins and Macfarlane, 2002; Banning, 2006). Toxins produced by the bacterium are also believed to stimulate the release of inflammatory cytokines (immune proteins), which increases the secretion and loss of fluid across the mucosal membrane and promotes inflammatory change within the intestinal mucosa (Banning, 2006; McFarland, 2005; Starr, 2005). This explains why many patients with *C. difficile* infection present with copious watery diarrhoea.

Salmonella is another bacterium that can cause diarrhoea but it is different to *C. difficile* because it is invasive (enters small intestine epithelial cells). Entry of salmonella into enterocytes leads to both an innate and specific immune response. Inflammation of intestinal tissue is caused by the accumulation of inflammatory cells (i.e. lymphocytes, macrophages and polymorphonuclear cells) in the infected epithelial cells. The arrival of these cells brings about cell activation with the release of various inflammatory mediators and cytokines into the intestinal lumen. This inflammatory secretion increases the volume of fluid in the intestine causing an inflammatory diarrhoea. Death or damage to the epithelial cells responsible for absorbing water and nutrients can also lead to an additional fluid volume in the intestine.

Other pathogens that can cause diarrhoea include viruses such as rotavirus and norovirus. Rotavirus diarrhoea is an illness that commonly affects young children. Rotavirus infection is the most common cause of severe diarrhoeal illness in children (Glass et al., 2006; Diggle, 2007). By the age of 5 years, nearly all children will have had rotavirus gastroenteritis (Parashar et al., 2003). Rotavirus gets its name from the wheel-like shape of the virus. Once ingested the virus attaches itself to the small intestine epithelial cells. It then enters the epithelial cells and produces a powerful enterotoxin (Glass et al., 2006; Diggle, 2007). This toxin destroys the epithelial lining causing blunting of villi, which in turn reduces the surface area for absorption and resulting in, among other symptoms, a profuse watery diarrhoea (Glass et al., 2006; Diggle, 2007).

Osmotic diarrhoea

Any factor that leads to the accumulation of excessive dietary nutrients in the intestinal lumen can lead to an osmotic diarrhoea. The absorption of water from the lumen of the intestines is reliant upon adequate absorption of nutrients. Malabsorption is a condition characterised by an inability to absorb certain nutrients. Carbohydrates have a major impact in osmotic diarrhoea. This condition is present in patients with coeliac disease where, as a result of damage to intestinal epithelial cells (caused by eating gluten), there is a lactose intolerance, in which damaged intestinal enterocytes (epithelial cells) fail to produce the enzyme lactase required to break down lactose (a disaccharide – too large to be absorbed) to glucose and galactose (monosaccharides – small enough to be absorbed). This means lactose stays within the intestinal lumen and exerts an osmotic effect, retaining water in the lumen and causing an osmotic diarrhoea. Damage to enterocytes by pathogens such as rotavirus and salmonella or inflammatory damage associated with autoimmune conditions such as Crohn's disease can reduce the ability of enterocytes to complete digestion and absorb nutrients. The corresponding buildup of unabsorbed nutrients in the intestine leads to retention of water in the intestinal lumen generating an osmotic diarrhoea.

An understanding of the causes and physiology of osmotic diarrhoea has led to the development of a number of laxatives designed to manage constipation. Osmotic laxatives work by retaining water in the intestinal lumen therefore helping to keep it soft. A commonly used osmotic laxative is lactulose. Lactulose is a sugar derivative which is broken down by bacteria in the large intestine into component sugars which cannot be absorbed and therefore function as an osmotic laxative, holding onto water in the lumen of the intestine (Chowdhury, 2006).

Motility disorders

Any factor that speeds up the transition time of chyme through the intestine can lead to diarrhoea. Increased motility means that water and nutrients do not remain in one place long enough for absorption to take place. The presence of chemicals and bacterial toxins can influence digestive motility through the stimulation of chemo-receptors which send nerve impulses to the enteric nervous system. Irritable bowel syndrome (IBS) can be characterised by frequent episodes of watery stool (Nunn, 2006). There seems to be a neurological component to IBS, and the condition seems to be aggravated by stress, though whether it plays a causative role is controversial. Emotions such as stress can influence digestive motility via the autonomic nervous system. Antibiotics and inappropriate use of laxative have also been shown to increase transit time.

Constipation

Normal bowel habit shows a great deal of variation among healthy adults. Bowel motions may vary from three times daily to three times weekly (Nazarko, 1996; Emmanuel, 2004). This has led to a range of definitions for constipation. Howie et al. (2003) define constipation as difficult and infrequent defaecation. Royle and Walsh (1992) define constipation as the existence of hard dry stools that are difficult to expel. Powell and Rigby (2000) define it as a sensation of incomplete evacuation of two or fewer bowel motions per week. Chowdhury (2006) define constipation as any factor that leads to a cessation or slowing of the transit time below what is considered normal which leads to more water being absorbed, the drying out of colon contents and the generation of a hard stool. One definition often used for research purposes is persistently difficult, infrequent or seemingly incomplete defaecation (Thompson et al., 1999).

Often constipation is wrongly considered to be a symptom of the ageing process. However, as argued by Harari (2002), this is a misconception as there is no evidence that healthy older people are any more constipated than younger people. Other factors and pathologies, commonly attributed to the older person, are the cause of constipation rather than age itself. A diverse range of risk factors have been identified for constipation which include both physical and psychological factors (Richmond, 2003; Prather, 2004). Stewart et al. (1992) describes additional potential risk factors for constipation in the older person which can increase incidence, and these include inadequate diet, immobility, dehydration, associated multiple drug use and concurrent illness (Table 7.1).

Constipation is associated with a number of pathophysiological diseases which can be grouped into two major types in the body. Constipation is therefore generally considered a symptom, rather than a disease in itself (Kamm, 2003; Duncan, 2004). The

Table 7.1 Some common causes of constipation

General	Drug induced
• Immobility	• Analgesics – codeine or opiates
• Neurological conditions – Parkinson's, multiple sclerosis, paraplegia disease	• Antacids – e.g. Aludrox (contains aluminium)
• Dehydration	• Antidepressants – amitriptyline, imipramine (tricyclic agents)
• Poor nutrition – poor fibre intake, weight loss diets	• Calcium antagonists – Nifedipine, verapamil
• Perianal discomfort	• Beta blockers – Propranolol, atenolol
• Anal fissure	• Iron supplements
• Haemorrhoids	• Diuretics (increased renal excretion)
• Pelvic floor muscle damage	• Antidiarrhoeals
• Obstruction – neoplasm, volvulus	
• Pregnancy	

Source: Adapted from Castledine G et al. 2007. *British Journal of Nursing* 16(18):1128–1131; Walker RD. 1997. *Practice Nursing* 8(4):20–22; Hicks A. 2001. *Journal of Orthopaedic Nursing* 5:208–211.

first pathophysiological type described is rectal outlet delay (also known as outlet obstruction or disordered defaecation) where the person has difficulty evacuating stool (Harari, 2002). Diseases and conditions that can lead to rectal outlet delay and chronic constipation include neurologic disorders such as Parkinson's disease or stroke (Wiesel and Bell, 2004). Also a condition called anismus which is characterised as a paradoxical (as opposed to a normal) contraction of the anal sphincter and pelvic floor (Preston and Lennard-Jones, 1985; Edwards et al., 1994). The second pathophysiological type described is slow colonic transit which occurs when colonic peristalsis is ineffective at facilitating the transport of stool to the rectum at a rate that prevents constipation (Müller-Lissner, 2002).

As well as the pathophysiological type, constipation can also be classified as either primary or secondary (Locke et al., 2000; Campbell et al., 2001; Smith, 2001). Primary constipation is characterised by extrinsic factors (causes are external to the body) such as reduced fibre and fluid intake or as a consequence of medications taken to manage other diseases. When constipation is the result of dysfunction in the body such as neurological, endocrine or obstructive disorders then the constipation is classed as secondary.

Primary constipation

Constipation in infants is rare and a common causative factor is diet. Constipation in childhood from year 1 onwards is most likely to be attributed to environmental factors or as a normal part of development. Reduced intake of food or a low fibre diet are common causes of constipation because they cause reduced stimulus for peristalsis and reduced stimulation of gastroileal and gastrocolic reflexes

leading to a slow colonic transit time (Norton, 1996, 2004; Müller-Lissner, 2002; Castledine et al., 2007). Reduced fluid intake or excessive loss of fluid can lead to dehydration which can exacerbate the absorption of water from the intestine causing drying out of food residues. Some medications such as codeine and stronger opiates have an effect on the muscles in the digestive tract, via the nervous system, slowing stool transit time. Normal peristalsis is achieved by contractions of the smooth muscle in the digestive tract, innervated by the autonomic nervous system. They slow down peristalsis and thus 'transit time'. Stool is therefore in the colon for longer and moves much more slowly through it. The longer it is there, the more water is absorbed and the more difficult it is to move and be expelled.

Secondary constipation

As explained earlier physiological abnormalities leading to constipation can be attributed to anorectal outlet obstruction and other obstructive disorders. Take for example a functional obstruction such as that seen in Hirschsprung's disease. Other obstructive disorders include imperforate anus which is a defect that is present from birth (congenital) where the opening to the anus is missing or blocked and intestinal strictures and other conditions like hypothyroidism. Constipation can also be caused by underlying pathology such as a tumour causing obstruction of the intestine or inflammation as seen with Crohn's and ulcerative colitis.

Possible causes of a neonate not passing meconium within the first 36 hours are Hirschsprung's disease, anal stenosis (or anal stricture) causing narrowing of the anal canal, intestinal atresia (a malformation causing a narrowing or absence of a portion of the intestine), hypothyroidism or a meconium plug. A slow transit time can also be caused by endocrine disorders such as Addison's disease (also known as primary adrenal insufficiency or hypoadrenalism), hypoparathyroidism where a lack of parathyroid hormone leads to decreased blood levels of calcium (hypocalcemia), hypothyroidism and phaeochromocytoma (a tumour of adrenal gland tissue causing excessive secretion of epinephrine and norepinephrine). Endocrine-induced constipation is also attributed to the changes associated with pregnancy (Müller-Lissner, 2002). Neurological conditions causing a slow transit time leading to chronic constipation include spinal cord injury, diabetic neuropathy, multiple sclerosis and Parkinson's disease.

Behavioural factors are also important contributors to constipation, for example individuals who ignore the 'call to stool' delay defaecation and extend the length of time dietary residues remain in the intestine. This delay provides more opportunity for water absorption and drying and hardening of stool. Constipation during pregnancy is common due to hormonal changes which have an impact upon the bowel. It is also common immediately after birth because of perineal trauma occurring in approximately 15%–20% of deliveries (Saurel-Cubizolles et al., 2000).

There are many potential complications associated with constipation. Common complications include abdominal distension and pain, nausea, vomiting, fatigue and headache. If undetected or left untreated constipation will progress on to more serious complications such as faecal impaction identified as a major cause of faecal incontinence in older people in long-term care (Barrett et al., 1989; Schaefer and Cheskin, 1998; Lamers, 2000; O'Mahony et al., 2002).

Diverticulosis

Diverticular disease is a general term that covers a number of conditions that include diverticulae, diverticulosis and diverticulitis. Diverticulosis is a condition which affects the mucosal layer of the colon, primarily affecting the older person and on the left side of the colon in Western populations. In Asian populations it has also been shown to affect younger people with the disease being more commonly located on the right side of the colon rather than left (Yang et al., 2004) suggesting both genetic and environmental causal factors. Recent research by Strate et al. (2013) has also strengthened the argument for both environmental and genetic causal factors by reporting that the pattern of disease changes among migrating populations and by reporting that twin studies show that 40%–53% of susceptibility to diverticular disease is due to inherited factors.

Diverticular disease is highly prevalent in Western countries with incidence rising with increasing age. According to Ferzoco et al. (1998) 5%–10% of the population over 45 years of age is affected and 80% of people above the age of 85% are affected. Whiteway and Morson (1985) reported that 30% of those aged over 60 years have the disease. Geographic regions with low fibre intake have been shown to have higher rates of diverticular disease (Burkitt et al., 1972; Brodribb and Humphreys, 1976; Gear et al., 1979). The incidences of diverticular disease continue to rise in the United Kingdom. According to Gaglia and Probert (2015) admission rates in the United Kingdom rose from 0.56 to 1.20/1000/year during the decade 1996–2006. In 2009 in the United States diverticular disease was found to be the most common inpatient digestive diagnosis with 283,355 hospitalisations (Shahedi et al., 2012).

Diverticular disease is therefore a multifactorial condition. Diverticula are pouch-like structures thought to develop from age-related degeneration of the mucosal wall and segmental increases in colon pressure that develop between the longitudinal muscle bands of the haustra at the site where the blood vessels move through the circular muscle layer bringing blood to the mucosal layer (Figure 7.13). This age-related degeneration also includes shortening of the taenia coli (longitudinal muscle layer), thickening of the circular muscle layer and neural degeneration leading to a reduction of neurons in the myenteric plexus. Diverticulosis describes the presence of multiple diverticula. It normally affects the sigmoid and descending colon but can occur anywhere in the colon. If there is a weakness in the colon wall any increase in pressure within the lumen of the colon can lead to the mucosal layer herniating through the muscularis layer. Until recently it was believed that the primary cause of the diverticula was a low fibre diet. It was believed that modern refined low-fibre diets can lead to hypertrophy of the colon wall which causes high intraluminal pressure leading to rigidity, fibrosis and eventually protrusion of the mucosa through the muscularis layer forming long and narrow pouches called diverticulae. This belief that the primary cause of diverticula is a low-fibre diet was

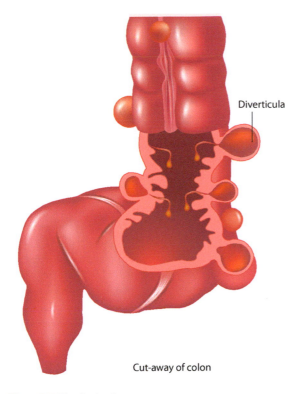

Diverticula

Cut-away of colon

Figure 7.13 Diverticular disease.

based upon observational data comparing the prevalence of diverticular disease in Western populations to that in rural Africa which showed that the prevalence in rural Africa was much lower than the West. This led to the assumption that the lack of dietary fibre predisposed the Western population to diverticulosis (Gaglia and Probert, 2015). However a large recent study by Peery et al. (2012) using colonoscopy screening on asymptomatic patients found that fibre intake was not correlated with the presence of diverticula. More importantly though, their research reported a positive association between diverticulosis and increased frequency of bowel movements and higher intake of fibre. Research carried out by Crowe et al. (2011) found that patients consuming more than 26 g/day of dietary fibre had a 42% lower risk of hospitalisation for diverticular disease compared with those consuming less than 14 g/day. This research suggests that the role played by fibre relates more to protection and prevention of diverticular disease rather than in the formation of diverticula.

Although, as shown, the mechanism of the formation of diverticula is poorly understood, the pathophysiological mechanisms for the chronic symptoms of diverticular disease are well known. Acute diverticulitis is believed to be caused by trapped faecal material within the diverticulum, causing irritation of the mucosa leading to inflammation. The inflammation may also be associated with a microperforation of the diverticula sac giving the faecal microbiota access to the lamina propria, leading to acute inflammation. Microperforation can also lead to the formation of an abscess and fistula formation. Perforation of the diverticula is potentially a life-threatening situation causing peritonitis. Prolonged or recurrent inflammation can lead to fibrosis and strictures. Alongside these complications patients with diverticulitis, in Western populations, generally present with left lower quadrant pain, leucocytosis (elevated white blood cell count), fever and diarrhoea. Dysuria may also be present secondary to the irritation of the bladder by the inflamed colon (Coyne and Kalbassi, 2014; Gaglia and Probert, 2015).

Adenomatous polyps

Adenomatous polyps are the most common type of neoplasm in the intestine and more than 80% of colorectal tumours develop from this type of polyp. A polyp or polypoid lesion consists of a mass of tissue that grows from the mucous membrane and protrudes into the colon of the intestine (Kudo et al., 2000; Schulmann et al., 2002; Geboes et al., 2005). Polyps are classified by the way they attach to the mucosa: pedunculated polyps are attached by a stalk and sessile polyps are raised nodules. Colorectal polyps are also classified as neoplastic (adenomatous) and non-neoplastic (hyperplastic) (Geboes et al., 2005). Adenomatous polyps develop when the crypt epithelial cells ignore inhibitory growth factor and start to replicate uncontrollably creating a mass of cells that may be benign or malignant. These new tumour cells grow in an erratic and uncoordinated way and there may be diminished apoptosis (cell death), persistence of cell replication, and failure of maturation and differentiation of the cells that migrate to the surface of the crypts. Alterations in cell differentiation can lead to dysplasia and the development of a malignant carcinoma (Kudo et al., 2000; Shulmann et al., 2002; Geboes et al., 2005). Adenomatous polyps are therefore premalignant lesions of colorectal cancer which can transform into malignant tumours. Adenomatous polyps are detected in 33% of the general population by age 50 and 50% of the population by age 70 (Shulmann et al., 2002). Research has established a relationship between colorectal adenomas and carcinomas. It can take between 5 and 10 years for an adenomatous polyp to develop into colon cancer.

Colorectal cancer

Colorectal cancer is the fourth most common cancer in males and the third most common in females in the world and represents between 11% and 17% of all new cancer cases. Approximately 1% are attributed to chronic inflammatory bowel disease such as ulcerative colitis and Crohn's disease where persistent tissue injury caused by inflammation can lead to cancerous changes (Geboes et al., 2005). And 5% are attributed to inherited genetic mutations such as familial adenomatous polyposis (FAP) (Shulmann et al., 2002). FAP is a rare inherited condition where during early adulthood multiple polyps (in some cases thousands) grow in the colon. If left untreated these polyps can develop into colon cancer (Geboes et al., 2005). The remaining 94% are believed to be spontaneous where environmental or other factors such as dietary factors (red meat, low fibre), alcohol, smoking and obesity can trigger genetic changes leading to cancer (Willett et al., 1990; Giovannucci et al., 1992; Heavey and Rowland, 2004). Colorectal cancer has also been shown to increase with age with 90% of cases being reported over the age of 50 (Smith et al., 2004).

The involvement of colonic bacteria in colorectal cancer has also been studied and increased numbers of bacteroides have been associated with increased risk of colon cancer (Heavey and Rowland, 2004). Bacteroides make up a major proportion of gut flora. Intestinal bacteria have also been shown to produce, from dietary components, substances which are carcinogenic (Moore and Moore, 1995; Heavey and Rowland, 2004).

Ulcerative colitis

Inflammatory bowel disease (IBD) is a general term that describes two related disorders: ulcerative colitis (UC) and Crohn's disease (CD). The two diseases have much in common: they both have patterns of familial inheritance, both cause inflammation of the bowel and both share similar systemic changes. Both UC and CD appear to be caused by an overly aggressive cell-mediated immune response to endogenous factors in genetically susceptible individuals. For a more in-depth examination of the pathogenesis of IBD read the section 'Crohn's disease' in Chapter 5. Although CD and UC share many characteristics there are also a wide range of immunological changes associated with each condition that require them to be identified separately (see Table 7.2 comparing CD and UC and Figure 7.14 comparing macro and micro

Table 7.2 Comparisons of various factors in Crohn's disease and ulcerative colitis.

	Crohn's disease	Ulcerative colitis
Terminal ileum involvement	Commonly	Seldom
Colon involvement	Usually	Always
Rectum involvement	Seldom	Usually
Involvement around the anus	Common	Seldom
Bile duct involvement	No increase in rate of primary sclerosing cholangitis	Higher rate
Distribution of disease	Patchy areas of inflammation (Skip lesions)	Continuous area of inflammation
Endoscopy	Deep geographic and serpiginous (snake-like) ulcers	Continuous ulcer
Depth of inflammation	May be transmural, deep into tissues	Shallow, mucosal
Fistulae	Common	Seldom
Autoimmune disease	Widely regarded as an autoimmune disease	No consensus
Cytokine response	Associated with T_h17	Vaguely associated with T_h2
Granulomas on biopsy	May have non-necrotising non-peri-intestinal crypt granulomas	Non-peri-intestinal crypt granulomas not seen
Surgical cure	Often returns following removal of affected part	Usually cured by removal of colon
Smoking	Higher risk for smokers	Lower risk for smokers

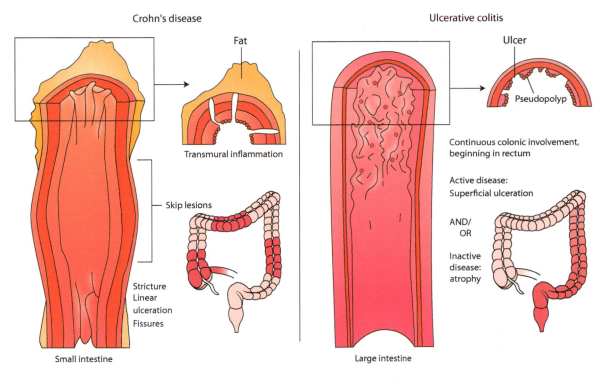

Figure 7.14 Comparison of the macro- and micro-histology of Crohn's disease and ulcerative colitis.

histology of CD and UC). This section focuses on the characteristics of ulcerative colitis.

Unlike Crohn's disease UC only affects the colon and rectum and is mainly confined to the mucosa although in some incidences it can progress to the submucosa. The disease is characterised by lesions that develop in the crypts of Lieberkühn. Inflammation of the mucosa causes small haemorrhages which can develop to become abscesses. These abscesses can become necrotic and lead to ulceration. Tongue-like structures can also develop from the mucosa and these are termed pseudopolyps. Repeated episodes of inflammation lead to the development of a thicker mucosa.

SUMMARY OF KEY POINTS

Large intestine (large bowel)
Receives the end products of digestion from the ileum which are predominantly water and cellulose.

The ileum terminates in a smooth muscle sphincter, the ileo-caecal valve. As this sphincter opens, chyme enters the caecum, a blind pouch at the beginning of the large intestine.

The large intestine consists of the following areas – the caecum, the ascending colon, the right colic flexure (hepatic flexure), the transverse colon, the left colic flexure (splenic flexure) and the descending colon. At the level of the iliac fossa, the colon curves to the right and at the body's midline curves again downward.

This curvaceous region is called the sigmoid colon (S-shaped). The appendix is a short, hollow extension from the caecum. Its walls are filled with lymphoid nodules.

The wall of the colon shows a number of variations from the rest of the digestive tract:

1. Haustra are pocket-like sacs in the wall of the colon.
2. Three longitudinal bands of smooth muscle, the taenia coli, are visible on the outer surface of the colon. The steady tone in this muscle is responsible for the pouch-like haustra.
3. The epiploic appendages are small, fat-filled pockets protruding through the serosa of the colon.

(Continued)

4. The mucosa is folded but has no villi.
5. The epithelium is simple columnar with a concentration of mucous cells.

Functions of the large intestine include the following:

1. Haustral churning, peristalsis and mass movement move the contents along the large intestine.
2. Bacteria digest protein and produce vitamins B and K.
3. The cells of the epithelium absorb water, ions and vitamins.
4. It forms faeces ready for defaecation.

Remaining portions of the digestive tract include the following:

1. The rectum is essentially the same structure as the colon.
2. At the end of the rectum, small longitudinal folds in the wall form the structures called rectal columns.
3. The anorectal canal is just distal to the rectal columns. Here the epithelium changes to stratified squamous.

Movement in the large intestine – two types:

1. Segmentation – the presence of food residues in the hausta produces segmenting-like contractions which move the contents backwards and forwards between the haustra (haustral shuttling).
2. Mass movement – powerful peristaltic contractions that occur three or four times a day, usually coinciding with mealtimes. Distension of the stomach by food brings about gastrocolic and duodenal colic reflexes, coordinated by nerve plexuses, these reflexes bring about a significant increase in colonic activity. Mass movement pushes faeces into the rectum, which is usually empty.

Defaecation – distension of the rectum stimulates the defaecation reflex, a spinal reflex mediated via the pelvic nerves and results in reflex relaxation of the internal anal sphincter followed by voluntary relaxation of the external anal sphincter.

The anus – the epithelium becomes keratinised stratified squamous.

The circular smooth muscle layer in this region forms the internal anal sphincter. Just distal to this structure is the external anal sphincter. The external sphincter is formed by the skeletal muscle of the perineal membrane and is under voluntary control.

CHECK ON LEARNING

Large intestine

What causes the colon to be puckered into pockets called haustra?
Answer – The cause includes three bands of smooth muscle called taeniae coli.

What are the functions of the internal and external anal sphincter?
Answer – The internal anal sphincter is under involuntary control (circular smooth muscle) and the presence of stool in the rectum causes a reflex which brings about relaxation of the sphincter and an urge to pass stool. The external anal sphincter is under voluntary control (circular skeletal muscle) and when the person relaxes this sphincter defaecation follows.

What type of epithelial cells is the anus lined with and why?
Answer – It is lined with stratified squamous epithelium – flattened, tightly packed cells designed to allow the smooth transition of faeces from the rectum out of the body.

CASE STUDY

Altered colorectal function

Ben is a 36-year-old man with learning difficulties. He had been admitted with generalised abdominal pain and is unable to give a clear history. His carers describe a recent flu-like illness during which Ben lost his appetite and was given analgesics to lower his temperature (2 weeks ago). He recovered after several days. During that time and since then, Ben has not regained his appetite fully and he was reluctant to drink while he was unwell. He spent several days in bed while he was poorly, but was not given antibiotics at any time. Since the flu-like illness Ben has been constipated but in the last few days appears to have developed incontinence of faeces, passing 'diarrhoea' several times a day. On examination his abdomen is generally tender and distended. His perineal area is excoriated.

Ben's problem is due to constipation. Look at the table below and see if you can work out why.

Explanation of normal and altered physiology

The following table sets out the normal and altered anatomy and physiology which explains the person's problems.

(Continued)

Related normal physiology	Altered anatomy/physiology and related problems
What reflexes trigger defaecation?	*How would large bowel reflexes be affected by Ben's loss of appetite?*

What reflexes trigger defaecation?

The gastrocolic reflex is initiated by eating and causes a mass wave of peristalsis through the colon, pushing the contents to the rectum.

Distention or stretch in the rectum initiates the defaecation reflex causing depolarisation of afferent fibres which synapse with spinal cord neurons. Parasympathetic efferent fibres cause contraction in the rectal muscularis and opening of the internal anal sphincter. The external sphincter is usually under voluntary control and is opened only when it is convenient to defaecate.

A regular, high-fibre diet, high fluid intake and physical exercise all contribute to colonic motility (peristalsis).

Explain the two types of movement in the large intestine.

1. Segmentation – the presence of food residues in the hausta produces segmenting-like contractions which move the contents backwards and forwards between the haustra (haustral shuttling).
2. Mass movement – powerful peristaltic contractions that occur three or four times a day, usually coinciding with mealtimes. Distension of the stomach by food brings about gastrocolic reflexes, coordinated by nerve plexuses, these reflexes bring about a significant increase in colonic activity. Mass movement pushes faeces into the rectum, which is usually empty.

The volume of stool residue entering the adult colon daily is approx. 500 mL. 150 mL is excreted.

Normal faeces bulk is made up of fibre and other food residue, bile pigments, bacteria and water and mucus secreted by the bowel wall.

The integrity of the anal sphincter and the semi-solid nature of faeces usually mean that the perineal and perianal areas are kept 'clean' and the skin intact.

How would large bowel reflexes be affected by Ben's loss of appetite?

While ill, Ben did not eat normally and so his gastrocolic reflex will have been muted at this time; thus the peristalsis will have been weaker. Without the usual gastrocolic reflexes the defaecation reflex is not stimulated and so a feeling of wanting to open the bowels is lost. If the defaecation reflex is ignored it will cease until the next peristaltic wave.

Which of these is Ben lacking and how have they contributed to the problem?

While ill Ben ate less, and drank less and will have lost fluid with his fever. While he was in bed he will not have taken any exercise. It might be that he did not have a particularly high fibre or fluid intake anyway which will have contributed to the problem.

Less food means less fibre and stimulus for peristalsis and reflexes.

Less fluid means dehydration and harder, drier stool.

Less exercise means less peristalsis and reduced reflexes.

Some antipyretics or analgesic drugs contain codeine. These and stronger opiate analgesics have an effect on the muscles in the gut via the nervous system.

What is this and how might it contribute to Ben's problem?

They slow down peristalsis and thus 'transit time'. Stool is in the colon for longer and moves much more slowly through it. The longer it is there, the more water is absorbed and the more difficult it is to move and expel.

How could Ben's pyrexia contribute to his constipation?

When pyrexial, more fluid is lost in sweating and an increased metabolic rate. This coupled with a reduced stimulus to empty the bowels means stool is in the colon for longer. As a result of this more water is absorbed and the stools get harder and harder.

Ben's diarrhoea is due to faecal impaction, not a true diarrhoea. His colon and rectum are full of hard stool which he now cannot pass. Secretion of *mucous* and the action of *bacteria* in the colon result in the liquefaction of the constipated faeces which leak out as 'spurious' diarrhoea.

Why is Ben's perineal skin excoriated?

Due to the 'overflow' diarrhoea he is incontinent. This is not unusual as the person cannot feel the fluid in the rectum or that it is leaking out due to the impaction with the solid faeces. The action of faeces on the skin is irritating due to enzymes and bile salts within the faeces. He needs to be kept clean to avoid this and to improve it despite the pain. It is basically like 'nappy rash' and needs to be avoided.

CLINICAL CHALLENGES

1. Find out how the patients' usual bowel habit is recorded and how and where their bowel actions are monitored while in your area.

2. If this does not happen ask why not and whether it should.
3. Find out how many patients are prescribed a laxative and why.
4. What factors can cause constipation – explain the mechanisms involved for each.

CASE STUDY

Hirschsprung's disease or congenital aganglionosis

A newborn infant was observed to have a distended abdomen. She had passed very little meconium in the two days since she had been born. The doctor examined the infant's rectum by inserting a finger. The examination revealed that the rectum was empty. However, when the doctor withdrew his finger there was a gush of meconium and decompression of the abdomen. The obstruction reoccurred within a day or so. By this time the child had started to vomit excessively. The symptoms were relieved by an enema. A biopsy of the rectum was performed and Hirschsprung's disease was diagnosed. An abdominal operation was arranged. The surgeon removed the distal large bowel and sutured the remaining colon to the lower rectum. The infant made a good recovery and her symptoms disappeared.

Explanation of normal and altered physiology

The following table sets out the normal and altered anatomy and physiology which explains the person's problems.

Normal anatomy/physiology	Altered anatomy/physiology and related problems
How is motility generated in the large intestine? 1. Segmentation – the presence of food residues in the hausta produces segmenting-like contractions which move the contents backwards and forwards between the haustra, 'haustral shuttling'. 2. Mass movement – powerful peristaltic contractions that occur three or four times a day, usually coinciding with meal times. Distension of the stomach by food brings about gastrocolic reflexes, coordinated by nerve plexuses, these reflexes bring about muscle contraction and a significant increase in colonic activity. Mass movement pushes faeces into the rectum, which is usually empty.	*How does Hirschsprung's disease affect motility in the colon?* The neonate has been diagnosed with Hirschsprung's disease. This is a condition where the nerves that regulate motility in a section of the colon are missing. This means that segmentation and peristalsis will not function in this section and therefore waste material cannot move through. *Why was the neonate's abdomen distended?* Without peristalsis the waste material remains in the affected section causing a blockage. The buildup of waste material leads to a distended bowel and abdomen. This also explains why the neonate did not pass any meconium after she was born.
What germ layer is responsible for the development of the enteric nervous system during embryonic development? Ectoderm layer – Both the myenteric plexus and the submucosal plexus are absent in Hirschsprung's disease. *What function do these nerve plexi perform in the colon?* 1. Myenteric plexus – regulates peristalsis (movement through the colon). 2. Submucosal plexus – regulates secretion of mucous from glands in the colon wall which help protect the epithelial lining and aid the movement of waste during peristalsis.	*What is the cause of Hirschsprung's disease?* Hirschsprung's disease is a congenital disorder. During embryonic development (5th–12th week) nerve cells form from the ectoderm layer of germ cells. The nerve cells start their growth in the mouth and finish in the anus. With Hirschsprung's disease nerve cells stop growing at a certain point in the colon. It is unclear why this growth stops.
What is the difference between defaecation in infancy and early childhood and defaecation in adults? In infancy and childhood defaecation is involuntary and in adults it is voluntary.	*Approximately 80% of children diagnosed with Hirschsprung's will have had symptoms within the first six weeks of life. List four of these symptoms.* 1. No bowel movement in the first 48 hours after birth 2. Distended abdomen 3. Vomiting 4. Fever caused by inflammation of the colon (enterocolitis)

(Continued)

What are the functions of the colon?
Transportation of waste material from the caecum to the rectum
Absorption of water and electrolytes
Microbial activity generates a number of important water-soluble vitamins. These include vitamin K (important for clotting), biotin (needed for glucose metabolism) and vitamin B_5 (needed for the synthesis of hormones and some neurotransmitters).

What is meconium and when does it appear in the foetal development?
It is a soft, greenish-black substance that consists of bile pigments, epithelial cell mucous, swallowed amniotic fluid and fatty acids. Meconium is produced in the immature intestines from about the 16th week of gestation.

After birth why does the stool change from greenish black to greenish-brown and then to soft yellow?
As the baby takes feeds, the colour of the stool changes from greenish-black to greenish-brown which indicates the whole of the digestive tract is patent. When lactation is fully established the stool is soft and yellow.

If only a small section of the colon is affected by Hirschsprung's disease the condition might not be diagnosed until many years later.

What affect could Hirschsprung's have on growth and development?
If Hirschsprung's disease is not diagnosed early on it can lead to worsening constipation, loss of appetite, problems absorbing nutrients, leading to weight loss and delayed or slowed growth.

Why is the absence of meconium after birth an indication of Hirschsprung's disease?
If there is no passing of meconium after birth this is an indication that the lower intestines are not patent. Normally, meconium is passed for approximately two days after birth.

Background – initial investigations

The table below provides the rationale behind the investigations that the neonate underwent to diagnose her condition.

Investigation	Result	Rationale
Abdominal x-ray	X-ray shows dilated segments of large and small intestine.	Absence of the nerve cells causes obstruction.
Barium enema	Narrowing of the large intestine shown on the x-ray suggests possible Hirschsprung's disease.	Absence of the nerve cells in the colon wall causes a narrowing of the lumen.
Manometry (test carried out only in older children)	An anal muscle that does not relax suggests possible Hirschsprung's disease.	Measures nerve reflexes that are missing in Hirschsprung's disease. Insertion and inflation of a balloon into the rectum normally cause the anal muscle to relax.
Biopsy (most accurate test for diagnosing Hirschsprung's disease)	Observation of tissue biopsy under microscope confirms Hirschsprung's disease.	Tissue biopsy under the microscope will show whether the nerve cells are missing or not. Absent nerve cells confirm Hirschsprung's disease.

References

Abramowicz S, Cooper M, Bardi K, Weyant R, Marazita M. 2003. Demographic and prenatal factors of patients with cleft lip and cleft palate – a pilot study. *Journal of the American Dental Association* 134:1371–1376.

Aerts R, Penninckx F. 2003. The burden of gallstone disease in Europe. *Alimentary Pharmacology and Therapy* 18(Suppl 3): 49–53.

Afdhal NH, Niu N, Nunes DP. 1995. Mucin-vesicle interactions in model bile: Evidence for vesicle aggregation and fusion before cholesterol crystal formation. *Hepatology* 22:856–865.

Agrawal S, Gupta A, Yachha SK, Muller-Myhsok B, Mehrotra P, Agarwal SS. 2000. Association of human leukocyte-DR and DQ antigens in celiac disease: A family study. *Journal of Gastroenterology and Hepatology* 15:771–774.

Ajit S, Midha V, Sood N, Avasthi G, Sehgal A. 2006. Prevalence of celiac disease among school children in Punjab, North India. *Journal of Gastroenterology and Hepatology* 21:1622–1625.

Allen B, Bernhoft R, Blanckaert N. 1981. Sludge is calcium bilirubinate associated with bile stasis. *American Journal of Surgery* 141:51–56.

Almond ML, Old O, Barr H. 2014. Strategies for the prevention of oesophageal adenocarcinoma. *International Journal of Surgery* 12:931–935.

Alter MJ, Kruszon-Moran D, Nainan OV, McQuillan GM, Gao F, Moyer LA, Kaslow RA, Margolis HS. 1999. The prevalence of hepatitis C virus infection in the United States, 1988 through 1994. *New England Journal of Medicine* 341(8):556–562.

Amano K, Adachi K, Katsube T, Watanabe M, Kinoshita Y. 2001. Role of hiatus hernia and gastric mucosal atrophy in the development of reflux oesophagitis in the elderly. *Journal of Gastroenterology and Hepatology* 16:132–136.

Amiel J, Lyonnet S. 2001. Hirschsprung disease, associated syndromes, and genetics: A review. *Journal of Medical Genetics* 38:729–739.

Angulo P. 2002. Nonalcoholic fatty liver disease. *New England Journal of Medicine* 346:1221–1230.

Annese V, Latiano A, Andriulli A. 2003. Genetics of inflammatory bowel disease: The beginning of the end or the end of the beginning? *Digestive and Liver Disease* 35:442–449.

Arendt T. 1989a. The pathogenesis of acute biliary pancreatitis: A controversial issue. Part I the concept of biliopancreatic reflux. *Gastroenterology* 49:50–53.

Arendt T. 1989b. The pathogenesis of acute biliary pancreatitis. Part II: The concepts of duodenopancreatic reflux and of obstruction of pancreatic exocrine secretion. *Gastroenterology* 49:98–101.

Arteel G, Marsano CM, Bentley F, Craig J. 2003. Advances in alcoholic liver disease. *Best Practice and Research Clinical Gastroenterology* 17(4):625–647.

Atherton JC. 2006. The pathogenesis of *Helicobacter pylori* induced gastro-duodenal diseases. *Annual Review of Pathology* 1:63–96.

Ayabe T, Satchell DP, Wilson CL. 2000. Secretion of microbicidal alpha-defensins by intestinal Paneth cells in response to bacteria. *Nature Immunology* 1(2):113–118.

Bairead E, Harmon DL, Curtis AM. 2003. Association of NOD2 with Crohn's disease in a homogeneous Irish population. *European Journal of Human Genetics* 11:237–244.

Baltazar U, Dunn J, Gonzalez-Diaz S, Browder W. 2000. Agenesis of the gallbladder. *Southern Medical Journal* 93:914–915.

Banning M. 2004. Functional dyspepsia: Aetiology, diagnosis and treatment. *Nurse Prescribing* 2(6):248–255.

Banning M. 2006. *Clostridium difficile*: Epidemiology, pathology, treatment and prevention. *Digestive Nursing* 4(6):20–27.

Barrett JA, Brocklehurst JC, Kiff ES, Ferguson G, Faragher EB. 1989. Anal function in geriatric patients with faecal incontinence. *Gut* 30:1244–1251.

Bartlett JG. 2006. Narrative review: The new epidemic of *Clostridium difficile* –associated enteric disease. *Annals of Internal Medicine* 145(10):758–764.

Behrman RE, Kliegman RM, Jenson HB (eds). 2000. *Nelson Textbook of Pediatrics*, 16th edn. Philadelphia: Saunders.

Bennett RA, Rubin PH, Present DH. 1991. Frequency of inflammatory bowel disease in offspring of couples both presenting with inflammatory bowel disease. *Gastroenterology* 100:1638–1643.

Bennion RS, Thompson JE, Tompkins RK. 1988. Agenesis of the gallbladder without extrahepatic biliary atresia. *Archives of Surgery* 123:1257–1260.

Bisschops R, Karamanolis G, Arts J. 2008. Relationship between symptoms and ingestion of a meal in functional dyspepsia. *Gut* 57:1495–1503.

Boeckxstaens GE. 2005. The lower oesophageal sphincter. *Neurogastroenterology and Motility* 17(Suppl 1):13–21.

Boeckxstaens GE, Zaninotto G, Richter JE. 2014. Achalasia. *The Lancet* 383:83–93.

Bootsma H, Spijkervet FK, Kroese FG, Vissink A. 2013. Towards a new classification criteria for Sjogrens disease. *Arthritis and Rheumatology* 65(1):21–23.

Bornschein J, Selgrad M, Warnecke M, Kuester D, Wex T, Malfertheiner P. 2010. *H. pylori* infection is a key risk factor for proximal gastric cancer. *Digestive Diseases and Sciences* 55(11):3124–3131.

Bouma G, Strober W. 2003. The immunological and genetic basis of inflammatory bowel disease. *Nature Reviews: Immunology* 3:521–528.

Brackbill S, Shi G, Birano I. 2003. Diminished mechanosensitivity and chemosensitivity in patients with achalasia. *American Journal of Physiology: Gastrointestinal and Liver Physiology* 285:G1198–G1203.

Bradshaw CJ, Thakkar H, Knutzen L, Marsh R, Pacilli M, Impey L, Lakhoo K. 2016. Accuracy of prenatal detection of tracheoesophageal fistula and oesophageal atresia. *Journal of Pediatric Surgery* 51(8):1268–1272.

Bredenoord AJ, Pandolfino JE, Smout AJPM. 2013. Gastro-oesophageal reflux disease. *The Lancet* 381:1933–1942.

Brodribb AJM, Humphreys DM. 1976. Diverticular disease: Three studies, part I - Relation to other disorders and fibre intake. *British Medical Journal* 1:424–430.

Brooks AS, Oostra BA, Hofstra RM. 2005. Studying the genetics of Hirschsprung's disease: Unraveling an oligogenic disorder. *Clinical Genetics* 67:6–14.

Bruha R, Dvorak K, Petrtyl J. 2012. Alcoholic liver disease. *World Journal of Hepatology* 4(3):81–90.

Burkitt DP, Wolker A, Painter NS. 1972. Effects of dietary fiber on stools and the transit time and its role in the causation of disease. *Lancet* 2:1408–1412.

Cabajo Caballero MA, Martin del Olmo JC, Blanco Alvarez JI, Atienza Sanchez R. 1997. Gallbladder and cystic duct absence. An infrequent malformation in laparoscopic surgery. *Surgical Endoscopy* 11:483–484.

Campbell T, Draper S, Reid J, Robinson L. 2001. The management of constipation in people with advanced cancer. *British Journal of Nursing* 7(3):110–119.

Cancer Research UK. 2016. http://www.cancerresearchuk.org/.

Carter MJ, Lobo AJ, Travis SP. 2004. Guidelines for the management of inflammatory bowel disease in adults, British Society of Gastroenterology. *Gut* 53(Suppl 5):V1–V16.

Castledine G, Grainger M, Wood N, Dilley C. 2007. Researching the management of constipation in long-term care: Part 1. *British Journal of Nursing* 16(18):1128–1131.

Cavanaugh JA, Adams KE, Quak EJ. 2003. CARD15/NOD2 risk alleles in the development of Crohn's disease in the Australian population. *Annals of Human Genetics* 67:35–41.

Chan G, Yuen S, Chu K, Ho J, Leung S, Ho J. 1999. *Helicobacter pylori* in Meckel's diverticulum with heterotopic gastric mucosa in a population with relatively high *H. pylori* prevalence rate. *Journal of Gastroenterol and Hepatology* 14:313–316.

Chen CP, Shin SL, Liu FF, Jan SW, Jeng CJ, Lan CC. 1997. Perinatal features of omphalocele-exstrophy-imperforate anus-spinal defects (OEIS complex) associated with large meningomyeloceles and severe limb defects. *American Journal of Perinatology* 14:275–279.

Chi Ho Y. 2012. 'Venous cut-off sign' as an adjunct to the 'whirl sign' in recognizing acute small bowel volvulus via CT scan. *Journal of Gastrointestinal Surgery* 16:2005–2006.

Chowdhury S. 2006. Exploring the science of laxatives: Mechanisms and modes of action. *Nurse Prescribing* 4(3):107–112.

Collen MJ, Abdulian JD, Chen YK. 1995. Gastroesophageal reflux disease in the elderly: More severe disease that requires aggressive therapy. *American Journal of Gastroenterology* 90:1053–1057.

Colquhoun A, Arnold M, Ferlay J, Goodman KJ, Forman D, Soerjomataram I. 2015. Global patterns of cardia and non-cardia gastric cancer incidence in 2012. *Gut* 64:1881–1888.

Coughlin JP, Rector FE, Klein MD. 1992. Agenesis of the gallbladder in duodenal atresia: Two case reports. *Journal of Pediatric Surgery* 27:1304.

Coyne PE, Kalbassi MR. 2014. Diverticular disease. *Surgery* 32(8):431–434.

Crowe FL, Appleby PN, Allen NE, Key TJ. 2011. Diet and risk of diverticular disease in Oxford cohort of European prospective investigation into cancer and nutrition (EPIC): Prospective study of British vegetarians and non-vegetarians. *BMJ* 343:d4131.

Cunliffe RN, Rose FR, Keyte J. 2001. Human defensin 5 is stored in precursor form in normal Paneth cells and is expressed by some villous epithelial cells and by metaplastic Paneth cells in the colon in inflammatory bowel disease. *Gut* 48(2):176–185.

Czinn SJ, Blanchard S. 2013. Gastro-oesophageal reflux disease in neonates and infants. *Pediatric Drugs* 15(19):19–27.

Darling JM, Wright TL. 2004. Immune responses in hepatitis C: Is virus or host the problem? *Current Opinion in Infectious Diseases* 17:193–198.

Dell'Abate P, Iosca A, Galimberti A, Faraci R, Soliani P, Foggi E. 2000. Agenesis of the gallbladder found at laparoscopy in an adult patient with cardiac congenital malformation. *Digestive Surgery* 17:284–286.

Dennery PA, Seidman DS, Stevenson DK. 2001. Neonatal hyperbilirubinemia. *New England Journal of Medicine* 344:581.

De Silva N, Fitzgerald R. 2015. Barrett's oesophagus and oesophageal adenocarcinoma. *Medicine* 43(4):202–209.

Diehl AM. 2002. Liver disease in alcohol abusers: Clinical perspective. *Alcohol* 27:7–11.

Dieterich W, Laag E, Schopper H. 1998. Autoantibodies to tissue transglutaminase as predictors of celiac disease. *Gastroenterology* 115:1317–1321.

Diggle L. 2007. Rotavirus diarrhoea and future prospects for prevention. *British Journal of Nursing* 6(16):970–974.

DiPalma J, Kirk CL, Hamosh M, Colon AR, Benjamin SB, Hamosh P. 1991. Lipase and pepsin activity in the gastric mucosa of infants, children, and adults. *Gastroenterology* 101:116.

Dixon MJ, Marazita M, Beaty T, Murray M. 2011. Cleft lip and palate: Understating genetic and environmental influences. *Nature Reviews* 12 March:167–178.

Drum BD, Rhoades JM, Stringer DA, Sherman PM, Ellis LE, Durie PR. 1988. Peptic ulcer disease in children: Etiology, clinical findings, and clinical course. *Pediatrics* 82:410–414.

D'Souza A. 2007. Ageing and the gut. *Postgraduate Medical Journal* 83(975):44–53.

Duncan J. 2004. The management of constipation by nurse prescribers. *Nurse Prescribing* 2(2):66–69.

Edmonds L, Boniface C, Alcock G, Stalewski H, Shi E. 2013. Congenital diaphragmatic hernia in Northern Queensland. *Journal of Paediatrics and Child Health* 49(6):475–479.

Edmunds J, Hazelbaker A, Murphy JG, Philipp BL. 2012. Tongue-tie. *Journal of Human Lactation* 28(1):14–17.

Edwards LL, Quigley EM, Harned RK, Hofman R, Pfeiffer RF. 1994. Characterization of swallowing and defecation in Parkinson's disease. *American Journal of Gastroenterology* 89:15–25.

Einarrson K, Nilsell K, Leijd B. 1985. Influence of age on secretion of cholesterol and synthesis of bile acids by the liver. *New England Journal of Medicine* 313:277.

Eland IA, Sturkenboom MJCM, Wilson HP. 2000. Incidence and mortality of acute pancreatitis between 1985 and 1995. *Scandinavian Journal of Gastroenterology* 35:1110–1116.

Elsharif M, Basu I, Phillips D. 2012. A case of triple volvulus. *Annals of the Royal College of Surgeons of England* 94(2):62–64.

Emmanuel A. 2004. Constipation. In: Norton C, Chelvanayagam S (eds). *Bowel Continence Nursing*. Beaconsfield, United Kingdom: Beaconsfield.

Emond A, Ingram J, Johnson D, Blair P, Whitelaw A, Copeland M, Sutcliffe A. 2014. Randomised controlled trial of early frenotomy in breastfed infants with mild-moderate tongue-tie. *Archives of Disease in Childhood: Fetal and Neonatal Edition*. 99(3):F189–F195.

Ertem D. 2013. Clinical practice: *Helicobacter pylori* infection in childhood. *European Journal of Pediatrics* 172:1427–1434.

Everhart JE, Khare M, Hill M, Maurer KR. 1999. Prevalence and ethnic differences in gallbladder disease in the United States. *Gastroenterology* 117:632–639.

Fagenholz PJ, Castillo CF, Harris NS. 2007. Increasing United States hospital admissions for acute pancreatitis, 1988–2003. *Annals of Epidemiology* 17:491–497.

Fanciulii C, D'Appello AR, Asmar EL. 2000. Antiendomysium versus antigliadin antibodies in screening the general population for celiac disease. *Scandanavian Journal of Gastrology* 35(7):732–736.

Fasano A, Berti I, Gerarduzzi T. 2003. Prevalence of celiac disease in at-risk and non-at-risk groups in the United States: A large multi-centre study. *Archives of Internal Medicine* 16:286–292.

Fasano A, Catassi C. 2001. Current approaches to diagnosis and treatment of celiac disease: An evolving spectrum. *Gastroenterology* 120:636–651.

Fasano A, Catassi C. 2012. Celiac disease. *New England Journal of Medicine* 367:2419–2426.

Feenstra B, Geller F, Krogh C, Hollegaard MV, Gortz S, Boyd H, Murray JC, Hougaard DM, Melbye M. 2012. Common variants near MBNLI and NKX"-5 are associated with idiopathic hypertrophic pyloric stenosis. *Nature Genetics* 44(3):334.

Feinle-Bisset C, Meier B, Fried M, Beglinger C. 2003. Role of cognitive factors in symptom induction following high and low fat meals in patients with functional dyspepsia. *Gut* 52:1414–1418.

Fellermann K, Wehkamp J, Herrlinger KR. 2003. Crohn's disease: A defensin deficiency syndrome? *European Journal of Gastroenterology and Hepatology* 15:627–634.

Ferzoco LB, Raptopoulos V, Silen W. 1998. Acute diverticulitis. *New England Journal of Medicine* 338:1521–1526.

Fike B, Mortellaro VE. 2011. Diagnosis of GERD in infants. *Pediatric Surgery International* 27(8):791–797.

Fitzgerald RC, Di Pietro M, Ragunath K, Ang Y, Kang, J-Y, Watson, P, Trudgill, N. 2014. British Society of Gastroenterology guidelines on the diagnosis and management of Barrett's oesophagus. *Gut* 63(1):7.

Flejou JF. 2005. Barrett's oesophagus: From metaplasia to dysplasia and cancer. *Gut* 54:i6–i12.

Fofaria RK, Morris DL. 2015. Hiatus hernia and gastro-oesophageal reflux disease. *Medicine* 43(4):192–196.

Ford AC, Marwaha A, Sood R, Moayyedi P. 2015. Global prevalence of, and risk factors for, uninvestigated dyspepsia: A meta-analysis. *Gut* 64:1049–1057.

Forsmark CE, Baillie J. 2007. AGA Institute technical review on acute pancreatitis. *Gastroenterology* 132:2022–2044.

Fortunato F, Deng X, Gates LK, McClain CJ, Bimmler D, Graf R, Whitcomb DC. 2006. Pancreatic response to endotoxin after chronic alcohol exposure: Switch from apoptosis to necrosis? *American Journal Physiological Digestive Liver Physiology* 290:G232–G241.

Fox RI. 2005. Sjögren's syndrome. *Lancet* 366(9482):321–331.

Frey CF, Zhou H, Harvey DJ. 2006. The incidence and case-fatality rates of acute biliary, alcoholic, and idiopathic pancreatitis in California, 1994–2001. *Pancreas* 33:336–344.

Gaglia A, Probert CS. 2015. Diverticular disease. *Medicine* 43(6):320–323.

Gamblin CT, Stephens RE Jr, Johnson RK, Rothwell M. 2003. Adult malrotation: A case report and review of the literature. *Current Surgery* 60(5):517–520.

Garg PK. 2012. Chronic pancreatitis in India and Asia. *Current Gastroenterology Reports* 14(2):118–124.

Gear JSS, Ware A, Fursdon P. 1979. Symptomless diverticular disease and intake of dietary fibre. *Lancet* 10:511–514.

Geboes K, Ectors N, Geboes KP. 2005. Pathology of early lower GI cancer. *Best Practice and Research Clinical Gastroenterology* 19(6):963–978.

Georgoula C, Gardiner M. 2012. Pyloric stenosis a 100 years after Ramstedt. *Archives of Disease in Childhood* 97:741–745.

Gilbert EW, Luna RA, Harrison VL, Hunter JG. 2011. Barrett's esophagus: A review of the literature. *Journal of Digestive Surgery* 15(5):708–718.

Giovannucci E, Stampfer MJ, Colditz G. 1992. Relationship of diet to risk of colorectal adenoma in men. *Journal of the National Cancer Institute* 84:91–98.

Gislason H, Horn A, Hoem D. 2004. Acute pancreatitis in Bergen, Norway. A study on incidence, etiology and severity. *Scandinavian Journal of Surgery* 93:29–33.

Glass RI, Parashar UD, Bresee JS, Turcios R, Fischer TK, Widdowson MA, Jiang B, Gentsch JR. 2006. Rotavirus vaccines: Current prospects and future challenges. *Lancet* 368:323–332.

Goel AK, Seenu V, Khosla NK, Gupta A, Sarda AK. 1994. Agenesis of gallbladder with choledochal cyst—an unusual combination. *Tropical Gastroenterology* 15(1):33–36.

Goldacre MJ, Roberts SE. 2004. Hospital admission for acute pancreatitis in an English population, 1963–98: Database study of incidence and mortality. *BMJ* 328:1466–1469.

Goudy S, Lott D, Canady J, Smith R. 2006. Conductive hearing loss and otopathology in cleft palate patients. *Otolaryngology-Head and Neck Surgery* 134:946–948.

Green PH, Jabri B. 2003. Coeliac disease. *Lancet* 362:383–391.

Groner JI, Zeigler MM. 2003. Cloacal exstrophy. In: Puri P (ed). *Newborn Surgery*, 2nd edn. London: Arnold, pp. 629–636.

Gukovskaya AS, Mareninova OA, Odinokova IV, Sung K, Lugea A, Fisher L, Wang Y, Guovsky I, Pandol SJ. 2006. Cell death in pancreatitis: Effects of alcohol. *Journal of Gastroenterology and Hepatology* 21:S10–S13.

Halabi WJ, Jafari MD, Kang CY, Nguyen VQ, Carmichael JC, Mills S, Pigazzi A, Stamos MJ. 2014. Colonic volvulus in the United States: Trends, outcomes, and predictors of mortality. *Annals of Surgery* 259(2):293–301.

Harari D. 2002. Epidemiology and risk factors for bowel problems in frail older people. In: Potter J, Norton C, Cottenden A (eds). *Bowel Care in Older People*. London: Royal College of Physicians, pp. 23–45.

Hassan N, Ng P. 2012. The management of reflux in infants. *InnovAiT* 5(2):69–75.

Hawkes N. 2012. 5m Pound UK study aims to discover what causes cleft lip and palate. *BMJ* 344:e2372.

Heavey PM, Rowland IR. 2004. Digestive cancer. *Best Practice and Research Clinical Gastroenterology* 18(2):323–336.

Hernanz-Schulman M. 2003. Infantile hypertrophic pyloric stenosis. *Radiology* 227:319–331.

Hicks A. 2001. The prevention and management of constipation. *Journal of Orthopaedic Nursing* 5:208–211.

Hilmer SN, Cogger VC, Fraser R, McLean AJ, Sullivan D, Le Couteur DG. 2005. Age-related changes in the hepatic sinusoidal endothelium impede lipoprotein transfer in the rat. *Hepatology* 42(6):1349–1354.

Hin H, Bird G, Fisher P. 1999. Coeliac disease in primary care case finding study. *BMJ* 318:164–167.

Hodgkinson PD, Brown S, Duncan D, Grant C, McNaughton A, Thomas P, Mattick CR. 2005. Management of children with cleft lip and palate; A review describing the application of multidisciplinary team working in this condition based upon the experiences of a regional cleft lip and palate centre in the United Kingdom. *Fetal and Maternal Medicine Review* 16(1):1–27.

Hollander WJ, Holster L, van Gilst B, van Vuuren AJ, Jaddoe VW, Hofman A, Perez-Perez GI, Kuipers EJ, Moll HA, Blaser MJ. 2015. Intergenerational change in *Helicobacter pylori* colonization in children living in a multi-ethnic Western population. *Gut* 64(8):1200–1208.

Hong P. 2013. Ankyloglossia (tongue–tie). *CMAJ* 185(2):E128.

Hopkins MJ, Macfarlane GT. 2002. Changes in predominant bacterial populations in human faeces with age and with *Clostridium difficile* infection. *Journal of Medical Microbiology* 51(5):448–454.

Homan M, Hojsak I, Kolacek S. 2012. *Helicobacter pylori* in paediatrics. *Helicobacter* 17(Suppl 1):43–48.

Hosie G, Gravens E. 2013. Oesophageal atresia. *Pediatric Surgery* 31(12):618–621.

Howie E, Miller MEA, Murchie MB. 2003. The digestive system, liver and biliary tract. In: Alexander MF, Fawcett JN, Runciman PJ (eds). *Nursing Practice: Home and Hospital*, 2nd edn. Edinburgh: Churchill Livingstone, pp. 87–133.

Hsu P, Klimek J, Nanan R. 2014. Infantile hypertrophic pyloric stenosis: Does size really matter? *Journal of Paediatrics and Child Health* 50(10):827–828.

Ishida H, Iwama T, Inokuma S, Takeuchi I, Hashimoto D, Miyaki M. 2002. APC gene mutations in a jejunal adenoma causing intussusception in a patient with familial adenomatous polyposis. *Journal of Gastroenterology* 39:1057–1061.

Isono S, Tanaka A, Ishikawa T, Nishino T. 2000. Developmental changes in collapsibility of the passive pharynx during infancy. *American Journal of Respiratory Critical Care Medicine* 162:832–836.

Iwashita T, Kruger GM, Pardal R. 2003. Hirschsprung disease is linked to defects in neural crest stem cell function. *Science* 301:972–976.

Iwuagwu O, Deans GT. 1999. Small bowel volvulus: A review. *Journal of the Royal College of Surgeons of Edinburgh* 44:150–155.

Jankowski J, Black J, Barr H, Wang K, Delaney B. 2010. Diagnosis and management of Barrett's oesophagus. *BMJ* 341:c4551.

Jankowski J, Harrison R, Perry I, Balkwill F, Tselepis C. 2000. Barrett's metaplasia. *Lancet* 356(9247):2079–2085.

Jansen PLM. 2002. Liver disease in the elderly. *Best Practice and Research Clinical Gastroenterology* 16(1):149–158.

Jarnagin WR. 2013. *Blumgart's Surgery of the Liver, Biliary Tract and Pancreas*, 5th edn. New York: Springer.

Jewell DP. 1998. Ulcerative colitis and Crohns disease: Susceptibility genes and clinical patterns. *Journal of Gastroenterology* 33:458–462.

Jones MP, Dilley JB, Drossman D, Crowells MD. 2006. Brain-gut connections in functional GI disorders: Anatomic and physiologic relationships. *Neurogastroenterology Motility* 18:91–103.

Jorge AM, Keswani RN, Veerappan A, Soper NJ, Gawron AJ. 2015. Non-operative management of symptomatic cholelithiasis in pregnancy is associated with frequent hospitalizations. *Journal of Gastrointestinal Surgery* 19:598–603.

Jupp J, Fine D, Johnson CD. 2010. The epidemiology and socioeconomic impact of chronic pancreatitis. *Best Practice and Research Clinical Gastroenterology* 24(3):219–231.

Kahrilas PJ. 2008. Gastro-oesophageal reflux disease. *New England Journal of Medicine* 359(16):1700–1707.

Kallen K, Castilla EE, Rober E, Mastroicovo P, Kallen B. 2000. OEIS complex – A population study. *American Journal of Medical Genetics* 92:62–68.

Kamisawa T. 2006. Is there a causal relation between pancreas divisum and pancreatic cancer? *Journal of Gastroenterology* 41:10881093.

Kamm MA. 2003. Constipation and its management. *BMJ* 327(7413):459–460.

Kapfer SA, Rappold JF. 2004. Intestinal malrotation—not just the pediatric surgeon's problem. *Journal of the American College of Surgeons* 199(4):628–635.

Kasapidis P, Vassilakis JS, Tzovaras G, Chrysos E, Xynos E. 1995. Effect of hiatus hernia on oesophageal manometry and pH-metry in gastroesophageal reflux disease. *Digestive Diseases and Sciences* 40:2724–2730.

Kassan SS, Moutsopoulos HM. 2004. Clinical manifestations and early diagnosis of Sjögren syndrome. *Archives of Internal Medicine* 164(12):1275–1284.

Kato S, Nishino Y, Ozawa K. 2004. *Helicobacter pylori* infection in childhood. *Journal of Gastroenterology* 39:809–810.

Kawanishi M. 2006. Will symptomatic digestive reflux disease develop into reflux oesophagitis? *Journal of Gastroenterology* 41:440–443.

Kemppainen E, Puolakkainen P. 2007. Non-alcoholic etiologies of acute pancreatitis – Exclusion of other etiologic factors besides alcohol and gallstones. *Pancreatology* 7:142–146.

Keppler-Noreuil KM. 2002. OEIS complex (Omphalocoele-Exstrophy-Imperforate anus-Spinal defects): A review of 14 cases. *American Journal of Medical Genetics* 107:72–76.

Keus F, Broeders IA, van Laarhoven CJ. 2006. Gallstone disease: Surgical aspects of symptomatic cholecystolithiasis and acute cholecystitis. *Best Practice and Research: Clinical Gastroenterology* 20:1031–1051.

Kline-Fath B. 2012. Congenital diaphragmatic hernia. *Paediatric Radiology Supplement* 42:74–90.

Kong SC. 2003. Understanding and managing coelic disease. *Nursing and Residential Care* 5(4):164–166.

Kopelman H, Corey M, Gaskin K. 1988. Impaired chloride secretion as well as bicarbonate secretion underlies the fluid secretory defect in cystic fibrosis pancreas. *Gastroenterology* 95:349–355.

Kotlow LA. 2013. Diagnosing and understanding the maxillary lip tie (superior labial, the maxillary labial frenum) as it relates to breast feeding. *Journal of Human Lactation* 29(4):458–464.

Kudo S, Kashida H, Tamura T. 2000. Early colorectal cancer: Flat or depressed type. *Journal of Gastroenterology and Hepatology* 15:66–70.

Kumar P, Clark M. 2000. *Clinical Medicine.* Philadelphia, PA: W.B. Saunders.

Lamah M, Karanjia ND, Dickson GH. 2001. Anatomical variations of the extrahepatic biliary tree: Review of the world literature. *Clinical Anatomy* 14:167–172.

Lamers W. 2000. Constipation can kill. *Journal of Pharmaceutical Care in Pain and Symptom Control* 8:69–73.

Lankisch PG, Assmus C, Maisonneuve P. 2002. Epidemiology of pancreatic diseases in Luneburg County. A study in a defined German population. *Pancreatology* 2:469–477.

Larché MJ. 2006. A short review of the pathogenesis of Sjögren's syndrome. *Autoimmunity Reviews* 5(2):132–135.

Lawson J, Sicklick J, Fanta P. 2011. Gastric cancer. *Current Problems in Cancer* 35(3):97–127.

Ledbetter DJ. 2006. Gastroschisis and omphalocele. *Surgical Clinics of North America* 86:246–260.

Lee JS, Kim HS, Jung JJ, Kim YB. 2002. Adenomyoma of the small intestine in an adult: A rare cause of intussusception. *Journal of Gastroenterology* 37:556–559.

Lee SP, Ko CW. 1999. Gallstones. In: Yamada T, Alpers DH, Laine L, Owyang C, Powel DH (eds). *Textbook of Gastroenterology*, 3rd edn. Philadelphia, PA: Lippincott Williams and Wilkins, pp. 2258–2280.

Lee W, Kirk JS, Shaheen KW, Romero R, Hodges AN, Comstock CH. 2000. Fetal cleft lip and palate detection by three-dimensional ultrasonography. *Ultrasound in Obstetrics and Gynecology* 16:314–320.

Lee YY, McColl KEL. 2013. Pathophysiology of gastro-oesophageal reflux disease. *Best Practice and Research: Clinical Gastroenterology* 27:339–351.

Lepage C, Drouillard A, Jouve JL, Faivre J. 2013. Epidemiology and risk factors for oesophageal adenocarcinoma. *Digestive and Liver Disease* 45:625–629.

Levitt MA, Pena A. 2007. Anorectal malformations. *Orphanet Journal of Rare Diseases* 2:33.

Lianos G, Ignatiadou E, Lianou E, Anastasiadi Z, Fatouros M. 2012. Simultaneous volvulus of the transverse and sigmoid colon: Case report. *Il Giornale di Chirurgia* 33(10):324–326.

Linde K, Boor PP, Houwing-Duistermaat JJ. 2003. CARD15 and Crohn's disease: Healthy homozygous carriers of the 3020insC frameshift mutation. *American Journal of Gastroenterology* 98:613–617.

Locke GR, Pemberton JH, Phillips SF. 2000. American Gastroenterological Association medical position statement: Guidelines on constipation. *Gastroenterology* 119(6):1761–1766.

Loffeld R, Van Der Putten A. 2002. Newly developing hiatus hernia: A survey in patients undergoing upper digestive endoscopy. *Journal of Gastroenterology and Hepatology* 17:542–544.

Lonnerdal B. 2003. Nutritional and physiologic significance of human milk proteins. *American Journal of Clinical Nutrition* 77(6):1537–1543.

Losty P. 2014. Congenital diaphragmatic hernia. *Seminars in Paediatric Surgery* 23:278–282.

Lourenço RL, Teixeira DNL, Costa B, Ribeiro GM. 2003. Dental anomalies of the permanent lateral incisors and prevalence of hypodontia outside the cleft area in complete unilateral cleft lip and palate. *Cleft Palate-Craniofacial Journal* 40:172–175.

Lu CL, Chen CY, Chiu ST, Chang FY, Lee SD. 2001. Adult intussuscepted Meckel's diverticulum presenting mainly lower digestive bleeding. *Journal of Gastroenterology and Hepatology* 16:478–480.

Lund DP, Hendren WH. 2001. Cloacal exstrophy: A 25 year experience with 50 cases. *Journal of Pediatric Surgery* 36:68–75.

MacDonald TT, Monteleone G, Pender SL. 2000. Recent developments in the immunology of inflammatory bowel disease. *Scandinavian Journal of Immunology* 51:2–9.

Mahadeva S, Goh K-L. 2006. Epidemiology of functional dyspepsia: A global perspective. *World Journal of Gastroenterology* 12:2661–2666.

Makharia G, Catassi C, Lee Goh, Mulder C. 2012. Celiac disease. *Gastroenterology Research and Practice* 2012:2.

Malik A, Shams-ul-Bari, Wani K, Khaja A. 2010. Meckel's diverticulum—Revisited. *Saudi Journal of Gastroenterology* 16(1):3–7.

Manzoni GM, Hurwitz RS. 1998. Cloacal exstrophy. In: Freeman NV, Burge DM, Griffiths M, Malone PSJ (eds). *Surgery of the Newborn*. Edinburgh: Churchill Livingstone, pp. 767–780.

Maringhini A, Marceno MP, Lanzarone F. 1987. Sludge and stones after pregnancy. *Journal of Hepatology* 5:218–223.

Marino CR, Matovcik LM, Gorelick FS, Cohn JA. 1991. Localisation of cystic fibrosis transmembrane conductance regulator in pancreas. *Journal of Clinical Investigation* 88:712–716.

Martigne L, Delaggage PH, Thomas-Delecourt F, Bonnelye G, Barthelemy P, Gottrand F. 2012. Prevalence and management of gastro-oesophageal reflux disease in children and adolescents; a nationwide cross sectional observational study. *European Journal of Pediatrics* 171:1767–1773.

Mavragani CP, Moutsopoulos HM. 2014. Sjogren syndrome. *Canadian Medical Association Journal* 186(15):E579–E586.

Mazen Jamal M, Morgan TR. 2003. Liver disease in alcohol and hepatitis C. *Best Practice and Research Clinical Gastroenterology* 17(4):649–662.

McFarland LV. 2005. Alternative treatments for *Clostridium difficile* disease: What really works. *Journal of Medical Microbiology* 54(Pt 2):101–111.

McFarlane XA, Marsham J, Reeves D, Bhalla AK, Robertson DAF. 1995. Subclinical nutritional deficiency in treated celiac disease and nutritional content of the gluten-free diet. *Journal of Human Nutrition and Dietetics* 8:231–237.

McGivern MR Best KE, Rankin J, Wellesley D, Greenlees R, Addor M-C, Arriola L et al. 2015. Epidemiology of congenital diaphragmatic hernia in Europe. *Archives of Disease in Childhood-Fetal and Neonatal Edition* 100(2):F137–F144.

McHoney M. 2014. Congenital diaphragmatic hernia. *Early Human Development* 90:941–946.

McPhillips J. 2000. Understanding coeliac disease: Symptoms and long-term risks. *British Journal of Nursing* 9(8):479–483.

Meza-Valencia BE, de Lorimier AJ, Person DA. 2005. Hirschsprung disease in the U.S. associated Pacific Islands: More common than expected. *Hawaii Medical Journal* 64(4):96–98, 100–101.

Milkiewicz P, Elias E, Williamson C, Weaver J. 2002. Obstetric cholestasis. *BMJ* 323:123–124.

Milkiewicz P, Gallagher R, Chambers J, Eggington E, Weaver J, Ellias E. 2003. Obstetric cholestasis with elevated gamma glutamyl transpeptidase: Incidence, presentation and treatment. *Journal of Gastroenterology and Hepatology* 18:1283–1286.

Mitchell RM, Byrne MF, Baillie J. 2003. Pancreatitis. *Lancet* 3(361):1447–1455.

Mittal R, Balaban D. 1997. The oesphagogastric junction. *New England Journal of Medicine* 336(13):924–933.

Moore WE, Moore LH. 1995. Intestinal floras of populations that have a high risk of colon cancer. *Applied and Environmental Microbiology* 61:3202–3207.

Morreale M, Marchione P, Giacomini P, Pontecorvo S, Marianetti M, Vento C, Tinelli E, Francia A. 2014. Neurological involvement in primary Sjogrens: A focus on central nervous system. *PLoS One* 9(1):e84605.

Mosahebi A, Kangesu L. 2006. Cleft lip and palate. *Surgery* 24(1):33–37.

Mossey PA, Little RG, Dixon MJ, Shaw WC. 2009. Cleft lip and palate. *Lancet* 374:1773–1785.

Mourad-Baars P, Hussey S, Jones NL. 2010. *Helicobacter pylori* infection and childhood. *Helicobacter* 15(Suppl 1):53–59.

Mu YP, Ogawa T, Kawada N. 2010. Reversibility of fibrosis, inflammation, and endoplasmic reticulum stress in the liver of rats fed a methionine-choline-deficient diet. *Laboratory Investigation* 90:245–256.

Müller-Lissner S. 2002. General geriatrics and gastroenterology: Constipation and faecal incontinence. *Best Practice and Research: Clinical Gastroenterology* 16:115–133.

Mustalahti K, Catassi C, Reunanen A. 2010. The prevalence of celiac disease in Europe: Results of a centralized, international mass screening project. *Annals of Medicine* 42:587–595.

Nakagawa H, Whelan K, Lynch JP. 2015. Mechanisms of Barrett's oesophagus: Intestinal differentiation, stem cells, and tissue models. *Best Practice and Research: Clinical Gastroenterology* 29:3–16.

Naruse S, Kitagawa M, Ishiguru H, Fujiki K, Hayakawa T. 2002. Cystic fibrosis and related diseases of the pancreas. *Best Practice and Research: Clinical Gastroenterology* 16(3):511–526.

Nazarko L. 1996. Preventing constipation in older people. *Journal of Professional Nursing* 11(12):816–818.

Neuschwander-Tetri BA, Caldwell SH. 2003. Nonalcoholic steatohepatitis: Summary of an AASLD single topic conference. *Hepatology* 37:1202–1219.

Newman TB, Liljestrand P, Jeremy RJ. 2006. Outcomes among newborns with total serum bilirubin levels of 25 mg per deciliter or more. *New England Journal of Medicine* 354:1889.

Nisell K, Angelin B, Liljeuist L. 1985. Biliary lipid output and bile acid kinetics in cholesterol gallstone disease. Evidence for an increased hepatic secretion of cholesterol in Swedish patients. *Gastroenterology* 287:293.

Noble KA. 2013. Gastro-oesophageal reflux disease. *Journal of PeriAnesthesia Nursing* 28(2):102–106.

Norton C. 1996. The causes and nursing management of constipation. *British Journal of Nursing* 5:1252–1258.

Norton C. 2004. Nurses, bowel continence, stigma and taboos. *Journal of Wound Ostomy and Continence Nursing* 31(2):85–94.

Not T, Horvath K, Hill ID. 1998. Celiac disease risk in the USA: High prevalence of antiendomysium antibodies in healthy blood donors. *Scandanavian Journal of Gastroenterology* 33:494–498.

Noto JM, Peek RM. 2012. *Helicobacter pylori*: An overview. *Methods in Molecular Biology* 92:7–10.

Nunn P. 2006. Irritable bowel syndrome: A common condition commonly misunderstood. *Digestive Nursing* 4(6):10–11.

Obermayr F, Hotta R, Enomoto H, Young HM. 2013. Development and developmental disorders of the enteric nervous system. *Nature Reviews Gastroenterology and Hepatology* 10:43–57.

O'Mahony DR, O'Leary P, Quigley E. 2002. Aging and intestinal motility: A review of factors that affect intestinal motility in the aged. *Drugs and Aging* 19(7):515–527.

Oppong P, Majumdar D, Atherton J, Bebb J. 2015. *Helicobacter pylori* infection and peptic ulcers. *Medicine* 43(4):215–222.

Orholm M, Sorensen TIA, Bentsen K, Hoybye G, Eghoje K, Christoffersen P. 1985. Mortality of alcohol abusing men prospectively assessed in relation to history of abuse and degree of liver injury. *Liver International* 5(5):253–260.

Orlando RC. 2006. Current understanding of the mechanisms of gastro-oesophageal reflux disease. *Drugs* 66(Suppl 1):1–5.

Orr WC. 2010. Review article: Sleep-related gastro-oesophageal reflux as a distinct clinical entity. *Alimentary Pharmacology and Therapeutics* 31(1):47–56.

O'Sullivan BP, Freedman SD. 2009. Cystic fibrosis – Review. *Lancet* 373(9678):1891–1904.

Oude Elferink R. 2003. Cholestasis. *Gut.* 52:42–48.

Oude Elferink RP, Paulusma CC, Groen AK. 2006. Hepatocanalicular transport defects: Pathophysiologic mechanisms of rare diseases. *Gastroenterology* 130:908–925.

Page M, Jeffery H. 2000. The role of gastro-oesophageal reflux in the etiology of SIDS. *Early Human Development* 59(2):127–149.

Palepu RP, Harmon CM, Goldberg SP, Clements RH. 2007. Intestinal malrotation discovered at the time of laparoscopic Roux-en-Y gastric bypass. *Journal of Gastrointestinal Surgery* 11:898–902.

Pang J, Broyles J, Redett R. 2013. Cleft lip and palate. www.eplasty.com.

Papachrisanthou MM, Davis RL. 2015. Clinical practice guidelines for the management of gastroesophageal reflux and gastroesophageal reflux disease: Birth to 1 year of age. *Journal of Pediatric Health Care* 29(6):558–564.

Papadimitriou G, Marinis A, Papakonstantinou A. 2011. Primary midgut volvulus in adults: Report of two cases and review of the literature. *Journal of Gastrointestinal Surgery* 15:1889–1892.

Parashar UD, Hummelman EG, Bresee JS, Miller MA, Glass RI. 2003. Global illness and deaths caused by rotavirus disease in children. *Emerging Infectious Diseases* 9:565–572.

Patti MG, Waxman I. 2010. Gastroesophageal reflux disease: From heartburn to cancer. *World Journal of Gastroenterology* 16(30):3743–3744.

Paumgartner G, Sauerbruch T. 1991. Gallstones: Pathogenesis. *Lancet* 338:1117–1121.

Peek RM, Crabtree JE. 2006. *Helicobacter* infection and gastric neoplasia. *Journal of Pathology* 208:233–248.

Peery AF, Barrett PR, Park D, Rogers AJ, Galanko JA, Martin CF, Sandler RS. 2012. A high-fiber diet does not protect against asymptomatic diverticulosis. *Gastroenterology* 142:266e72.

Pena A, Levitt MA. 2006. Anorectal malformations. In: Grosfeld JL, O'Neill JA, Fonkalsrud EW, Coran AG (eds). *Pediatric Surgery*, 6th edn. Philadelphia: Mosby Elsevier, pp. 1566–1589.

Pennathur A, Gibson MK, Jobe BA, Luketich JD. 2013. Oesophageal carcinoma. *Lancet* 381:400–412.

Pickhardt PJ, Bhalla S. 2002. Intestinal malrotation in adolescents and adults: Spectrum of clinical and imaging features. *American Journal of Roentgenology* 179(6):1429–1435.

Powell M, Rigby D. 2000. Management of bowel dysfunction: Evacuation difficulties. *Nursing Standard* 14(47):47–54.

Power RF, Murphy JF. 2015. Tongue tie and frenotomy in infants with breast feeding difficulties; achieving a balance. *Archives of Disease in Childhood* 100:489–494.

Poynard T, McHutchison J, Davis GL, Esteban-Mur R, Goodman Z, Bedossa P, Albrecht J. 2000. Impact of interferon alfa-2b and ribavirin on progression of liver fibrosis in patients with chronic hepatitis C. *Hepatology* 32:1131–1137.

Prather CM. 2004. Subtypes of constipation: Sorting out the confusion. *Reviews in Gastroenterological Disorders* 4(Suppl 2):S11–S16.

Preston DM, Lennard-Jones JE. 1985. Anismus in chronic constipation. *Digestive Diseases and Sciences* 30:413–418.

Probert CSJ, Jayanthi V, Hughes AO. 1993. Prevalence and family risk of ulcerative colitis and Crohn's disease: An epidemiological study among Europeans and South Asians in Leicestershire. *Gut* 34:1547–1551.

Ramos-Casals M, Brito-Zeron P, Siso-Almirall A. 2012. Primary Sjogren syndrome. *BMJ* 344(e3821):1–7.

Rampton DS, Shanahan F. 2006. *Fast Facts: Inflammatory Bowel Disease*, 2nd edn. Oxford: Health Press.

Rampton, DS, Shanahan, F. 2008. *Fast Facts Inflammatory Bowel Disease*, 3rd edn. Oxford: Health Press.

Ranells JD, Carver JD, Kirby RS. 2011. Infantile hypertrophic pyloric stenosis: Epidemiology, genetics, and clinical update. *Advances in Pediatrics* 58(1):195–206.

Reeves HL, Burt AD, Wood S, Day CP. 1996. Hepatic stellate cell activation occurs in the absence of hepatitis in alcoholic liver disease and correlates with the severity of steatosis. *Journal of Hepatology* 25:677–683.

Reider F, Biancani P, Harnett K, Yerian L, Falk GW. 2010. Inflammatory mediators in gastro-oesophageal reflux disease: Impact on esophageal motility, fibrosis and carcinogenesis. *American Journal of Physiology. Gastrointestinal and Liver Physiology* 298:G571–G581.

Ribeiro LL, Das Neves LT, Costa B, Gomide MR. 2003. Dental associations of the permanent lateral incisors and prevalenc of hypodontia outside the cleft eare in complete unilateral cleft lip and palate. *Cleft Palate-Craniofacial Journal* 40(2):172–174.

Richards RJ, Taubin H, Wasson D. 1993. Agenesis of the gallbladder in symptomatic adults. A case and review of the literature. *Journal of Clinical Gastroenterology* 16:231–233.

Richmond J. 2003. Prevention of constipation through risk management. *Nursing Standard* 17:39–46.

Richter JE. 2013. Achalasia and lower oesophageal sphincter anatomy and physiology: Implications for peroral esophageal myotomy technique. *Techniques in Digestive Endoscopy* 15:122–126.

Riordan JR, Rommens JM, Kerem B, Alon N, Rozmahel R, Grzelczak Z et al. 1989. Identification of the cystic fibrosis gene: Cloning and characterization of complementary DNA. *Science* 245(4922):1066–1073.

Roberts EA. 2002. Steatohepatitis in children. *Best Practice and Research: Clinical Gastroenterology* 16(5):749–765.

Roggo A, Ottinger LW. 1992. Acute small bowel volvulus in adults. *Annals of Surgery* 216(2):135–141.

Rogler G. 2004. Update in inflammatory bowel disease pathogenesis. *Current Opinion in Gastroenterology* 20:311–317.

Roman S, Kahrilas PJ. 2015. Mechanisms of Barrett's oesophagus (clinical); LOS dysfunction, hiatal hernia, peristaltic defects. *Best Practice and Research: Clinical Gastroenterology* 29:17–28.

Rommens JM, Iannuzzi MC, Kerem B, Drumm ML, Melmer G, Dean M et al. 1989. Identification of the cystic fibrosis gene: Chromosome walking and jumping. *Science* 245(4922):1059–1065.

Roosendaal R, Kuipers EJ, Buitenwerf J, Uffelen C, Meuwissen SGM, Kamp GJ. 1997. *Helicobacter pylori* and the birth cohort effect: Evidence of a continuous decrease of infection rates in childhood. *American Journal of Gastroenterology* 92:1480–1482.

Rothenbacher D, Inceoglu J, Bode G, Brenner H. 2000. Acquisition of *Helicobacter pylori* infection in a high risk population occurs within the first 2 years of life. *Journal of Pediatrics* 136:744–748.

Royle J, Walsh M. 1992. *Watson's Medical-Surgical Nursing and Related Physiology*, 4th edn. London: Baillière Tindall.

Russell MB, Russell CA, Niebuhr E. 1994. An epidemiological study of Hirschsprung's disease and additional anomalies. *Acta Paediatrica* 83(1):68–71.

Ryan ET, Ecker JL, Christakis NA, Folkman J. 1992. Hirschsprung's disease: Associated abnormalities and demography. *Journal of Pediatric Surgery* 27(1):76–81.

Sakamoto N, Kono S, Wakai K, Fukuda Y, Satomi M, Shimoyama T; Epidemiology Group of the Research Committee on Inflammatory Bowel Disease in Japan. 2005. Dietary risk factors for inflammatory bowel disease: A multicenter case-control study in Japan. *Inflammatory Bowel Diseases* 11:154–163.

Sakurai M, Toshinari T, Tsuguhito O, Hitoshi A, Kyosuke K, Motoko S, Yasuni N, Katsuyuki M, Shuichi K. 2007. Liver steatosis, but not fibrosis, is associated with insulin resistance in nonalcoholic fatty liver disease. *Journal of Gastroenterology* 42:312–317.

Salmon P. 2007. Barrett's oesophagus foundation. *Digestive Nursing* 5(6):36–39.

Sandler RS, Everhart JE, Donowitz M. 2002. The burden of selected digestive diseases in the United States. *Gastroenterology* 122:1500–1511.

Sands BE. 2007. Inflammatory bowel disease: Past, present, and future. *Journal of Gastroenterology* 42:16–25.

Sanyal AJ. 2002. AGA technical review on nonalcoholic fatty liver disease. *Gastroenterology* 123:1705–1725.

Sartor R. 1994. Cytokines in intestinal inflammation: Pathophysiological and clinical considerations. *Gastroenterology* 106:533–539.

Sartor RB. 1997. Pathogenesis and immune mechanisms of chronic inflammatory bowel diseases. *American Journal of Gastroenterology* 92:5S–11S.

Sartor RB. 1999. Microbial factors in the pathogenesis of Crohn's disease, ulcerative colitis and experimental intestinal inflammation. In: Kirsner JB. (ed). *Inflammatory Bowel Disease*, 5th edn. Philadelphia: Saunders, pp. 153–178.

Sartor RB. 2001. Intestinal microflora in human and experimental inflammatory bowel disease. *Current Opinion in Gastroenterology* 17:324–330.

Satsangi J, Rosenberg WMC, Jewell DP. 1994. The prevalence of inflammatory bowel disease in relatives of patients with Crohn's disease. *European Journal of Gastroenterology and Hepatology* 6:413–416.

Saurel-Cubizolles MJ, Romito P, Lelong N, Ance PY. 2000. Women's health after childbirth: A longitudinal study in France and Italy. *British Journal of Obstetrics and Gynaecology* 107:1202–1209.

Scaparrotta A, Di Pillo S, Attanasi M, Consilvio NP, Cingolani A, Rapino D et al. 2012. Growth failure in children with cystic fibrosis. *Journal of Pediatric Endocrinology and Metabolism* 25(5–6):393–405.

Schaefer DC, Cheskin LJ. 1998. Constipation in the elderly. *American Family Physician* 58:907–914.

Schechter R, Torfs CP, Bateson TF. 1997. The epidemiology of infantile hypertrophic pyloric stenosis. *Paediatric Perinatal Epidemiology* 11:407–427.

Schneider J, Corley DA. 2015. A review of the epidemiology of Barrett's oesophagus and oesophageal carcinoma. *Best Practice and Research: Clinical Gastroenterology* 29:29–39.

Schulmann K, Reiser M, Schmiegel W. 2002. Colonic cancer and polyps. *Best Practice and Research: Clinical Gastroenterology* 16(1):91–114.

Seeff LB. 2002. Natural history of chronic hepatitis C. *Hepatology* 36(S1):S35–S46.

Shaffer EA. 2005. Epidemiology and risk factors for gallstone disease: Has the paradigm changed in the twenty-first century? *Current Gastroenterology Reports* 7(2):132–140.

Shaffer EA. 2006. Gallstone disease: Epidemiology of gallbladder stone disease. *Best Practice and Research: Clinical Gastroenterology* 20:981–996.

Shahedi K, Fuller G, Bolus R, Snyder BJ, Cohen ER, Vu M et al. 2012. Progression from incidental diverticulosis to acute diverticulitis. *Gastroenterology* 142(Suppl 1):S144.

Shaker JL, Brickner RC, Findling JW, Kelly TM, Rapp R, Rizk G et al. 1997. Hypocalcemic and skeletal disease as presenting features of coeliac disease. *Archives Internal Medicine* 157:1013–1016.

Shaw-Smith C. 2006. Oesophageal atresis, trachea-oesophageal fistula and the VACTERL association: Review of genetics and epidemiology. *Journal of Medical Genetics* 43(7):545–554.

Sheahan P, Miller, I, Sheahan JN, Earley MJ, Blayney AW. 2003. Incidence and outcome of middle ear disease in cleft lip and/or cleft palate. *Inernational Journal of Paediatric Otorhinolaryngology* 67:785–793.

Sherman PM. 1994. Peptic ulcer disease in children: Diagnosis, treatment, and the implications of *Helicobacter pylori*. *Gastroenterology Clinics of North America* 23:707–725.

Shiffman ML, Sugerman HJ, Kellum JM. 1991. Gallstone formation after rapid weight loss: A prospective study in patients undergoing gastric bypass surgery for treatment of morbid obesity. *American Journal of Gastroenterology* 86:1000–1005.

Silvester J, Duerksen D. 2013. Five things to know about celiac disease. *Canadian Medical Association Journal* 185(1):60.

Singh B, Satyapal KS, Moodley J, Haffejee AA. 1999. Congenital absence of the gall bladder. *Surgical and Radiologic Anatomy* 21:221–224.

Sipponen P. 2002. Gastric cancer: Pathogenesis, risks, and prevention. *Journal of Gastroenterology* 37:39–44.

Siurala M, Sipponen P, Kekki M. 1985. Chronic gastritis: Dynamic and clinical aspects. *Scandanavian Journal of Gastroenterology* 20:69–76.

Skopouli FN, Dafni U, Ioannidis JP, Moutsopoulos HM. 2000. Clinical evolution, and morbidity and mortality of primary Sjögren's syndrome. *Seminars in Arthritis and Rheumatism* 29(5):296–304.

Slater BJ, Rothnberg SS. 2016. Tracheoesophageal fistula. *Seminars in Pediatric Surgery* 25:176–178.

Smith N. 2014. Oesophageal atresis and trachea-oesophageal fistula. *Early Human Development* 90:947–950.

Smith NM, Chambers HM, Furness ME, Haan EA. 1992. The OEIS complex (Omphalocoele-Exstrophy-Imperforate anus-Spinal defects): Recurrence in sibs. *Journal of Medical Genetics* 29:730–732.

Smith RA, Cokkinides V, Eyre HJ. 2004. Guidelines for the early detection of cancer. *American Cancer Society* 54(1):41–52.

Smith S. 2001. Evidence-based management of constipation in the oncology patient. *European Journal of Oncology Nursing* 5(1):18–25.

Sørensen HT, Nørgård B, Pedersen L, Larsen H, Johnsen P. 2002. Maternal smoking and risk of hypertrophic infantile pyloric stenosis: 10 year population based study. *BMJ* 325:1011–1012.

Spanier BWM, Dijkgraaf MG, Bruno MJ. 2008. Epidemiology, aetiology and outcome of acute and chronic pancreatitis: An update. *Best Practice and Research: Clinical Gastroenterology* 22(1):45–63.

Spechler SJ, Souza RF. 2014. Barrett's esophagus. *New England Journal of Medicine* 371:836–845.

Spicak J, Poulova P, Plucnarova J, Rehor M, Filipova H, Hucl T. 2007. Pancreas divisum does not modify the natural course of chronic pancreatitis. *Journal of Gastroenterology* 42:135–139.

Spitz L. 2007. Oesophageal atresia. *Orphanet Journal of Rare Diseases* 2:24.

Sriram PV, Rao GV, Das G, Sharma PP, Reddy DN. 2001. Gall bladder agenesis, pancreas divisum and undescended testes: A rare association. *Indian Journal of Gastroenterology* 20:71–72.

Stanier P, Moore GE. 2004. Genetics of cleft lip and palate: Syndromic genes contribute to the incidence of non-syndromic clefts. *Human Molecular Genetics* 13(S1): R73–R81.

Starr J. 2005. *Clostridium* difficilie associated diarrhoea: Diagnosis and treatment. *BMJ* 331(7515):498–501.

Stewart RB, Moore MT, Marks RG, Hale WE. 1992. Correlates of constipation in an ambulatory elderly population. *American Journal of Gastroenterology* 87:859–864.

Stewart SF, Day CP. 2004. Alcoholic liver disease. In: Boyer TD, Wright TL, Manns MP (eds). *Zakim and Boyer's Hepatology. A Textbook of Liver Disease.* Philadelphia, PA: Elsevier, pp. 579–623.

Stoll C, Alembik Y, Dott B, Roth MP. 2008. Omphalocele and gastroschisis and associated malformations. *American Journal of Medical Genetics Part A* 146(10):1280–1285.

Strate LL, Erichsen R, Baron JA et al. 2013. Heritability and familial aggregation of diverticular disease: A population-based study of twins and siblings. *Gastroenterology* 144:736e42.

Strong TV, Boehm K, Collins FS. 1994. Localisation of cystic fibrosis transmembrane conductance regulator mRNA in the human digestive tract by *in situ* hybridisation. *Journal of Clinical Investigation* 93:347–354.

Sulkanen S, Halttunen T, Laurila K. 1998. Tissue transglutaminase autoantibody enzyme-linked immunosorbent assay in detecting celiac disease. *Gastroenterology* 115:1322–1328.

Talley N, Wiklund I. 2005. Patient reported outcomes in gastro-oesophageal reflux disease: An overview of available measures. *Quality of Life Research* 14:21–33.

Talley NJ, Ford AC. 2015. Functional dyspepsia. *New England Journal of Medicine* 373(19):1853–1863.

Talley NJ, Axon A, Bytzer P, Holtmann G, Lam SK, Zanten SV. 1999. Management of uninvestigated and functional dyspepsia: A working party report for the *World Congresses of Gastroenterology Alimentary Pharmacology & Therapeutics* 13:1135–1148.

Tan KG, Roberts-Thomson IC. 2006. Gastrointestinal: Meckel's diverticulum. *Journal of Gastroenterology and Hepatology* 21(2):475.

Taylor ND, Cass DT, Holland AJA. 2013. Infantile hypertrophic pyloric stenosis: Has anything changed? *Journal of Paediatrics and Child Health* 49(1):33–37.

Teli MR, Day CP, Burt AD et al. 1995a. Determinants of progression to cirrhosis or fibrosis in pure alcoholic fatty liver. *Lancet* 346:987–990.

Teli MR, James OF, Burt AD, Bennett MK, Day CP. 1995b. The natural history of nonalcoholic fatty liver: A follow-up study. *Hepatology* 22:1714–1719.

Thompson WG, Longstreth GF, Drossman DA, Heaton KW, Irvine EJ, Müller-Lissner SA. 1999. Functional bowel disorders and functional abdominal pain. *Gut* 45(Suppl 2):II43–II47.

Trynka G, Hunt KA, Bockett NA. 2011. Dense genotyping identifies and localizes multiple common and rare variant association signals in celiac disease. *Nature Genetics* 43:1193–1201.

Tsujikawa T, Ohta N, Nakamura T. 2001. Medium-chain triglyceride-rich enteral nutrition is more effective than low-fat enteral nutrition in rat colitis, but is equal in enteritis. *Journal of Gastroenterology* 36:673–680.

Tysk C, Riedesel H, Lindberg E et al. 1991. Colonic glycoproteins in monozygotic twins with inflammatory bowel disease. *Gastroenterology* 100:419–423.

Vallino L, Zuker R, Napoli J. 2008. A study of speech, language, hearing and dentition in children with cleft lip only. *Cleft Palate-Craniofacial Journal* 45(5):485–494.

Van Cutsem E, Sagaert X, Topal B, Haustermans K, Prenen H. 2016. Gastric cancer. *Lancet* 388(10060):2654–2664.

VanDevanter DR, Kahle JS, O'Sullivan AK, Sikirica S, Hodgkins PS. 2016. Cystic fibrosis in young children: A review of disease manifestation, progression, and response to early treatment. *Journal of Cystic Fibrosis* 15:147–157.

Vijay KT, Kocher HH, Koti RS, Bapat RD. 1996. Agenesis of gall bladder: A diagnostic dilemma. *Journal of Postgraduate Medicine* 42:80–82.

Volzke H, Baumeister SE, Alte D. 2005. Independent risk factors for gallstone formation in a region with high cholelithiasis prevalence. *Digestion* 71:97–105.

Walker MM, Powell N, Talley NJ. 2014. Atopy and the digestive tract – A review of a common association in unexplained digestive disease. *Expert Review of Gastroenterology and Hepatology* 8(3):289–299.

Walker RD. 1997. Diagnosis and treatment of constipation. *Practice Nursing* 8(4):20–22.

Wallander MA, Johansson S, Ruigómez A, Rodríguez G, Alberto L, Jones R. 2007. Dyspepsia in general practice: Incidence, risk factors, comorbidity and mortality. *Family Practice* 24(5):403–411.

Wang AY, Peura DA. 2011. The prevalence and incidence of *Helicobacter pylori* associated peptic ulcer disease and upper gastrointestinal bleeding throughout the world. *Gastrointestinal Endoscopy Clinics of North America* 21:613–635.

Wang F, Meng W, Wang B, Qiao L. 2014. *Helicobacter pylori*-induced gastric inflammation and gastric cancer. *Cancer Letters* 345:196–202.

Wang LW, Li ZS, Li SD, Jin ZD, Zou DW, Chen F. 2009. Prevalence and clinical features of chronic pancreatitis in China: A retrospective multicenter analysis over 10 years. *Pancreas* 38(3):248–254.

Warner BW, Ziegler MM. 2000. Exstrophy of the cloaca. In: Ashcraft KW (ed). *Pediatric Surgery*, 3rd edn. Philadelphia, PA: W.B. Saunders, pp. 493–501.

Watson A, Bowling T. 2004. Acid reflux and gastro-oesophageal reflux disease. *British Journal of Community Nursing* 9(8):326–330.

Weaver LT, Laker MF, Nelson R. 1986. Neonatal intestinal lactase activity. *Archives of Disease in Childhood* 61:896–899.

Whitcomb DC. 2006. Acute pancreatitis. *New England Journal of Medicine* 354:2142–2150.

Whiteway J, Morson BC. 1985. Pathology of the ageing—Diverticular disease. *Clinics in Gastroenterology* 14:829–846.

WHO. 2015. *Guidelines for the Prevention, Care and Treatment of Persons with Chronic Hepatitis B Infection*. Geneva: World Health Organization.

Wiesel P, Bell S. 2004. Bowel dysfunction: Assessment and management in the neurological patient. In: Norton C, Chelvanayagam S (eds). *Bowel Continence Nursing*. Beaconsfield: Beaconsfield Publishers.

Willett WC, Stampfer MJ, Colditz GA. 1990. Relation of meat, fat, and fibre intake to the risk of colon cancer in a prospective study among women. *New England Journal of Medicine* 323:1664–1672.

Wilson JE, Deitrick JE. 1986. Agenesis of the gallbladder: Case report and familial investigation. *Surgery* 99:106–109.

Wilson RD, Johnson MP. 2004. Congenital abdominal wall defects: An update. *Fetal Diagnosis and Therapy* 19:385–398.

World Health Organisation. 2004. The Molecular Genetic Epidemiology of Cystic Fibrosis, Report of a Joint Meeting of WHO/ECFTN/ICF(M)A/ECFS. http://tinyurl.com/.csog2ye (accessed 12 April 2016).

Yadav D. 2011. Incidence, prevalence and survival of chronic pancreatitis: A population-based study. *American Journal of Gastroenterology* 106(12):2192–2199.

Yamamoto C, Okada Y, Nakano H. 2003. A case of Meckel's diverticulum adherent to the posterior abdominal wall: The efficacy of small-bowel radiography coupled with barium enema examination. *Journal of Gastroenterology* 38:194–196.

Yang JY, Melville D, Maxwell JD. 2004. Epidemiology and management of diverticular disease of the colon. *Drugs and Aging* 4:211e28.

Yoldas O, Yazıcı P, Ozsan I, Karabuga T, Alpdogan O, Sahin E, Aydın U. 2014. Coexistence of gallbladder agenesis and cholangiocarcinoma. *Journal of Gastrointestinal Surgery* 18:1373–1376.

Young LS, Thomas DJ. 2004. Celiac spruce treatment in primary care. *Nurse Practitioner* 29(7):42–45.

Zmijewska C, Surdyk-Zasada J, Zabel M. 2003. Development of innervation in primary incisors in the foetal period. *Archives of Oral Biology* 48:745–752.

Appendix

Systems Association Table

Body system	System association
Digestive system	The digestive system provides nutrients for all the systems in the body through the processes of chemical and mechanical digestion, breaking down macromolecules in ingested food to basic nutrients small enough to be absorbed. The digestive system, via blood and lymph, supplies all of the cells of the body with nutrients so cells can carry out functions of metabolism, growth and repair.
Reproductive	Conception and the normal development of the embryo and foetus are dependent upon the regular supply of adequate nutrients. Conception is dependent upon active nutrition. Embryological and foetal development is dependent on the placenta, passive nutrition.
Immunity/lymphatic	The lacteals, which are a component of the lymphatic system, play an important role in transporting absorbed fats (fatty lymph) from villi in the small intestine to blood where it can then be circulated to cells around the body. Peyer's patches are collections of lymphoid tissue which can be found in the small intestine. These patches contain immune cells that help prevent the invasion of bacteria into the blood supply from the small intestine lumen.
Muscular	Muscles, co-ordinated by the nervous system, facilitate movement along the digestive tract through the processes of mastication, deglutition, peristalsis, churning, segmentation and defaecation.
Skeletal	The hard palate and other bony structures in the oral cavity assist with mastication. The digestive system supplies calcium needed for bone growth and repair.
Nervous	Normal functioning of the digestive system is dependent upon communication between the central nervous system (CNS), the autonomic nervous system (ANS) and the enteric nervous system (ENS). The digestive system provides nutrients which are the building blocks for neurotransmitters. The CNS regulates eating and drinking behaviour. The presence of nutrients in blood circulation stimulates receptors in the brain that regulate satiety.
Endocrine	In association with the nervous system entero-endocrine cells lining the stomach, pancreas and small intestine produce hormones which regulate digestive activity. Hepatocytes in the liver remove and inactivate hormones produced by entero-endocrine cells.
Cardiovascular	The circulatory system transports absorbed nutrients to all cells in the body. It also transports hormones produced by enteroendocrine cells that regulate digestive activity. The digestive system absorbs iron and vitamin B_{12} needed for healthy red blood cells and water to provide blood volume. Hepatocytes in the liver remove bilirubin (blood pigment) which is then excreted in bile.
Respiratory	The specialist cells of the digestive system rely upon the respiratory system to provide the oxygen needed for metabolic processes and to remove carbon dioxide, a waste product of cellular metabolism.
Renal/urinary	The kidneys, in association with the liver, activate vitamin D which is needed for the absorption of calcium from the intestine. The specialist cells of the digestive system produce metabolic waste. The kidneys filter and remove the waste products from blood and excrete it as urine.
Integumentary	Vitamin D is activated in the skin by sunlight which is needed for the absorption of calcium from the intestine.

References for Age-Related Changes in the Digestive System

Digestive system	Normal changes: anatomical	Normal changes: physiological
Oral cavity	• Reduced saliva production • Atrophy of taste buds	• Reduced taste sensation
Oesophagus	• Degenerative changes in smooth muscle lining of lower oesophagus • Slower and weaker peristalsis • Reduced resting pressure of lower oesophageal sphincter	• Increasing potential for stomach content reflux into lower oesophagus
Stomach	• Reduced elasticity • Reduced motility • Reduced gastric surface area • Reduced gastric secretions • Atrophy of gastric mucosa • Slowing of stomach emptying	• Reduced digestion • Reduced absorption
Small and large intestine	• Reduced secretion of digestive enzymes • Reduced elasticity of rectal wall • Reduced internal anal sphincter tone • Reduced mucus secretion • Atrophy of muscle and mucosal surfaces • Thinning of villi and reduced number of epithelial cells	• Potential reduced absorption of fats and vitamin B_{12} • Slower and dulled neural impulses that sense urge to defaecate
Liver	• Reduced overall weight and liver mass • Reduced number of hepatic cells • Reduced regenerative capacity • Reduced blood flow to liver • Reduced hepatic enzymes	• Reduced drug clearance • Reduced hormone metabolism
Gallbladder, bile ducts	• No significant changes to structure of gallbladder • Reduced bile storage • Reduced bile salt pool • End of common bile duct narrows	• No significant changes to physiology of gallbladder – potential for reduced fat digestion
Pancreas	• Pancreatic ductal hyperplasia fibrosis • Reduced pancreatic enzyme secretion	• Potential reduced digestion • Potential reduced absorption

Glossary of Terms

Abdomen area between the chest and the hips that contains the stomach, small intestine, large intestine, liver, gallbladder, pancreas and spleen.

Absorption to move a substance into the body, such as the absorption of nutrients in the digestive tract.

Accessory organs organs that help with digestion but are not part of the digestive tract.

Achalasia failure of the lower esophageal sphincter to relax.

Adenocarcinoma malignant tumour of glandular epithelial tissue.

Adipose tissue fatty tissue.

Adventitia outermost connective tissue covering.

Aetiology cause.

Afferent nerves nerve fibres (usually sensory) that carry impulses from an organ or tissue toward the brain and spinal cord (central nervous system), or the information processing centres of the enteric nervous system, which is located within the walls of the digestive tract.

Afferent pathways nerve structures through which impulses are conducted from a peripheral part (e.g. the gut or intestines) towards a nerve centre (e.g. the central nervous system).

Aganglionosis absence of nerve cells.

Alimentary canal the digestive tract, extends from the mouth to the anus.

Alveolar ridge ridged area of the maxilla and mandible situated behind the teeth.

Amino acids a group of 20 different kinds of small molecules that link together in long chains to form proteins. Often referred to as the 'building blocks' of proteins.

Amniotic fluid fluid surrounding the foetus within the amniotic sac.

Amylase enzyme produced by acini cells in the pancreas and salivary glands that helps in the digestion of starches.

Angular chelitis inflammatory condition of one or both corners of the mouth.

Anorectal atresia absence of a normal opening between the anus and the rectum.

Anorectal malformation congenital birth defect in which the anus and rectum do not develop properly.

Anorectal manometry a test that can be used to measure resting and squeezing anal sphincter pressures, rectal sensation and compliance and sphincter response.

Anus the opening of the rectum.

Apoptosis programmed cell death.

Appendix (vermiform appendix) small 'wormlike' structure, made of lymphoid tissue, projecting out from the base of the caecum at the start of the ascending colon.

Ascending colon first section of the large intestine that is on the right side of the abdomen.

Atrophic gastritis chronic inflammation of the stomach mucosa.

Auditory tubes (eustachian tubes or pharyngotympanic tube) tube linking the middle ear to the nasopharynx.

Autoimmune disease an inherited genetic defect causing a number of conditions characterised by dysfunction of the immune system where the body's immune system attacks and destroys its own cells.

Autonomic nervous system the part of the nervous system that controls involuntary actions of internal organs such as the bowel.

Bacteria very small organisms (microbes) that are normally in the gut (intestines). There are over 500 different kinds known to live in the gut; most (up to several billion) bacteria are in the large intestine (colon). 'Normal' bacteria have important functions in life and health. Bacteria that can cause infection are called 'pathogens'. Normal bacteria protect against pathogens.

Barium a metallic, chemical, chalky, liquid used to coat the inside of organs so that they will show up on an x-ray.

Barium enema investigative procedure that examines the rectum, large intestine and lower part of the small intestine.

Bifid uvula a cleft in the uvula.

Bile a yellow-green fluid, made by the liver, stored in the gallbladder and passes through the common bile duct into the duodenum where it emulsifies fats.

Bile duct duct that transports bile.

Biliary atresia congenital birth defect in which the bile ducts do not have normal openings, preventing bile from leaving the liver.

Biliary tract gallbladder and the bile ducts.

Bilirubin pigment produced when red blood cells are broken down. Bilirubin is a constituent of bile and is excreted by the liver.

Biopsy removal of a sample of tissue for study, usually under a microscope.

Bowel another name for the intestines.

Buccal cavity oral cavity.

Buccinator muscle large muscle forming the cheek.

Buccopharyngeal membrane (oral membrane) membrane which forms the external upper membrane limit (cranial end) of the early digestive tract (GIT). This membrane develops during gastrulation by ectoderm and endoderm without a middle (intervening) layer of mesoderm. The membrane lies at the floor of the ventral depression (stomadeum) where the oral cavity will open and will break down to form the initial 'oral opening' of the digestive tract. The equivilant membrane at the lower end of the digestive tract is the cloacal.

Call to stool feeling the need to have a bowel movement.

Cancer group of diseases that cause cells in the body to change and grow out of control. Can be benign or malignant.

Carbohydrates constitute one of the three principal types of nutrients used as energy sources (calories) by the body. Consist of mainly sugars and starches.

Cartilage a mesenchymal derivative (connective tissue).

Cell the basic unit of any living organism. It is a small, watery compartment filled with chemicals and a complete copy of the organism's genome.

Central arch (fauces) passage at the back of the mouth leading to the oropharynx.

Cephalic relating to the head.

Chemical digestion action of chemicals to breakdown bonds of complex molecules.

Central nervous system (CNS) constitutes the brain and spinal cord.

Chemoreceptors sensory nerves that detect changes in chemical composition.

Choanal atresia a congenital disorder where there is narrowing or blockage of the nasal airway by tissue.

Cholesterol a lipid that is important in cell membrane structure and hormone synthesis. Found in food but also manufactured by the body. Excess cholesterol is excreted in bile.

Chronic symptoms occurring over a long period of time.

Cirrhosis progressive disease in which healthy liver tissue is replaced with scar tissue eventually disrupting liver function.

Cleft lip congenital birth defect in which the tissues forming the lip do not completely fuse.

Cleft palate congenital birth defect in which the roof of the mouth does not completely fuse, leaving an opening that can extend into the nasal cavity.

Cloacal membrane forms the external lower membrane limit (caudal end) of the early digestive tract (GIT). Formed during gastrulation by ectoderm and endoderm without a middle (intervening) layer of mesoderm. The membrane breaks down to form the initial 'anal opening' of the digestive tract.

Clostridium difficile (C. difficile) a gram-positive anaerobic bacterium. *C. difficile* is recognised as the major causative agent of colitis (inflammation of the colon) and diarrhoea that may occur following antibiotic intake.

Coeliac disease inability to digest and absorb the protein gliadin (a component of gluten). Gliadin is found in wheat, rye, barley and oats. Coeliac disease is also called coeliac sprue, and gluten intolerance.

Coelom term used to describe a space. There are extraembryonic and intraembryonic coeloms that form during vertebrate development. The single intraembryonic coelom will form the three major body cavities: pleural, pericardial and peritoneal.

Colitis inflammation of the colon.

Colon part of the large intestine that runs from the caecum to the rectum.

Colonic inertia delayed colonic action. Symptoms include long delays in the passage of stool accompanied by lack of urgency to move the bowels.

Colonoscopy a fiberoptic (endoscopic) procedure in which a thin, flexible, lighted viewing tube (a colonoscope) is threaded up through the rectum for the purpose of inspecting the entire colon and rectum and, if there is an abnormality, taking a tissue sample of it (biopsy) for examination under a microscope, or removing it.

Colostomy a surgically created opening of the colon to the abdominal wall, allowing the diversion of faecal waste.

Common bile duct tube that transports bile from the liver to the duodenum.

Congenital anomaly health problem or abnormality present at birth (not necessarily genetic). Conditions existing at birth, but not through heredity.

Connective tissue mesenchymal derivatives, a type of tissue consisting of cells and an extracellular matrix of fibres.

Contrast radiology a test in which a contrast material (i.e. barium) is used to coat the rectum, colon and lower part of the small intestine so they show up on an x–ray.

Constipation reduced stool frequency, or hard stools, difficulty passing stools, or painful bowel movements.

Cotransport the movement of two substances across a membrane using one transporter.

Cranial nerves 12 pairs of nerves originating directly from the brain.

Crohn's disease a chronic form of inflammatory bowel disease. Can occur anywhere along the digestive tract from the mouth to the anus but most commonly found in the ileum and colon.

Cystic fibrosis inherited genetic condition involving many of the body's systems and characterised by thick secretions in ducts and glands of the body leading to obstructive conditions.

Cytokines a type of protein released by cells of the immune system, which act through specific cell receptors to regulate immune responses.

Descending colon section of the large intestine located on the left side of the abdomen.

Dehydration an excessive loss of fluids in the body.

Diabetes a disease in which blood glucose (blood sugar) levels are above normal. Type 2 diabetes, also known as adult-onset or non-insulin-dependent diabetes mellitus (NIDDM), is the most common form of diabetes.

Diarrhoea increase in frequency of stools compared to normal, or looser bowel movements than usual.

Differentiate development of specific cell types from stem cells by gene activation and repression.

Diffusion random movements that lead to a uniform distribution of molecules both within a solution and on the two sides of a membrane.

Digestive system organs responsible for ingesting, digesting and absorbing nutrients: include the salivary glands, the mouth, oesophagus, stomach, small intestine, liver, gallbladder, pancreas, colon, rectum and anus.

Distention an uncomfortable swelling in the intestines.

Diverticula small pouches in the colon.

Diverticulitis a term used to describe a condition in which (one or more) small pouches in the large intestine (called a diverticulum) become irritated or infected.

Diverticulosis a condition of having multiple diverticula in the walls of the colon. Also called uncomplicated diverticular disease.

Diverticulum singular of diverticula.

Duodenal ulcer a break in the integrity (open sore) of the duodenal mucosa.

Duodenum first part of the small intestine and extends from the pylorus at the bottom of the stomach to the jejunum. The duodenum secretes hormones and receives enzymes from the pancreas and bile from the gallbladder.

Dysphagia difficulty swallowing.

Ectomesenchymal a form of mesenchyme, in the embryo, consisting of neural crest cells.

Edwards's syndrome (trisomy 18) a genetic condition caused by an additional copy of chromosome 18 in some or all of the cells in the body.

Efferent nerves nerve fibres that carry impulses away from the brain and spinal cord (central nervous system), which cause a muscle or gland to contract, or which modify or inhibit its contraction.

Electrolytes chemicals that break down into ions (atoms) in the body's fluids and are essential to regulating many body functions.

Embryogenesis development of an embryo.

Embryonic disc flattened circular bilaminar plate of cells derived from the embryoblast in the second week of embryonic development.

Encopresis involuntary defaecation.

Endodermal cells embryonic cells derived from the endoderm.

Endoscope a thin, flexible tube with a light and a lens on the end used to look into the oesophagus, stomach, duodenum, small intestine, colon or rectum.

Endoscopic retrograde cholangiopancreatography (See ERCP)

Endoscopy a procedure that uses an endoscope to diagnose or treat a condition. There are many types of endoscopy; examples include colonoscopy, sigmoidoscopy, gastroscopy, enteroscopy and oesophago-gastro-duodenoscopy (EGD).

Enteral nutrition food provided through a tube placed in the nose, stomach or small intestine.

Enteric nervous system (ENS) autonomic nervous system within the walls of the digestive tract. The ENS regulates digestion and the muscle contractions that eliminate solid waste.

Enteritis an irritation of the small intestine.

Enterocolitis inflammation of the intestines.

Enterocytes small intestine epithelial cell.

Entero-endocrine cells hormone-producing cells of the intestine.

Enzymes proteins that act as catalysts in mediating and speeding a specific chemical reaction.

Epidemiology the study of the distribution of health-related states or events in specified populations and the application of this study to the control of health problems.

Epithelium the inner and outer tissue covering digestive tract organs.

ERCP (endoscopic retrograde cholangiopancreatography) investigation that allows examination of the bile ducts (biliary tree) and pancreatic ducts that combines the use of x-rays and an endoscope.

Faeces waste eliminated from the bowels.

Failure to thrive (paediatric) a condition that occurs when a baby does not grow normally.

Familial tending to occur in more members of a family than expected by chance alone.

Fibrosis process by which inflamed tissue becomes scarred.

Fistula an abnormal passage between two organs or between an organ and the outside of the body.

Foecal incontinence the involuntary loss of solid liquid stool in children.

Foetus term used to describe an unborn baby from the eighth week after fertilisation until delivery.

Food allergy an immune system response by which the body creates antibodies as a reaction to certain food. Studies show that true food allergies are present in only 1%–2% of adults.

Foregut the first of the three divisions (foregut-midgut-hindgut) of the early forming digestive tract. The foregut runs from the buccopharyngeal membrane to the midgut.

Gallbladder pear-shaped organ that stores bile secreted by the liver.

Gallstone solid matter that develops in the gallbladder when substances in the bile, primarily cholesterol, and bile pigments form hard, crystal-like particles.

Ganglion (Plural: ganglia) – usually, a group of nerve cell bodies lying outside of the central nervous system (CNS); also used for one group of nerve cell bodies within the CNS – the basal ganglia.

Gastric related to the stomach.

Gastric secretions liquids produced in the stomach to help break down food and kill bacteria.

Gastrin hormone that stimulates the stomach to produce acid.

Gastritis an inflammation of the stomach lining.

Gastroenteritis an infection or irritation of the stomach and intestines.

Gastroenterologist a doctor who specialises in digestive diseases or disorders.

Gastroenterology the field of medicine concerned with the function and disorders of the digestive system.

Gastrointestinal (GI) tract the muscular tube from the mouth to the anus, also called the alimentary canal or digestive tract.

Gastroschisis a congenital birth defect in a baby's abdominal wall that allows the infant's intestines to protrude through to the outside.

Gastroscopy examination of the inside of the oesophagus, stomach, and duodenum using an endoscope.

Gene the functional and physical unit of heredity passed from parent to offspring. Genes are pieces of DNA, and most genes contain the information for making a specific protein.

Gestation the period of time from conception to birth. A pregnancy with multiple foetuses is referred to as a multiple gestation.

Gingival tissue gums.

Glossopharyngeal nerve the ninth (IX) of the 12 pairs of cranial nerves.

Gluten protein found in grains such as wheat, oats, rye and barley.

Gluten intolerance see Coeliac disease.

Goblet cells mucous-producing cells.

GOR (gastroesophageal reflux) also called acid reflux, a condition where the contents of the stomach regurgitate (or back up) into the oesophagus (food pipe), causing discomfort.

GORD (gastroesophageal reflux disease) condition characterised by the chronic movement of food, fluids and digestive juices from the stomach into the oesophagus causing irritation of the oesophageal lining by acid, resulting in discomfort.

H_2-blockers medicines that reduce the amount of acid the stomach produces.

Haemorrhoids veins around the anus or lower rectum that are swollen and inflamed.

Heartburn painful burning sensation in the chest associated with reflux of gastric contents into the oesophagus.

Helicobacter pylori (H. pylori) spiral-shaped bacterium found in the stomach, which helps cause inflammation and can damage stomach and duodenal tissue, causing ulcers.

Hepatic related to the liver.

Hepatitis inflammation of the liver caused by viruses, drugs, alcohol or parasites.

Hepatitis Chepatitis caused by the hepatitis C virus.

Heredity the passing of a trait from parent to offspring through genetically coded information.

Hereditary genetically transmitted or transmittable from parent to offspring.

Hernia section of intestine or other internal organ which has pushed its way through an opening in the abdominal muscle.

Hiatus hernia a small opening in the diaphragm that allows the upper part of the stomach to move up into the chest.

Hindgut last of the three divisions (foregut–midgut–hindgut) of the early forming digestive tract. The hindgut forms all the tract from the distal transverse colon to the cloacal membrane and extends into the connecting stalk (placental cord) as the allantois.

Hirschsprung's disease a rare congenital birth defect that is caused by absence of nerve cells (ganglion) in the rectum and/or colon.

Homeostasis maintenance of a relatively stable or balanced internal body state despite environmental fluctuations. The tendency in an organism toward maintenance of physiological and psychological stability.

Hormones a substance, made and released by cells in a specific organ or structure, that moves throughout the body and exerts specific effects on specific cells in other organs or structures.

Hypersensitivity an increased or exaggerated response to stimuli.

Hypobrachial eminence an embryogenic structure which forms the third posterior part (copula) of the adult tongue during embryonic development.

Hypoglossal nerve 12th paired cranial nerve.

Ileostomy a surgically created opening of the abdominal wall to the ileum, allowing the diversion of faecal waste.

Ileum last third of the small intestine, adjoining the colon.

Imperforate anus a congenital birth defect in which the anal canal fails to develop. The opening at the end of the rectum or anus is absent.

Incidence describes the occurrence of a disease or disorder in a population. It is a rate, showing how many new cases of a disease occurred in a population (typically a susceptible population called the 'at-risk population') during a specified interval of time (usually expressed as number of new cases per unit time per fixed number of people; e.g. number of new cases per 1000 persons in 1 year).

Inflammation redness, swelling, pain and/or a feeling of heat in an area of the body. This is a protective reaction to injury, disease or irritation of the tissues.

Inflammatory bowel disease (IBD) chronic inflammation of the digestive tract, thought to be caused by an unusual immune response to bacteria normally found in the intestines. Causes inflammation, scarring and ulcers in the digestive tract (common disorders are ulcerative colitis and Crohn's disease).

Ingestion taking into the body by mouth.

Inherited transmitted through genes from parents to offspring.

Innervated a structure supplied with intact nerves.

Interneurons association neurons; neurons that are neither sensory nor motor.

Interstitial cells of Cajal a type of interstitial cell found in the gastrointestinal tract.

Intervention anything meant to change the course of events for someone (e.g. drug, surgery, test, treatment, counseling, etc.).

Intestinal relating to or occurring in the intestines.

Intestinal mucosa the surface lining of the intestines where the cells absorb nutrients.

Intestinal permeability the barrier properties of the lining of the intestines, which prevent harmful substances from passing through into the body.

Intestines also known as the gut or bowels, is the long, tube-like organ in the human body that completes digestion or the breaking down of food. They consist of the small intestine and the large intestine.

Intussusception occurs when a section of the intestine (most commonly terminal ileum) folds like a telescope, with one section slipping inside another section.

Irritable bowel syndrome a functional bowel disorder in which abdominal discomfort or pain is associated with defaecation or a change in bowel habit, and with features of disordered defaecation.

Ischemic colitis inflammation of the large intestine (colon) caused by decreased blood flow to the colon. Symptoms may include abdominal pain, fever, vomiting, blood in the stool, diarrhoea, low back pain.

Isotonic a solution having the same osmotic pressure as some other solution.

Jaundice buildup of yellow bilirubin pigment (produced from the breakdown of haemoglobin) in the skin, eyes and mucous membranes.

Jejunum second part of the small intestine. Lies between the duodenum and ileum. Main site for the absorption of nutrients.

Keratinised stratified squamous epithelium epithelium with added intermediate filament protein in which the cells are arranged in multiple layers.

Lactase enzyme, produced by enterocytes, in the small intestine needed to digest lactose (carbohydrate found in milk and milk products).

Lactose a sugar found commonly in milk and dairy products.

Lactose intolerance the inability to digest or absorb lactose.

Lamina propria a thin layer of connective tissue which lies beneath the epithelium.

Large intestine tube-like organ, connected to the small intestine at the ileo-caecal valve and the anus distally. The large intestine comprises four parts: caecum, colon, rectum and anal canal.

Lateral away from the midline of the body, to the side.

Laxative a compound that increases faecal water content.

Limbic system a network of brain regions involved in the regulation of the function of internal organs, emotions and the maintenance of homeostasis.

Lipase a lipid-digesting enzyme.

Lipid fatty substance.

Liver largest organ in the body. Located in the upper abdomen and assists in the process of digestion through the production of bile.

Lower oesophageal sphincter thick band of smooth circular muscle at the top portion of the stomach that relaxes to allow food to pass from the oesophagus to the stomach.

Lymphatic system specialist tissues and organs of the immune system that produce white blood cells to protect the body from infection.

Lymphocytes white blood cells that fight infection and disease. A type of white blood cell.

Macromolecules large molecules.

Malabsorption incomplete absorption of nutrients in the intestine.

Mandibular prominences in head and face development, lower part and majority of pharyngeal arch 1 which forms the lower jaw (mandible) of the face. The smaller upper parts of pharyngeal arch 1 are the maxillary processes.

Manometry a test that measures pressure or contractions in the intestinal tract.

Mast cell a type of immune system cell present in blood and tissue.

Mast cell degranulation the release from within the cell of granules, or small sacs, containing chemicals that can digest microorganisms and activate other cells to fight infection.

Mastication (or chewing) the process by which food is crushed and ground by teeth.

Maxillary prominences in head and face development, upper part of pharyngeal arch 1 which forms as a pair of small lateral swellings which contributes the upper jaw and forms the palatal shelves. Larger lower part of pharyngeal arch 1 is the mandibular process.

Mechanoreceptors a sensory receptor that responds to mechanical pressure.

Meckel's diverticulum a congenital birth defect that occurs during embryonic development in which a small pouch (or sac) forms in the ileum (the lower end of the small intestine).

Meconium viscous greenish-black substance that forms in the intestines during foetal development and is the first bowel movement of a newborn.

Mediators substances within the body, such as hormones, that can transmit messages to nerve or muscle tissue to stimulate a response.

Meissner's plexus (or submucosal plexus) collection of nerve fibres (nerve plexus) found in the submucosa in the lower oesophagus, stomach and intestines.

Mesenchyme tissue term used to describe the cellular organisation of undifferentiated embryonic connective tissue. Mainly derived from mesoderm and neural crest, which will form most of the adult connective tissues.

Mesentery membranous tissue supporting blood vessels, nerves and lymph glands, connects abdominal organs and is continuous with the abdominal wall (peritoneum).

Mesoderm the middle layer of the three germ cell layers of the embryo.

Metaplasia a change of cells to a form that does not normally occur in the tissue in which it is found.

Micromolecules small molecules.

Midgut middle of the three divisions (foregut-midgut-hindgut) of the early forming digestive tract. The midgut forms all the tract from beneath the stomach (duodenum, small intestine and large intestine) to the distal transverse colon.

Migration the movement of cells, etc. from one position to another.

Monosaccharides the smallest unit of carbohydrate, consisting of a single ring-shaped structure of carbon, hydrogen and oxygen with a 2:1 hydrogen-to-oxygen ratio.

Morbidity a disease or the incidence of disease within a population. Morbidity also refers to adverse effects caused by a treatment.

Motility spontaneous movement. A term used to describe the motor activity of smooth muscles in the digestive (GI) tract.

Mucosa first layer in the wall of a tubular organ that lines the lumen; usually consists of the epithelium and the lamina propria.

Mucosal epithelium the layer in the wall of a tubular organ that lines the lumen.

Muscularis mucosae thin muscular layer in the mucosal wall of the alimentary canal.

Myenteric (or Auerbach's) plexus collection of nerve fibres (nerve plexus) situated between the circular muscle layer and the longitudinal muscle layer in the lower oesophagus, stomach and intestines.

Myogenic originating in muscle tissue.

Neonate newborn.

Nerve(s) cells in the human body that are the building blocks of the nervous system (the system that records and transmits information chemically and electrically within a person). Nerve cells, or neurons, are made up of a nerve cell body and various extensions from the cell body that receive and transmit impulses from and to other nerves and muscles.

Neural having to do with nerves or the nervous system, including the brain and the spinal cord.

Neural crest a cell region at edge of neural plate, can differentiate into many different cell types. Those that remain on the dorsal neural tube form the sensory spinal ganglia (DRG).

Neuroendocrine interaction between hormones, glands and the nervous system.

Nociceptors pain receptors.

Nutrients a chemical compound (such as protein, fat, carbohydrate, vitamins or minerals) that make up foods.

Nutrition the taking in and use of food and other nourishing material by the body.

Oesophageal atresia congenital birth defect in which the neonate's oesophagus does not develop properly, and ends before reaching the stomach. Food cannot pass from the mouth into the stomach.

Oesophagitis an irritation of the oesophagus, usually caused by acid that flows up from the stomach.

Oesophago-gastro-duodenoscopy (OGD) insertion of a flexible tube with a small camera, via the mouth, to visualise the oesophagus, stomach and duodenum.

Oesophagus tube connecting the pharynx (throat) with the stomach. Facilitates the transport of a bolus from the mouth to the stomach.

Omphalocele a congenital birth defect of the abdominal wall that allows some of the abdominal organs to protrude through it.

Oropharynx middle part of the pharynx (throat).

Osmolarity the concentration of osmotically active particles in a solution expressed in osmoles per litre (Osm.L^{-1}) of the solution.

Osmosis the tendency of a fluid, usually water, to pass through a semipermeable membrane into a solution where the solvent concentration is higher.

Palate roof of the mouth. The front section is bony (hard palate), and the rear section is muscular (soft palate).

Pancreas pink elongated organ that extends across the abdomen behind the stomach. Performs an important exocrine (enzymes) and endocrine (hormones) role.

Pancreatitis inflammation of the pancreas.

Papillae involved in the sensations of taste and have taste buds embedded in their surfaces.

Parenteral nutrition the slow infusion of a solution of nutrients into a vein through a catheter, which is surgically implanted. This may be partial, to supplement food and nutrient intake, or total (TPN, total parenteral nutrition), providing the sole source of energy and nutrient intake for the patient.

Pathogenesis the origin and development of a disease or disorder.

Pathogens disease-causing microorganisms.

Pathological disease related.

Pathology the study of the fundamental nature, causes and development of abnormal conditions and the structural and functional changes that result.

Pathophysiology changes or alterations in function that accompany a particular syndrome or disease, generally as distinguished from structural defects.

Pepsin enzyme (protease) that breaks down proteins into smaller peptides released in the stomach.

Peptic ulcer a sore in the lining of the oesophagus, stomach or duodenum, usually caused by the bacterium *Helicobacter pylori* (*H. pylori*).

Perineum the area of the body between the anus and the vulva in females, and between the anus and the scrotum in males.

Peristalsis synchronised or coordinated contraction of the muscles that propel food content through the digestive (GI) tract to facilitate normal digestion and the absorption of nutrients. Peristalsis is dependent upon the coordination between the muscles, nerves and hormones in the digestive tract.

Peritoneal cavity space between the parietal peritoneum and visceral peritoneum.

Peritoneum serous membrane lining the walls of the abdominal and pelvic cavities (parietal peritoneum) and surrounding abdominal organs (visceral peritoneum).

Peritonitis infection within the abdominal cavity.

Pharynx hollow tube comprising three structures: nasopharynx, oropharynx and laryngopharynx. Through the process of deglutition (swallowing) the pharynx facilitates the transport of a bolus from the mouth to the oesophagus.

Physiology the study of how the body functions at the levels of organs, cells and molecules.

Prevalence the proportion of people in the entire population who are found to be with a disease or disorder at a certain point in time (sometimes called a 'cross section'), without regard to when they first got the disease.

Primary lactase deficiency when a person is born with the inability to digest lactose, a sugar found in milk and milk products. Lactose cannot be digested because there is not enough of an enzyme, called lactase, in the body. Consuming milk and dairy products causes diarrhoea, bloating, gas and discomfort. This deficiency can also develop over time, as the amount of lactase in the body decreases with age.

Protease a protein that digests other proteins.

Protein a large complex molecule made up of one or more chains of amino acids.

Proton pump inhibitor (PPI) a drug that limits acid secretion in the stomach.

Pseudo-obstruction (intestinal) a motility disorder with symptoms like those of a bowel blockage, but with no physical evidence of blockage or obstruction. Symptoms may include cramps, stomach pain, nausea, vomiting, bloating, fewer bowel movements than usual and loose stools. May be chronic or acute (Ogilvie's syndrome).

Pyloric sphincter thickened band of smooth circular muscle between the stomach and the small intestine.

Receptor a structure in each cell that selectively receives and binds a specific substance, such as a neurotransmitter.

Rectum dilated section of the large intestine leading to the anus.

Reflex involuntary reaction innervated by the nervous system.

Reflux (regurgitation) backward movement of food into the oesophagus.

Reflux oesophagitis inflammation of the oesophageal epithelium which can lead to erosion and ulceration.

Saliva secretion from three salivary glands: parotid, sublingual and submandibular, into the mouth that assists with mechanical and chemical digestion.

Salivary glands glands that discharge a fluid secretion (especially saliva) into the mouth cavity.

Secretin a hormone released into the bloodstream by entero-endocrine cells lining the duodenum (especially in response to acidity) to stimulate secretion by the liver and pancreas.

Segmentation alternating forward and backward movements of chyme in the intestines designed to aid chemical and mechanical digestion.

Sensitisation enhancement of a response by an organism that is produced by delivering a strong, generally noxious, stimulus. A neuron becomes more excitable or responsive; it may respond more intensely to naturally occurring stimuli, either peripherally (in the viscera) or centrally (in the brain).

Serosa (serous membrane) membrane lining organs and cavities within the body.

Sigmoid colon S-shaped lower section of the colon that connects to the rectum.

Sigmoidoscopy examination of the inside of the sigmoid colon and rectum using an endoscope – a thin, lighted tube (sigmoidoscope).

Samples of tissue or cells may be collected for examination under a microscope. Also called proctosigmoidoscopy.

Simple columnar epithelium single layer of columnar-shape cells often found lining structures within the digestive tract.

Small intestine long tube-like structure joined to the stomach via the pyloric sphincter and large intestine via the ileo-caecal valve. Consists of three sections: duodenum, jejunum and ileum. Important for digestion and absorption.

Smooth muscle involuntary non-striated muscle.

Soft palate muscular part of the roof of the mouth located directly behind the hard palate.

Somatic layers skin and muscle.

Sphincter ring of muscle that opens and closes.

Sphincter of Oddi a muscle at that juncture of the bile and pancreatic ducts and the small intestine. It functions by opening and closing these ducts.

Spinal cord a column of nerve tissue that runs from the base of the skull down the back. It is surrounded by three protective membranes and is enclosed within the vertebrae (back bones). The spinal cord and the brain make up the central nervous system, and spinal cord nerves carry most messages between the brain and the rest of the body.

Splanchnic relating to viscera or organs of digestive tract.

Squamocolumnar junction (SCJ) or Z-line the point of transition between squamous epithelium and columnar epithelium.

Squamous cell a flat cell that looks like a fish scale under a microscope. Squamous cells cover internal and external surfaces of the body.

Squamous cell carcinoma a cancer that develops in squamous epithelial cells.

Stomach J-shaped digestive organ that is located in the upper abdomen, under the diaphragm. Upper part of the stomach connects to the oesophagus and the lower part connects to the duodenum via the pyloric sphincter.

Stomadeum an ectodermal depression in the embryo that is the precursor of the mouth.

Stool solid waste matter to be eliminated from the body through the process of defaecation.

Stratified squamous epithelium epithelium in which the cells are arranged in multiple layers.

Stress neurophysiological and subjective response to stimuli.

Stricture abnormal narrowing of a body opening.

Submucosa dense connective tissue layer supporting the mucosa.

Submucosal (Meissner's) plexus network of nerve fibres within the submucosa of the digestive tract.

Substance P neurotransmitter that stimulates pain.

Sulcus terminalis V-shaped groove pointing posteriorly, on the surface of the tongue.

Superior above.

Sympathetic pathway pathway of a division of the autonomic nervous system.

Synapse a junction between two nerves.

Syndrome a set of symptoms or conditions that occur together and suggest the presence of a certain disease or an increased chance of developing the disease.

Systemic affecting the entire body.

Taenia coli longitudinal ribbons of smooth muscle tissue in the large intestine.

Taste one of the senses. Taste buds translate chemical substances into nerve impulses which are interpreted by the brain.

Taste buds specialised nerve endings in the mouth and tongue that sense taste.

Thermoreceptors sensory receptor that senses temperature changes.

Tongue powerful muscle anchored to the floor of the mouth. Plays an important role in chemical and mechanical digestion and taste.

Tonsils a pair of small lymphoid masses on each side of the throat within the pharynx.

Trachea tube-like structure for breathing.

Transient lower oesophageal relaxations (TLOSRs) short relaxations of lower oesophageal sphincter that occur.

Transverse horizontal plane.

Trigeminal nerve cranial nerve (V).

Tuberculum impar an embryonic swelling that contribute to the development of the tongue.

Ulcerative colitis a form of inflammatory bowel disease that causes ulcers and inflammation in the inner lining of the colon and rectum.

Ultrasound an imaging method in which high-frequency sound waves are used to outline a part of the body.

Uvula an extension of the soft palate that hangs at the entrance to the oropharynx.

Vagus nerve the primary communication pathway between the brain and the digestive organs, controlling much of the activity of the oesophagus, stomach, intestine and pancreas.

Vestibule area between the lips and teeth/gums.

Villi tiny finger-like projections on the surface of the small intestine that help absorb nutrients.

Viscera internal organs such as the gut/intestines or bladder.

Visceral relating to the internal organs, such as the gut/intestines or bladder.

Visceral peritoneum thin membrane which covers organs within the peritoneum.

Voluntary conscious action (the opposite of involuntary).

Volvulus twisting of the stomach or large intestine that leads to obstruction of the digestive tract.

Z line see squamocolumnar junction (SCJ).

INDEX